First Edition

Respiratory Protection for Fire and Emergency Services

Fred Stowell, Project Manager/Writer
Barbara Adams, Editor
Lynne Murnane, Editor

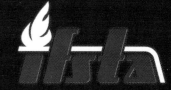

**Validated by the
International Fire Service Training Association**

**Published by
Fire Protection Publications
Oklahoma State University**

The International Fire Service Training Association

The International Fire Service Training Association (IFSTA) was established in 1934 as a "nonprofit educational association of fire fighting personnel who are dedicated to upgrading fire fighting techniques and safety through training." To carry out the mission of IFSTA, Fire Protection Publications was established as an entity of Oklahoma State University. Fire Protection Publications' primary function is to publish and disseminate training texts as proposed and validated by IFSTA. As a secondary function, Fire Protection Publications researches, acquires, produces, and markets high-quality learning and teaching aids as consistent with IFSTA's mission.

The IFSTA Validation Conference is held the second full week in July. Committees of technical experts meet and work at the conference addressing the current standards of the National Fire Protection Association and other standard-making groups as applicable. The Validation Conference brings together individuals from several related and allied fields, such as:

- Key fire department executives and training officers
- Educators from colleges and universities
- Representatives from governmental agencies
- Delegates of firefighter associations and industrial organizations

Committee members are not paid nor are they reimbursed for their expenses by IFSTA or Fire Protection Publications. They participate because of commitment to the fire service and its future through training. Being on a committee is prestigious in the fire service community, and committee members are acknowledged leaders in their fields. This unique feature provides a close relationship between the International Fire Service Training Association and fire protection agencies which helps to correlate the efforts of all concerned.

IFSTA manuals are now the official teaching texts of most of the states and provinces of North America. Additionally, numerous U.S. and Canadian government agencies as well as other English-speaking countries have officially accepted the IFSTA manuals.

ISBN 0-87939-204-5   Library of Congress Control Number: 2002100558

First Edition, First Printing, March 2002
Printed in the United States of America   2   3   4   5   6   7   8   9 10

If you need additional information concerning the International Fire Service Training Association (IFSTA) or Fire Protection Publications, contact:
Customer Service, Fire Protection Publications, Oklahoma State University
930 North Willis, Stillwater, OK 74078-8045
800-654-4055   Fax: 405-744-8204

For assistance with training materials, to recommend material for inclusion in an IFSTA manual, or to ask questions or comment on manual content, contact:
Editorial Department, Fire Protection Publications, Oklahoma State University
930 North Willis, Stillwater, OK 74078-8045
405-744-4111   Fax: 405-744-4112   E-mail: editors@osufpp.org

Table of Contents

Administrative Topics

Preface

This first edition of IFSTA **Respiratory Protection for Fire and Emergency Services** provides information for firefighters and emergency responders who are required to wear respiratory protection while performing their assigned duties. While constructed on the strong foundation of the IFSTA **Self-Contained Breathing Apparatus** manual, this new publication contains changes necessitated by changes in NFPA 1500, *Standard on Fire Department Occupational Safety and Health Program* (2002 Edition); NFPA 1404, *Standard for Fire Service Respiratory Protection Training* (2002 Edition); and NFPA 1852, *Standard on Selection, Care, and Maintenance of Open-Circuit Self-Contained Breathing Apparatus* (2002 Edition).

Acknowledgments and special thanks are extended to the members of the IFSTA Validation Committee who contributed their time, wisdom, and talents to the creation of this manual.

IFSTA Respiratory Protection for Fire and Emergency Services Validation Committee

Committee Chair
Tom Ruane
Fire Marshal
Peoria Fire Department
Peoria, Arizona

Committee Secretaries
Kevin Roche
Health and Safety Officer
Phoenix Fire Department
Phoenix, Arizona

Richard A. Dunn
Captain
Columbia Fire Department
Columbia, South Carolina

Committee Members
Maura Casey
Respiratory Protection Program Coordinator
Emergency Services Training Institute
Texas A&M University System
College Station, Texas

Robert Giorgio
Fire Chief
Cherry Hill Fire Department
Cherry Hill, New Jersey

Todd W. Haines
Hazardous Materials Engineer
Austin Fire Department
Austin, Texas

Richard Hofmeister
National Service Manager
Scott Health and Safety
Monroe, North Carolina

David Hyland
Battalion Chief
County Fire District No. 2
Roseburg, Oregon

Kirk Johnson
Captain
Valdosta Fire Department
Valdosta, Georgia

Ed Kirtley
Fire Chief
Guymon Fire Department
Guymon, Oklahoma

Lloyd Lees
Captain
Justice Institute of British Columbia
New Westminster, British Columbia, Canada

Steve Saksa
Firefighter/Paramedic
Columbus Division of Fire
Columbus Ohio

Doug Sanders
Office of the Fire Commissioner
Regina, Saskatchewan, Canada

Miles Schuler
Captain
Mid Carmel Valley Fire Protection District
Carmel, California

Tim Stemple
Fire Chief
Lockheed Martin Fire Department
Fort Worth, Texas

The following individuals and organizations contributed information, photographs, and other assistance that made the completion of this manual possible:

Texas A&M University System, Emergency Services Training Institute Staff:
    Maura Casey, Respiratory Protection Program Coordinator
    John Franceschi, Assistant Training Specialist
    Jeffery Joubert, Breathing Apparatus Technician
    Chris Masterson, Breathing Apparatus Technician
    Antone Nemec, Breathing Apparatus Technician
    Caleb Young, Student Technician

Tulsa (Oklahoma) Fire Department:
    Mike Mallory, Health and Safety Officer
    Jennie Teeter, Assistant Health and Safety Officer
    Frank Mason, Audio Visual Officer
    Walt Ringer, Audio Visual Technician

Casco Industries, Inc.
    Jeff Davenport
    Jerry Yort
    Charles Zurmehly

Denny Atchley, Oklahoma City (Oklahoma) Fire Department
Kenneth Baum, Cherry Hill (New Jersey) Fire Department
R. J. Bennett
Captain Jack Photo Services
Clemens Industries
Neil Constantine, Broughton Firefighters, Manchester, United Kingdom
Federal Emergency Management Agency
Dennis Hawkins
Ron Jeffers
Lloyd Lees
John F. Lewis
Joe Marino, Massachusetts Fire Research Institute
Howard Meile
Chris E. Mickal, New Orleans (Louisiana) Fire Department
Mike Nixon, Portland (Maine) Fire Department
Bob Parker, Austin (Texas) Fire Department
Scott Aviation
Bill Tompkins
Chris Tompkins
United States Navy Archives
Michael Watiker

Additionally, gratitude is extended to the following members of the Fire Protection Publications **Respiratory Protection for Fire and Emergency Services** Project Team whose contributions made the final publication of this manual possible:

Project Manager/Writer
Fred Stowell, Senior Technical Editor

Editors
Barbara Adams, Associate Editor
Lynne Murnane, Senior Editor

Staff Liaison
Richard Hall, Manager
International Fire Service Accreditation Congress

Technical Reviewer
Mike Wieder, Acting Managing Editor and IFSTA Projects Manager

Proofreader
Cynthia Brakhage, Associate Editor

Production Coordinator
Don Davis, Coordinator, Publications Productions

Illustrators and Layout Designers
Ann Moffat, Graphic Design Analyst
Desa Porter, Senior Graphic Designer
Ben Brock, Senior Graphic Designer
Brien McDowell, Graphic Technicion

Library Researchers
Susan F. Walker, Librarian
Shelly Magee, Library Assistant
Nathan Traunicht, Library Assistant

Editorial Assistant
Tara Gladden

Introduction

This is the first edition of the IFSTA **Respiratory Protection for Fire and Emergency Services** manual. It takes the place of **Self-Contained Breathing Apparatus** (2nd edition), a manual that was specific to the fire service and limited to the use of self-contained breathing apparatus (SCBA). In developing this new manual, the IFSTA material review committee and the writer/editor worked to include all types of respiratory hazards faced by personnel during emergency responses and the appropriate respiratory protection equipment that must be worn when operating in those hazardous environments. The committee recognized the fact that changes in respiratory hazards, technology, and regulations required a totally new approach to the subject and therefore adopted a new format for the manual. The manual is divided into two sections: The first (Chapters 1 through 7) deals with administrative topics, and the second (Chapters 8 through 10) deals with operational topics. While all the information is needed for a comprehensive understanding of respiratory protection, the first section may be of greater value to personnel who are assigned the task of developing a respiratory protection program and selecting, evaluating, purchasing, and maintaining respiratory protection equipment. The operational section is directed toward the topics of operational care, cleaning, maintenance, wearing, and use of respiratory equipment at emergency incidents. Emergency responders may be more interested in these particular topics.

The use of respiratory protection is mandated by the United States Occupational Safety and Health Administration (OSHA) and in National Fire Protection Association (NFPA) standards when they are adopted into law. Beyond the requirements of law, the use of respiratory protection makes just plain good sense. Data maintained by the United States Federal Emergency Management Agency (FEMA), United States Centers for Disease Control (CDC), and Canadian occupational health and safety (OH&S) agencies have established direct relationships between smoke inhalation and heart disease and cancer in addition to long-term injuries

and deaths caused by the inhalation of toxic gases. Respiratory protection must be worn whenever there is the slightest indication that chemically or biologically contaminated or oxygen-deficient atmospheres are present.

Fire and emergency services organizations, public or private, must have an established respiratory protection program, including guidelines for respiratory equipment selection, care, use, maintenance, facepiece fit testing, and training. It is the intent of this manual to provide the necessary direction for such organizations in meeting the requirements for a respiratory protection program.

Purpose

The purpose of this first edition of **Respiratory Protection for Fire and Emergency Services** is to provide both fire department administrations and emergency services personnel with information necessary to meet changes in respiratory protection standards and technology. The manual is, therefore, divided into two sections. The administrative section (Chapters 1 through 7) provides guidelines for the development of a comprehensive respiratory protection program, an overview of regulations and standards for respiratory protection, training requirements, product evaluation and procurement procedures, and operational policy development procedures. The operational section (Chapters 8 through 10) includes practical instruction in the use, care, cleaning, storage, and maintenance of respiratory protection equipment plus cylinder refilling techniques and safety practices.

Scope

The scope of this manual covers the regulatory requirements for a respiratory protection program, the process for developing such a program, medical requirements, facepiece fit-testing procedures, training requirements, operational and safety requirements, and selection process procedures for respiratory protection equipment. Additionally, operational information in respiratory equipment donning and doffing, inspection, maintenance, care and cleaning, safety, storage, cylinder refilling, and emergency scene use are included.

The material in this manual will assist fire and emergency services administrations and individual members in meeting the respiratory protection requirements of the following NFPA documents:

- NFPA 1500, *Standard on Fire Department Occupational Safety and Health Program* (2002 edition)

- NFPA 1404, *Standard for Fire Service Respiratory Protection Training* (2002 edition)

- NFPA 1852, *Standard on Selection, Care, and Maintenance of Open-Circuit Self-Contained Breathing Apparatus* (2002 edition)

This manual also refers to some of the respiratory protection requirements found in the following NFPA, OSHA, American National Standards Institute (ANSI), National Institute for Occupational Safety and Health (NIOSH), and Canadian OH&S documents:

- NFPA 1521, *Standard for Fire Department Safety Officer*

- NFPA 1582, *Standard on Medical Requirements for Fire Fighters*

- NFPA 1001, *Standard for Fire Fighter Professional Qualifications*

- NFPA 1003, *Standard for Airport Fire Fighter Professional Qualifications*

- NFPA 472, *Standard on Professional Competence of Responders to Hazardous Materials Incidents* (2002 edition)

- NFPA 1403, *Standard on Live Fire Training Evolutions* (2002 edition)

- NFPA 1981, *Standard on Open-Circuit Self-Contained Breathing Apparatus for the Fire Service*

- OSHA Title 29 (Labor) *CFR* 1910.120, *Hazardous Waste Operations and Emergency Response Requirements*

- OSHA Title 29 (Labor) *CFR* 1910.134, *Respiratory Protection Requirements*

- OSHA Title 29 (Labor) *CFR* 1910.156, *Fire Brigades*

- OSHA Title 29 (Labor) *CFR* 1910.134, Appendix A, *Fit Testing Procedures (Mandatory)*

- OSHA Title 42 (Public Health) *CFR* 84 *Certification for Particulate Respirators*

- ANSI Z88.2-1992, *Practices for Respiratory Protection*

- ANSI Z88.5-1981, *Practices for Respiratory Protection for the Fire Service*

- ANSI Z88.6-1984, *For Respiratory Protection — Respirator Use — Physical Qualifications for Personnel*

- ANSI Z88.7-2001, *Color Coding of APR Canisters, Cartridges, and Filters*

- ANSI Z88.8-2001, *Performance Criteria and Test Methods for APRs*

- ANSI Z88.10-2001, *Fit Testing Methods*

- NIOSH 87-108, *Respirator Decision Logic*

- NIOSH 87-116, *Guide to Industrial Respiratory Protection*

- Canadian OH&S regulations (where different from OSHA)

Introduction to Respiratory Protection

This chapter provides information that will assist the reader in meeting the following job performance requirements from NFPA 1404, *Standard for Fire Service Respiratory Protection Training*, 2002 Edition, and NFPA 1500, *Standard on Fire Department Occupational Safety and Health Program*, 2002 Edition.

NFPA 1500

7.9.7 When engaged in any operation where they could encounter atmospheres that are immediately dangerous to life or health (IDLH) or potentially IDLH or where the atmosphere is unknown, the fire department shall provide and require all members to use SCBA that has been certified as being compliant with NFPA 1981, *Standard on Open-Circuit Self-Contained Breathing Apparatus for the Fire Service*.

7.9.8 Members using SCBA shall not compromise the protective integrity of the SCBA for any reason when operating in IDLH, potentially IDLH, or unknown atmospheres by removing the facepiece or disconnecting any portion of the SCBA that would allow the ambient atmosphere to be breathed.

7.11.1.1 Fire service SCBA shall meet the 1987 edition or later of NFPA 1981, *Standard on Open-Circuit Self-Contained Breathing Apparatus for the Fire Service*.

7.11.1.2 Closed-circuit SCBA shall be permitted when long-duration SCBA is required.

7.11.1.3 Closed-circuit SCBA shall be NIOSH certified with a minimum rated service life of at least 2 hours and shall operate in the positive-pressure mode only.

7.11.2.1 Supplied-air respirator units used shall be of the type and manufacture employed by the authority having jurisdiction.

7.11.2.2 Supplied-air respirators shall not be used in IDLH atmospheres unless equipped with a NIOSH-certified emergency escape air cylinder and a pressure-demand facepiece.

7.11.2.3 Supplied-air respirator, Type C Pressure-Demand Class shall not be used in IDLH atmospheres unless they meet manufacturer's specifications for that purpose.

7.11.3.1 Full facepiece air-purifying respirators shall be used only in non-IDLH atmospheres for those contaminants that NIOSH certifies them against.

7.11.3.2 The authority having jurisdiction shall provide NIOSH-certified respirators that protect the user and ensure compliance with all other OHSA requirements.

7.11.3.3 The authority having jurisdiction shall establish a policy to ensure canisters and cartridges are changed before the end of their service life.

NFPA 1404

5.1.7 Training policies shall include, but shall not be limited to the following:

(1) Identification of the various types of respiratory protection equipment

(2) Responsibilities of members to obtain and maintain proper facepiece fit

(3) Responsibilities of members for proper cleaning and maintenance

(4) Identification of the factors that affect the duration of the air supply

(5) Determination of the point of no return for each member

(6) Responsibilities of members for using respiratory protection equipment in a hazardous atmosphere

(7) Limitations of respiratory protection devices

5.2 Requirements of the Respiratory Protection Training Component. The authority having jurisdiction shall ensure that each employee can demonstrate knowledge of the following:

(1) Why the respirator is necessary and how improper fit, usage, or maintenance can compromise the protective effect of the respirator

(2) What are the limitations and capabilities of the respirator

(3) How to use the respirator effectively in emergency situations, including situations in which the respirator malfunctions

(4) How to inspect, don and doff, use, and check the seals of the respirator

(5) What the procedures are for maintenance and storage of the respirator

(6) How to recognize medical signs and symptoms that can limit or prevent the effective use of respirators

(7) General requirements of Section 5.2

6.5.1 Recruit training shall include the identification of SCBA, SAR, and FFAPR components, terminology, and equipment specifications through the following:

(1) Operation of SCBA, SAR units, and FFAPR, and related equipment

(2) Inspection and maintenance of equipment

(3) Donning methods employed by the authority having jurisdiction

(4) Performance of related emergency scene activities, such as advancing hose lines, climbing ladders, crawling through windows and confined spaces, and performing rescues, while wearing respiratory protection

(5) Comprehension of organizational policies and procedures concerning safety procedures, emergency operations, use, inspection, and maintenance

(6) Performance of activities under simulated emergency conditions

(7) Compliance with all performance standards of the authority having jurisdiction

6.6.1 The training program of the authority having jurisdiction shall evaluate the ability of personnel to identify the following:

(1) Hazardous environments that require the use of respiratory protection

(2) Primary gases produced by combustion

(3) Primary characteristics of gases that are present or generated by processes other than combustion

(4) Any toxic gases that are unique to the particular authority having jurisdiction resulting from manufacturing or industrial processes

(5) Shipping labels of hazardous materials

6.7.2 Understanding the Safety Features and Limitations of SCBA. The training program of the authority having jurisdiction shall evaluate the ability of members to perform the following skills:

(1) Describe the operational principles of warning devices required on a SCBA

(2) Identify the limitations of the SCBA used by the authority having jurisdiction

(3) Describe the limitations of the SCBA's ability to protect the body from absorption of toxins through the skin

(4) Describe the procedures to be utilized if unintentionally submerged in water while wearing a SCBA

(5) Demonstrate the possible means of communications when wearing a SCBA

(6) Describe the emergency bypass operation

(7) Describe how to recognize medical signs and symptoms that could prevent the effective use of respirators

6.8.4 Practical Application in SAR Training. The training program of the authority having jurisdiction shall evaluate the ability of members to perform the following skills:

(1) Demonstrate knowledge of the components of the SAR System

(2) Understand that the use of SAR is prohibited for fire fighting

(3) Demonstrate the use of SAR utilized by the authority having jurisdiction under conditions of obscured visibility

(4) Demonstrate the emergency operations that are required when the SAR fails

(5) Demonstrate the use of SAR when using hazardous materials personal protective equipment if utilized by the authority having jurisdiction

(6) Demonstrate the use of SAR in limited or confined spaces

(7) Demonstrate the proper cleaning and sanitizing of the facepiece

6.9.1 Understanding the Components of FFAPR units. The training program of the authority having jurisdiction shall evaluate the ability of members to perform the following skills:

(1) Identify the components of facepieces, canisters, and cartridges used by the authority having jurisdiction

(2) Describe the operation of the FFAPR used by the authority having jurisdiction

(3) Describe the limitations of the FFAPR

(4) Demonstrate the operation of the FFAPR used by the authority having jurisdiction

(5) Describe how a selected FFAPR must be appropriate for the chemical state and physical form of the contaminate

(6) Determine when to replace canisters and cartridge units

(7) Demonstrate proper procedures for inspection, cleaning, and storage of FFAPR

6.9.2 Understanding the Safety Features and Limitations of FFAPR. The training program of the authority having jurisdiction shall evaluate the ability of members to perform the following skills:

(1) Describe the operational principles of the FFAPR

(2) Identify the limitations of the FFAPR used by the authority having jurisdiction

(3) Describe the limitations of the FFAPR's ability to protect the body from absorption of toxins through the skin

(4) Describe the procedures for determining canister and cartridge selection by color-coded as well as NIOSH-approved labeling

(5) Understand labels are not to be removed from canisters or cartridges

(6) Understand that the use of FFAPR is prohibited for fire fighting

(7) Describe the limitations of FFAPR in fire ground activities

Reprinted with permission from NFPA 1404, *Standard for Fire Service Respiratory Protection Training*, and NFPA 1500, *Standard on Fire Department Occupational Safety and Health Program*, Copyright © 2002, National Fire Protection Association, Quincy, MA 02269. This reprinted material is not the complete and official position of the National Fire Protection Association on the referenced subject, which is represented only by the standard in its entirety.

Chapter 1
Introduction to Respiratory Protection

Immediately following the Second World War, the fire and emergency services in North America and around the world expanded their concerns over respiratory protection for its members. Prior to the war, respiratory protection had limited use by emergency responders. It was, however, utilized in very specialized circumstances, including deep-tunnel work, mining, and poisonous atmospheres. During the late 1960s with the introduction of plastics in consumer products and the use of synthetic materials in residences and offices, respiratory protection saw an increase in acceptance and use by the fire and emergency services. Today, respiratory protection use has expanded to include postsuppression activities such as loss control, overhaul and cause determination, hazardous materials incidents, and emergency medical incidents. These changes in attitude and policy resulted from an increase in the types of hazards faced by firefighters and emergency responders, an increased awareness of the hazards posed by toxic atmospheres and infectious diseases, and improvements in the types of respiratory protection available to the fire and emergency services. In addition, federal, state/provincial, and local occupational safety and health regulations now mandate specific types of respiratory protection for specific fire and emergency service functions. It is no longer considered courageous for a firefighter or rescuer to attempt a rescue or enter a toxic atmosphere without first donning respiratory protection (**Figure 1.1**).

This chapter provides a general background of respiratory protection and includes the following topics:

- Brief history of the development of respiratory protection

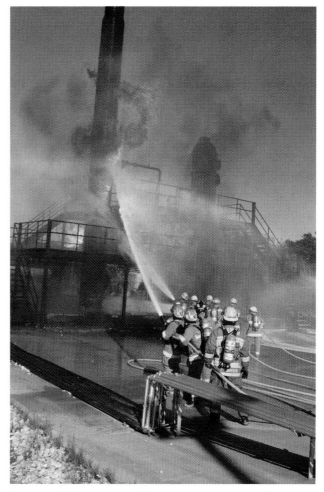

Figure 1.1 Modern fire fighting requires the use of full personal protective clothing and respiratory equipment.

- Overview of the physiology of the human body that creates the demand for respiratory protection

- Overview of the hazards to the respiratory system

- Various types of respiratory protection currently available to the fire and emergency services

History and Background of Respiratory Protection

Historical records indicate that the recognition of the need for respiratory protection dates back close to 2,000 years. In 50 C.E., Pliny, a Roman writer, made reference to the use of loose-fitting animal bladders to protect Roman miners against inhalation of red oxides of lead. While doing his analysis of human anatomy, Italian artist/inventor Leonardo da Vinci (1452–1519) recognized the need for respiratory protection against hazardous atmospheres. Italian Bernardino Ramazzini (1633–1714), the founder of the discipline of occupational medicine, recognized the need for respiratory protection in such occupations as mining, stone cutting, and milling. During the 1700s, the original ancestors of modern respiratory protection devices were developed (**Figure 1.2**). Although the designs have changed drastically in the past 300 years, the performance of the respirators is still based on the following two basic principles:

- Purifying the ambient air by removing contaminants
- Providing clean breathing air from an uncontaminated source

These two principles were applied in Europe and North America during the 19th century to protect workers against hazardous atmospheres. In 1814, the first air-purifying filter (a filter in a rigid container) was developed. Activated charcoals began to be used as a filtration medium in 1854. The concept of oxygen rebreathing was developed by Galibert, and he applied it to his design for a respiratory protection device in 1864 in England (**Figure 1.3**). An early patent for an air-purifying mask in the U.S. was issued in 1872 to Peter Ackerman of Bangor, Maine. For several years the London Fire

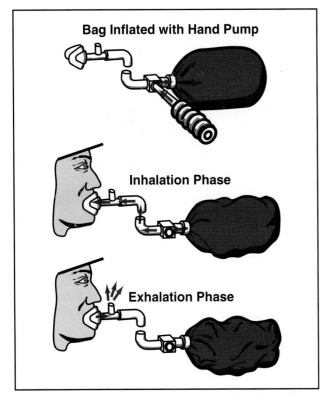

Figure 1.2 Illustration of the first self-contained breathing apparatus designed by Alexander Humboldt in 1795.

Bag Inflated with Hand Pump

Inhalation Phase

Exhalation Phase

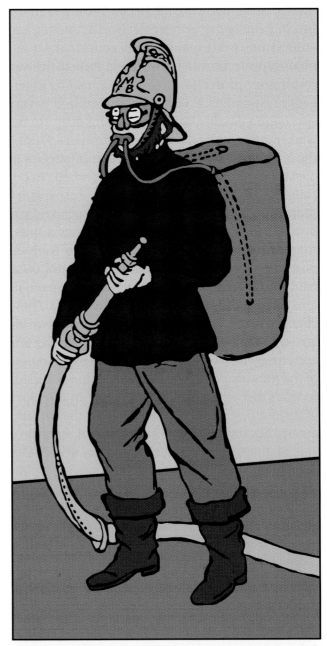

Figure 1.3 The Galibert breathing apparatus was an early oxygen rebreather.

Chronological History of the Development of Respiratory Protection in the Fire and Emergency Services

50 C.E.	Roman miners use animal bladders to prevent the inhalation of lead oxides.
1500 C.E.	Italian Leonardo da Vinci determines the need for protection of the respiratory system from hazardous atmospheres.
1700 C.E.	Italian Bernardo Ramazzini determines the need for respiratory protection in mining, milling, and stone cutting.
1795 C.E.	Alexander Humboldt invents the first self-contained breathing apparatus (SCBA) in Germany.
1814 C.E.	An air-purifying respirator (APR) is developed in Europe.
1830 C.E.	The Vienna Fire Brigade in Austria uses a primitive SCBA made of sheet iron.
1830 C.E.	Chief Paulin of the Paris (France) Fire Department invents a smoke jacket that is supplied with air from a pump through a hose.
1854 C.E.	Activated charcoal is first used to purify breathing air.
1864 C.E.	Galibert develops the concept of the rebreather in England.
1872 C.E.	A patent is issued to American Peter Ackerman in Maine for an air-purifying mask.
1877 C.E.	Fayol develops the concept of a pressure-demand respirator in England.
1877 C.E.	A patent is issued for the LaCour SCBA in the United States.
1877 C.E.	Use of smoke hoods becomes popular in the United States.
1877 C.E.	The Nealy Smoke Mask is developed in the United States.
1890 C.E.	E. M. Shaw and John Tyndall develop a canister and facepiece rebreather in England.
1892 C.E.	The Merriman Smoke Mask is developed in the United States.
1914 C.E.	The use of chemical warfare in World War I forces development of more effective respiratory protection devices.
1920 C.E.	Mine Safety Appliances Company produces SCBA for the deep-mining industry. It was the first such unit approved by the Bureau of Mines.
1930 C.E.	Resin-impregnated dust filters are produced in the United States for protection against dust and fibrous contaminates.
1930s C.E.	The British Fire Service provides two breathing apparatus per fire apparatus.
1940 C.E.	The U.S. Navy develops an oxygen-generating canister mask.
1960 C.E.	Britain provides breathing apparatus (BA) training for all fire service personnel who have 18 months of service.
1960 C.E.	The British Fire Service establishes age and physical fitness requirements.
1969 C.E.	Ultralightweight air cylinders are placed in service in Britain.
1970 C.E.	The Occupational Safety and Health (OSH) Act is passed, initiating the creation of workplace safety regulations by the U.S. Government.
1970 C.E. to present	Technological advances in lightweight and fire-retardant materials increase the safety and durability of respiratory protection equipment.

Brigade used a facepiece designed by Captain E. M. Shaw with a canister designed by Professor John Tyndall in 1890. The design was the forerunner of the Type N, Universal gas mask canister used by many fire departments until the late 1960s.

The introduction of mustard gas and other toxic agents to the battlefields of World War I caused inventors/engineers in England, Germany, and France and later the United States to develop more suitable respiratory protection devices. These gas masks were full facepiece, oxygen-rebreathing units that provided limited protection when donned quickly.

The 1930s saw the development of resin-impregnated dust filters for industrial use. The filters were efficient, inexpensive, and provided good protection against particulates in the atmosphere.

In the United States, oxygen-generating or oxygen breathing apparatus (OBA) were initially developed for the mining and tunneling industry. The units provided breathing air to workers in areas that lacked ventilation and for escape and rescue purposes. Further development of the oxygen-generating canister occurred through a United States Navy contract during World War II. OBAs (also called Chemox™ units were used for shipboard fire fighting and escape and rescue from toxic atmospheres within the ships (**Figure 1.4**). The moisture from the wearer's exhaled breath reacted with the chemicals in the canister, which produced oxygen and absorbed carbon dioxide (CO_2). The product of exchange was mixed well in the breathing bag and then inhaled by the wearer. A collapsible breathing bag connected to the canister served as a reservoir to store the oxygen as it was generated. Because pure oxygen was involved, firefighters were warned to keep oil, grease, or open flame from entering the canister; otherwise rapid oxidation or explosion of the canister could result. Oxygen-generating canisters were designed to last for 45 to 60 minutes, but

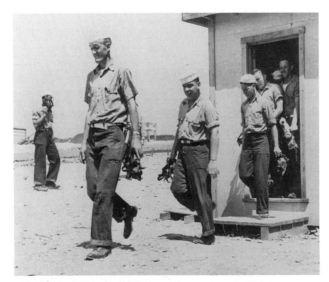

Figure 1.4 During World War II, the United States Navy trained personnel in the use of oxygen breathing apparatus (OBA) for protection during shipboard fire fighting. *Courtesy of U. S. Navy Archives.*

once the chemical process started, there was no way to turn it off. These units remained in limited service with the U.S. Navy into the 1990s.

Further improvements in air-purifying masks, both particulate filter and oxygen rebreathers, have been made since the end of World War II. Most changes have been generated by workplace safety regulations such as those resulting from the Occupational Safety and Health Act. Respiratory protections in industry, construction, emergency services, and agriculture have been addressed in various federal and state/provincial regulations. To address these requirements, manufacturers of respiratory protection equipment have developed filter systems and masks to meet the specific hazards outlined in the regulations. The same technology that created some hazards has also helped create types of protection against these hazards. For instance, fine glass fibers that can create a breathing hazard have made the construction of high-efficiency filters possible. Other developments include smaller, better fitting facepieces with improved fields of vision, lower profile masks that interface with other types of head and eye protection, and filters that provide specific levels of protection.

The development of air-supplied systems began in the late 1700s. The first known self-contained breathing apparatus (SCBA) was developed in Germany in 1795. About 1830, the Vienna Fire Brigade began using a container made of sheet iron that carried atmospheric air. In 1877 in England, Fayol developed an apparatus that may have been the first pressure-demand device. The unit had a bellows-type air bag filled with clean air capped with a lead lid. The weight of the lid forced air to the user's mouthpiece for breathing and also supplied air to a lamp to keep it burning in an oxygen-deficient atmosphere (**Figure 1.5**).

An example of another type of breathing apparatus was Paulin's Smoke Jacket, developed by the Chief of the Paris Fire Department in 1830. A hand-operated pump supplied air to a cowhide blouse. The air was discharged at the wrists and waist. An attachment to provide air to a lamp was also provided.

In Britain, the use of breathing apparatus (BA) increased in the 1930s and 1940s. At that time, two BAs were carried on all fire service apparatus, and two men on each crew were trained in their use. The BAs were used primarily for search and rescue but were also to be worn "if the smoke is thick" or there is "burning electrical insulation." By 1960, BA training was provided for all personnel with 18 months service. Age restrictions and fitness standards were also in place. Ultralightweight air cylinders were introduced into service in 1969.

The United States had very few, if any, dependable manufacturers of protective breathing devices before World War I. As late as 1910, many cities required firefighters to have beards at least 6 inches (150 mm) long. Firefighters would dip their beards into buckets of water, fold them into their mouths, and use them as smoke filters for breathing.

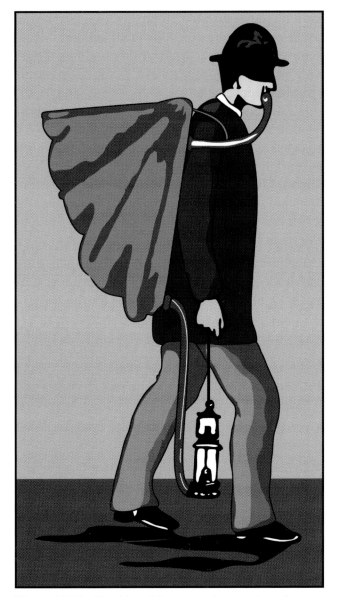

Figure 1.5 The Fayol breathing apparatus may have been the first true pressure-demand apparatus.

The earliest known American-made SCBA was LaCour's device in 1877 (**Figure 1.6**). This apparatus was similar to Galibert's SCBA. LaCour's device used a leather air bag containing two tubes leading from the bag to the mouth. One tube went into the top of the bag for inhaling oxygen and the other tube went into the bottom of the bag for exhaling carbon dioxide. Smoke hoods containing compressed air or oxygen were also manufactured during this time period.

Supplied-air equipment was developed for the U.S. fire service in the late 1800s and saw limited use at fires until the adoption of SCBA for respiratory protection. For instance, in 1892, Merriman's Smoke Mask featured an air hose located inside a water hose. Moistened-sponge devices for cooling and filtering inhaled air were also commonly used. The Nealy Smoke Mask of 1877 had sponges that were kept moist from water contained in a boat on the user's chest.

The first SCBA to be approved in the United States was the Gibbs closed-circuit oxygen breathing apparatus developed by the Mine Safety Appliances Company. The device was approved for deep mine

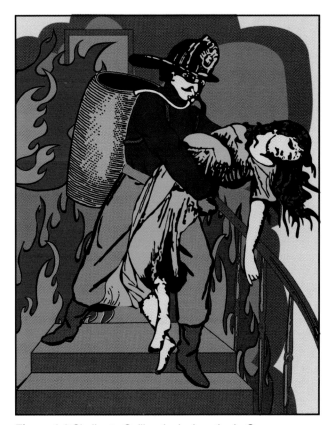

Figure 1.6 Similar to Galibert's design, the LaCour apparatus was developed in the United States in 1877.

operations by the Bureau of Mines (known since 1978 as the Mine Safety and Health Administration [MSHA]). This device, the forerunner of today's equipment, was the first to use a completely lung-governed principle of operation. The Gibbs apparatus was widely used in the early 1920s.

The use of air-supplied respiratory protection equipment in the fire service in North America dates from the 1950s. The early SCBAs were expensive and not viewed as necessary by fire department administrations. Units were usually placed on ladder trucks and used only for search, rescue, and ventilation. Engine companies were rarely equipped with SCBAs and then only with one or two units (**Figure 1.7**).

The need for air-supplied respiratory protection equipment only became apparent with the increase in hazardous materials in the environment. Plastics and synthetic materials in homes, chemicals and petroleum products in warehouses and on highways, and the use of flammable and toxic materials in manufacturing led to the creation of government regulations for their manufacture, han-dling, and disposal. These regulations, intended to create a safe work environment culminated in the creation of the Occupational Safety and Health Administration (OSHA) in 1970. Although originally intended to regulate private industry, the laws have been applied subsequently to the public sector and to the fire and emergency services.

With the increasing hazards and the new government regulations, the fire and emergency services began to increase its use of air-supplied systems, in particular SCBA. Fire departments equipped all fire apparatus with one SCBA per crew member during a given work shift. Training in respiratory protection was provided, first for existing employees and then for new personnel in recruit classes. Annual medical evaluations and physical fitness programs were also inaugurated to ensure that personnel could operate in hazardous environments while using SCBA. By the 1990s, individual facepieces were issued to fire department members, spare air cylinders were carried on all apparatus, and protocols were in place that required the wearing of respiratory protection whenever personnel were engaged in interior fire fighting or when entering a potentially hazardous or unknown atmosphere (**Figure 1.8**). In some areas National Fire Protection Association (NFPA) standards became the basis for respiratory protection programs in the fire and emergency services.

Technological changes paralleled the increasing use of air-supplied respiratory protection equipment. Equipment changes include the following:

- Use of fire-retardant material on the harness system and hoses
- Increased capacity air cylinders
- Use of lightweight materials to reduce weight and bulkiness
- Integrated personal alert safety system (PASS) devices
- Heat- and fire-resistant material for facepieces
- Integrated facepiece and helmet systems
- Shift from negative-pressure to positive-pressure type regulators
- Development of quick-fill systems
- Development of buddy-breathing adapters
- Improved communications systems integrated with the breathing air system

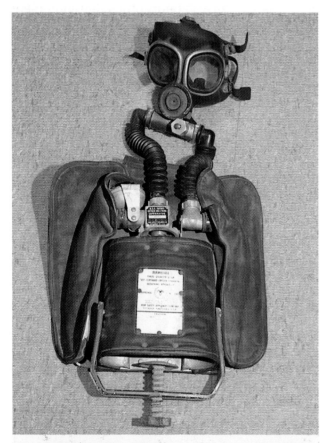

Figure 1.7 During the 1950s, many firefighters wore the Mine Safety Appliances Company (MSA) Chemox™ three-quarter-hour self-contained breathing apparatus.

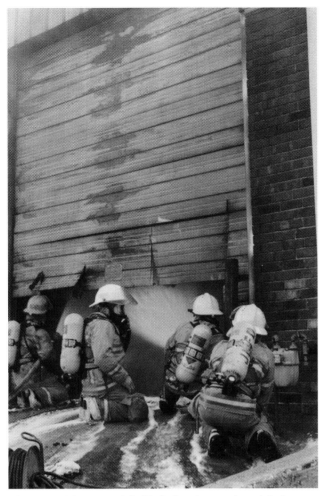

Figure 1.8 The potential of lethal toxins produced during interior fires has created awareness of the need for respiratory protection by firefighters. *Courtesy of Chris Mickal.*

These changes, and many more, have increased the respiratory protection of emergency responders. Changes occur rapidly in respiratory protection technology. Because changes inevitably make the respiratory protection equipment safer and easier to use, the fire and emergency services must take an active role in making certain that their equipment is state of the art — capable of ensuring user safety and performing effectively under the diverse conditions in which firefighters/emergency responders are required to work. This role includes participation in the standards-writing process and working directly with manufacturers to improve respiratory protection equipment designs.

Physiology

The body is a remarkable system with great capabilities; however, it obviously has its limitations. Our bodies can be adversely affected by injury, disease and age, exposure to hazardous materials, and inactivity or lack of physical conditioning. Because firefighters and emergency response personnel depend on their physical abilities to perform their duties, they must understand the body's capabilities and limitations. This information will help them realize the importance of wearing proper respiratory protection equipment (such as self-contained breathing apparatus and air-purifying respirators [APRs]) and of taking other safety precautions to protect their bodies (particularly their respiratory and cardiovascular systems). Besides the need for respiratory protection, fire and emergency services personnel must be aware of the importance of physical fitness, good nutrition, annual medical evaluations and examinations, and the effects of smoking and stimulants on the body. In addition, firefighters and emergency responders must be aware of the physiological and psychological effects of respiratory protection use, the body's defense mechanisms that protect it from respiratory hazards, and methods of controlled breathing that can be used when respiratory protection equipment fails.

Respiratory and Cardiovascular Systems

Body cells need a continuous supply of oxygen to live and convert food to energy. Oxygen is supplied to the body by the respiratory system. The respiratory system consists of the nose, pharynx, larynx, trachea, bronchi, and lungs, which contain bronchioles and alveolar ducts and sacs (alveoli) (**Figure 1.9**). The respiratory system enables gas exchange to occur through external and internal respirations. The body takes in oxygen and removes carbon dioxide by breathing, or external respiration. Internal respiration refers to the exchange of oxygen and carbon dioxide between the blood and body cells and use of oxygen by the cells.

The cardiovascular, or circulatory, system serves as the body's transportation system. Included in the cardiovascular system are the heart, blood, and blood vessels. One function of the cardiovascular system is to transport oxygen-rich blood from the respiratory system and deliver it to cells.

Oxygen, supplied through the respiratory system, is passed to the circulatory system and delivered to

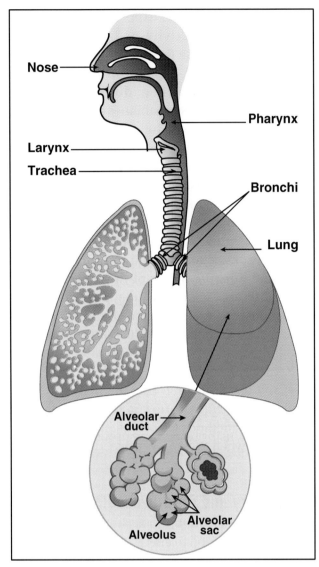

Figure 1.9 The principle structure of the body's respiratory system includes the nose, pharynx, larynx, trachea, bronchi, and lungs.

Nose
Pharynx
Larynx
Trachea
Bronchi
Lung
Alveolar duct
Alveolar sac
Alveolus

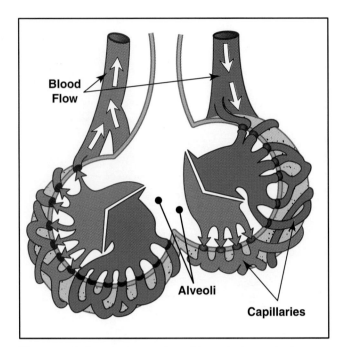

Blood Flow
Alveoli
Capillaries

Figure 1.10 Oxygen is transferred from the lungs to the blood stream by way of the alveolus.

body cells, and carbon dioxide is removed from body cells. To enable body cells to exchange gases, the respiratory system first exchanges gases with blood, the blood circulates, and then blood cells and body cells exchange gases. The blood, which travels through the heart, arteries, and veins, carries oxygen to all the cells. Blood cells perform other functions as well, including carrying nutrients to cells and waste from them. In terms of respiration, the most important cells are the red blood cells because they contain hemoglobin. Hemoglobin carries the oxygen, which chemically bonds to the hemoglobin (**Figure 1.10**). An important note about hemoglobin is that it has a great affinity for carbon monoxide (CO), which means that the blood would

rather carry it than oxygen. Carbon monoxide is present in large quantities at fires. Therefore, an emergency responder who is not wearing respiratory protection can very rapidly develop problems because of carbon monoxide poisoning.

Exposure to smoke and/or toxic gases can result in serious injury or death because the body cannot live for more than 4 to 6 minutes without a constant supply of oxygen. By learning how the body functions, the firefighter/emergency responder should have a better understanding of the consequences of not wearing respiratory protection. Entering a hazardous atmosphere without respiratory protection exposes the body to smoke, toxic gases, and an atmosphere deficient in oxygen. Toxic gases that reach the alveoli can cause irreparable and permanent damage to them, preventing normal gas exchange from occurring. If toxic gases burn the lung tissue, the alveoli fill with fluids and the gas exchange cannot occur. Undamaged alveoli exposed to high concentrations of toxic gases pass these gases to the blood cells through diffusion. Because blood cells have a high affinity for carbon monoxide and other gases, they absorb them rapidly (**Figure 1.11**). Once toxic gases are in the blood cells, they go on to destroy them. Toxic substances capable of passing through the alveoli and into the bloodstream have the quickest effect on the body.

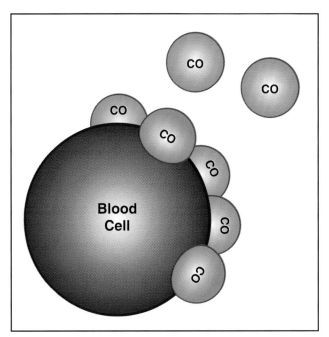

Figure 1.11 The same blood cells that carry oxygen throughout the body also attract carbon monoxide and other toxic gases.

Body's Defense Mechanisms

The body has defense mechanisms to help protect it and the respiratory system from invasion by foreign particles and injury. The primary level of protection is found in the mucous membranes of the nasal passage. The secondary level of protection consists of special cells in the alveoli of the lungs that act as filters to remove the particles before they enter the bloodstream. An important factor affecting these protection systems is the size of the particle entering the body: the smaller the particle, the more easily it can penetrate the body's defenses. While large foreign particles are trapped by nasal hair in the nose, gases, vapors, and small particulates can still reach the alveoli. Once the alveoli are damaged, they are not only unable to repair themselves but can no longer perform oxygen exchange. Also, gases reaching this area of the lungs could pass directly into the bloodstream and may attack the vital organs of the body (liver, heart, brain, etc.). Wearing respiratory protection is necessary to protect these delicate parts of the body from these hazards.

Body's Reaction While Wearing Respiratory Protection

Most fire and emergency service personnel must perform strenuous work that requires using great amounts of energy during short periods of time.

The use of respiratory protection equipment can have both positive and negative effects on the wearer's body.

The currently approved positive-pressure respiratory breathing apparatus supplies breathing air to the facepiece under a greater pressure than that found in the external atmosphere. This positive pressure prevents the external atmosphere from entering the facepiece through the exhalation valve or an incomplete face seal and thus keeps out a toxic atmosphere (**Figure 1.12**). Also when a positive-pressure facepiece is worn, a positive pressure of 1/27 psi (0.255 kPa) is found throughout the lungs as well as in the facepiece. This positive pressure in the lungs causes the lungs to become hyperinflated; that is, the amount of air left in the lungs is greater than normal due to exhaling against resistance. With more air in the lungs, the alveoli exchange gases more efficiently.

However, wearing respiratory protection has some negative effects on the body as well (**Figure 1.13**). No matter how physically fit an emergency responder is, using respiratory protection generally causes a 20-percent decrease in physical performance. Also, when an emergency responder exhales

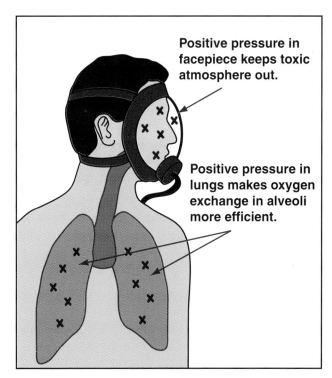

Figure 1.12 A positive-pressure facepiece causes an increase in the pressure within the lungs, which makes the exchange of oxygen and gases more efficient.

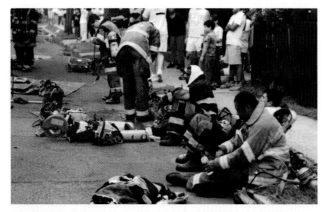

Figure 1.13 The use of respiratory protection equipment can place additional stresses on the body of the wearer, reducing physical performance by as much as 20 percent. *Courtesy of Bill Tompkins.*

into the facepiece of an open-circuit SCBA (one in which exhaled air is normally vented to the outside of the facepiece), some of that air is brought in on the next inhalation. This inhaled air contains more CO_2 than normal, and increased levels of CO_2 cause respirations to increase. Design changes in the facepiece, including the use of nose cups, cross-lens ventilation, and improved circulation patterns, have reduced this problem.

In the past, a problem also developed when the respiratory cycle increased beyond a certain air-flow rate. Older positive-pressure regulators could not meet the wearer's peak flow demands when the inhalation rate exceeded 40 L/min, which is the consumption rate established by National Institute for Occupational Safety and Health (NIOSH) for 1,200 liters of air in 30 minutes. When this flow rate was exceeded, it caused negative pressure within the facepiece. However, newer NFPA performance standards require a more realistic minimum flow rate of 100 L/min. The 100 L/min ventilation rate is based on studies indicating that 98 percent of the firefighters who participated breathed at this rate. Beginning in 1987, positive-pressure regulators intended for use by emergency responders have all been manufactured to meet NFPA standards and to sustain an air-flow rate of 100 L/min with maximum capabilities of 400 to 500 L/min. At present, SCBA that comply with the current NFPA 1981, *Standard on Open-Circuit Self-Contained Breathing Apparatus for the Fire Service*, provide enough flow to maintain a positive pressure within the facepiece even under extreme increased breathing. Although all new SCBA manufactured in the United States and

intended for fire service use must meet the current standard, older units that may not meet this criterion are still in service. As long as they meet the standard in effect at the time of manufacture, those units may still be used as certified.

Physiological and Psychological Factors

An emergency responder must not only be physically prepared for an emergency incident, but also mentally and emotionally ready. Challenges and frightening experiences can produce fear and anxiety that trigger an autonomic response commonly known as the *fight-or-flight syndrome*. This response increases heart and respiration rates. The body reacts by releasing adrenaline, which chemically causes the breathing rate to increase. Fear can also trigger sweating and dry mouth. Anticipating increased work levels, the brain also causes the liver to release extra sugar for energy. Tense or fearful emergency responders use their air supplies faster than personnel who remain calm. Some people may feel claustrophobic or "closed in" when they first put on a breathing apparatus facepiece. This feeling increases the mental stress and fight-or-flight response.

Proper training, confidence in one's abilities, and knowledge of the equipment can reduce fear, thereby improving the rate of air consumption. A trained emergency responder in good physical condition should also be able to override some of the increased breathing rates and gain efficient respiration through controlled breathing techniques (**Figure 1.14**). *Controlled breathing* is a

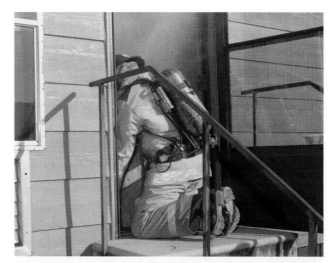

Figure 1.14 Smoke-room training provides the trainee with an opportunity to experience the limitations created in actual structural fires including restricted vision and communications.

conscious effort to reduce air consumption by forcing exhalation from the mouth and allowing natural inhalation through the nose. Emergency responders should practice and perfect controlled breathing methods in training sessions until using such methods becomes second nature. Detailed descriptions of these methods are found in Chapter 10, Emergency Scene Use.

Monitoring the Degree of Physical Exertion

During emergency operations that require the use of self-contained breathing apparatus, emergency response personnel should be medically evaluated whenever they expend one cylinder of breathing air. Medical personnel or the incident safety officer should evaluate them every 30 to 45 minutes, depending on environmental conditions (**Figure 1.15**). Evaluations established by the department's emergency medical services (EMS) protocol should

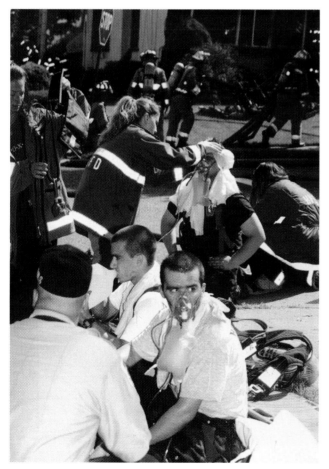

Figure 1.15 Medical personnel should monitor the conditions of emergency personnel during rehabilitation by checking body temperature, heart rate, blood pressure, and signs of fatigue. *Courtesy of Chris Tompkins.*

include recording temperature readings, heart rates, blood pressure readings, and signs of fatigue. The incident commander or incident safety officer should keep track of the conditions of emergency personnel during an incident.

Physical Fitness

The physical fitness of emergency responders is an increasing concern in the fire and emergency services. Emergency response tasks may tax a responder to his or her physical limits; therefore, above-average strength and endurance are required. Being in good physical condition lessens the chances of fatigue, and thus a responder will be less likely to make mental errors or become injured.

Extra physical work requires extra oxygen for the muscles. Depending on their physical conditions, individuals performing the same work may require different levels of exertion and oxygen use. An emergency responder in poor physical condition has to work harder and thus consumes a supply of air faster than a responder in good physical condition. Duration rating tests do not fully take into account the extra oxygen needed by the obese or otherwise physically unfit responder.

The two greatest risks to emergency responder fitness and performance are being obese and smoking tobacco products. Excessive body weight strains the body's cardiovascular system. During extreme exertion, this strain can lead to heart failure. Cigarette, cigar, and pipe smoking greatly compounds the effects of fire fighting and emergency responses by reducing lung capacity and by leading to the development of chronic lung diseases. To address these two risks, the emergency services organization should establish a health and wellness program for employees. To be effective, it should provide a physical fitness regimen, a nutrition element, and a smoking secession and prohibition policy. The IFSTA **Fire Department Safety Officer** manual provides a guide for a health and wellness program (**Figure 1.16**).

Standards established by NFPA and the American National Standards Institute (ANSI) address the physical fitness issue. ANSI Z88.5, *Practices for Respiratory Protection for the Fire Service,* recommends that firefighters be physically fit. ANSI Z88.6, *For Respiratory Protection — Respirator Use — Physical*

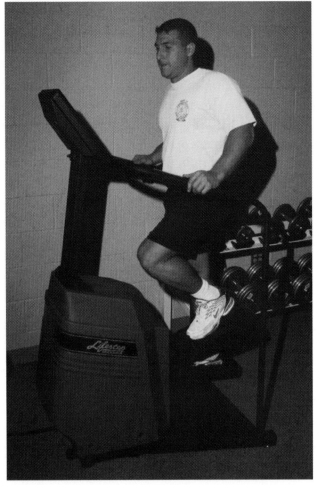

Figure 1.16 An effective health and wellness program including a physical fitness program can help to improve individual stamina.

Qualifications for Personnel, gives guidelines for departments and physicians to use in determining whether a firefighter is physically qualified to use a respirator. In Canada, Canadian Standards Association (CSA) Z94.4-93, *Selection, Use, and Care of Respirators*, provides similar guidelines. If adopted by the local authority having jurisdiction, OSHA Title 29 (Labor) *Code of Federal Regulations (CFR)* 1910.134 (Respiratory Protection) and both NFPA 1500, *Standard on Fire Department Occupational Safety and Health Program* (2002 edition), and NFPA 1404, *Standard for Fire Service Respiratory Protection Training* (2002 edition), require that firefighters/emergency responders be checked annually by physicians before they are allowed to use respiratory protection equipment such as SCBA and supplied-air respirators (SARs). Therefore, accurate records of physical fitness and medical examinations of each firefighter/emergency responder must

be kept. NFPA 1500 also lists guidelines for departments to follow in regard to establishing, implementing, and maintaining firefighter/emergency responder safety and health programs. Breathing consumption ratios are addressed later in this manual.

Respiratory Hazards

Fire and emergency services personnel must be familiar with the different types of respiratory hazards they will encounter. Although the body is amazing in its scope of possible activities, its ability to adapt to environmental change is limited by the narrow range of permissible oxygen concentration in the air breathed. This limitation is clearly demonstrated by the body's extremely low tolerance to a variety of foreign substances in the air. Firefighters and emergency services personnel routinely encounter situations that tax or even exceed this adaptive capacity (**Figure 1.17**). Without respiratory protection, the body can sustain fatal injuries when exposed to respiratory hazards. Wearing respiratory protection is the most effective way to protect the body from these hazards.

This section covers hazards from both fires and nonfire incidents. Respiratory hazards from structural fires are separated into oxygen-deficient atmospheres, thermal hazards (including elevated temperatures, rollovers, flashovers, and backdrafts), smoke, and toxic fire gases. Other hazardous atmo-

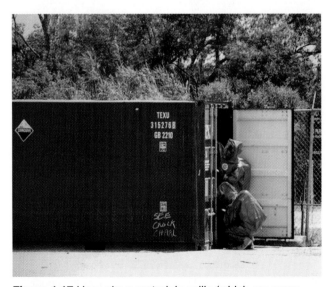

Figure 1.17 Hazardous materials spills (which are sometimes restricted to containers) pose a variety of respiratory hazards for emergency responders.

spheres not associated with structural fire fighting are also discussed such as exposures to asbestos, polychlorinated biphenyl, oxygen deficiency, hazardous materials, biological/medical pathogens, and weapons of mass destruction. The short- and long-term effects of respiratory hazards are also addressed.

Respiratory Hazards Encountered During Emergency Responses

Respiratory Hazards Associated with Fire
    Oxygen Deficiency
    Thermal Hazards
        Elevated Temperatures
        Rollover
        Flashover
        Backdraft
    Smoke
    Toxic Fire Gases
        Carbon Monoxide
        Hydrogen Chloride
        Hydrogen Cyanide
        Carbon Dioxide
        Phosgene
        Oxides of Nitrogen
        Acrolein
        Formaldehyde
        Hydrogen Sulfide
        Sulfur Dioxide
        Benzene
Respiratory Hazards Not Associated with Fire
    Asbestos
    Polychlorinated Biphenyl
    Oxygen-Deficient Atmospheres
    Hazardous Materials
    Biological/Medical Pathogens
    Exposure to Weapons of Mass Destruction

Respiratory Hazards Associated with Fire

[NFPA 1500: 7.9.7, 7.9.8]
[NFPA 1404: 5.1.7 (4) (6) (7), 5.2 (1) (2), 6.6.1, 6.7.2 (2) (3)]

Fires, whether interior or exterior, present a respiratory hazard to emergency responders. The lack of oxygen, the increases in temperature, and the cre-

ation of smoke and toxic gases contribute to the potential for illness, injury, or death if respiratory protection is inadequate or not used.

Oxygen Deficiency

Oxygen deficiency during fires occurs in two ways: through consumption and displacement. Because the combustion process requires oxygen, fires consume large amounts of oxygen from the air. Fires also produce toxic gases in large quantities that displace the oxygen in the atmosphere. OSHA and NFPA define an *oxygen-deficient atmosphere* as one that contains less than 19.5 percent oxygen per volume. **Table 1.1** shows the physiological effects of hypoxia (lack of oxygen) on the human body due to reduced percentages of oxygen in the atmosphere.

Table 1.1
Physiological Effects of Reduced Oxygen (Hypoxia)

Oxygen in Air (Percent)	Symptoms
21	None — normal conditions
17	Some impairment of muscular coordination; increase in respiratory rate to compensate for lower oxygen content
12	Dizziness, headache, rapid fatigue
9	Unconsciousness
6	Death within a few minutes from respiratory failure and concurrent heart failure

NOTE: The information in this table cannot be considered absolute because it does not account for differences in breathing rate or length of time exposed.

These symptoms occur only from reduced oxygen. If the atmosphere is contaminated with toxic gases, other symptoms may develop.

Thermal Hazards

Thermal hazards associated with fires include elevated temperatures, rollovers, flashovers, and backdrafts. These hazards have characteristic warning signs, and fire and emergency responders must recognize these indicators. Each of these thermal hazards can have irreparable damage on the respiratory system and exposed areas of the body. The responder wearing respiratory protection and complete protective clothing is likely to be in an area where these situations may occur. Therefore, it is important for the responder to be aware that current protective equipment may not adequately protect the wearer from these thermal hazards.

Elevated temperatures. Fire creates elevated temperatures especially within a confined area. Ceiling temperatures in a burning room can reach over 1,000°F (538°C) (**Figure 1.18**). Inhaling superheated air, especially moist superheated air (which happens after water is applied to a fire), causes intense burns of the respiratory tract. Pulmonary edema (accumulation of fluid in the lungs), which can completely block the airways, results quickly. When this condition occurs, edema in the alveoli can occur, interrupting respiratory gas exchange. Physiologically, the excessive heat may cause both a larynx spasm and bronchial spasm that completely block the airways of the lungs, causing imminent death.

> # WARNING!
> ### Inhaling superheated air can cause serious injury or death.

Excessive heat conducted to the lungs can also very quickly result in a serious drop in blood pressure. This situation can lead to cardiovascular collapse through shock. Inhalation injuries are often fatal, so prompt medical attention is essential.

Wearing respiratory protection not only keeps out toxic gases, but it also protects the respiratory system from temperatures that the body cannot withstand.

Rollover. *Rollover* is a condition that occurs when flames move through or across unburned gases. The flames of a fire, like smoke or water, seek the path of least resistance. When obstructed in their vertical movement, they try to proceed by moving horizontally; thus they "roll" across the ceiling. Rollover is a phenomenon that occurs prior to flashover and is often confused with it (see following paragraph). See **Figure 1.19** for illustrations of rollover, flashover, and backdraft.

Flashover. *Flashover* is the simultaneous ignition of all combustible contents in a compartment. It is caused by excessive accumulation of heat from a fire. As a fire burns, all the combustible contents in the area are heated and release flammable gases. As the heat becomes more intense, the flammable gases are raised to their ignition temperatures. While no exact temperature is associated with flashover, a range of approximately 900°F to 1,200°F (483°C to 649°C) is widely accepted. Carbon monoxide, for example, ignites at 1,200°F (649°C). When the ignition temperatures are reached, all the combustible gases ignite simultaneously and the area is suddenly fully involved in fire. The fire spreads rapidly, producing great amounts of toxic gases. Respiratory protection must be used to protect against the intense heat and toxic gases associated with flashover.

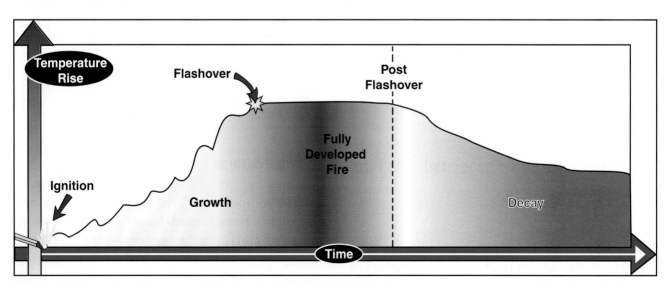

Figure 1.18 Illustration of the stages of the development of an interior fire.

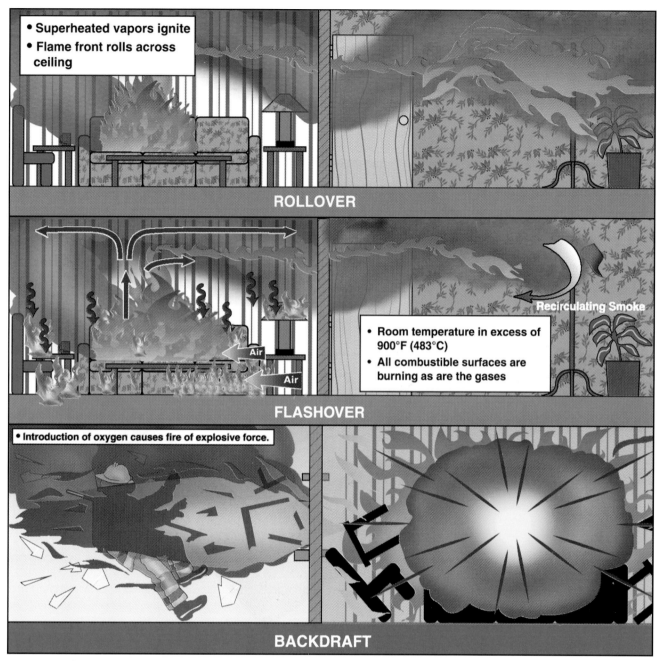

ROLLOVER
- Superheated vapors ignite
- Flame front rolls across ceiling

FLASHOVER
- Room temperature in excess of 900°F (483°C)
- All combustible surfaces are burning as are the gases

Recirculating Smoke

Air

Air

BACKDRAFT
- Introduction of oxygen causes fire of explosive force.

Figure 1.19 Rollover, flashover, and backdraft are three of the most dangerous fire situations responders can face.

Backdraft. *Backdraft* is an explosive ignition of gases. Even though backdraft is a rare occurrence, it can occur in the decay or late stages of a fire. When a fire has reached the smoldering stage, most of the available oxygen in the compartment has been used, but heat and fuels are still present in large quantities. All that is necessary to create a backdraft is the introduction of oxygen into an area that has not been properly ventilated. The result is very rapid oxidation, resulting in an explosion. Proper fire-suppression tactics and full personal protective equipment with SCBA reduce the possibility of in-

juries. The following conditions (**Figure 1.20**) indicate the possibility of backdraft:

- Pressurized smoke exiting small openings
- Black smoke becoming dense gray-yellow
- Confinement and excessive heat in a windowless structure
- Little or no visible flame
- Smoke leaving the building in puffs or at intervals
- Smoke-stained windows with heat-induced cracking of glass
- Inwardly drawn smoke (sucking phenomenon)

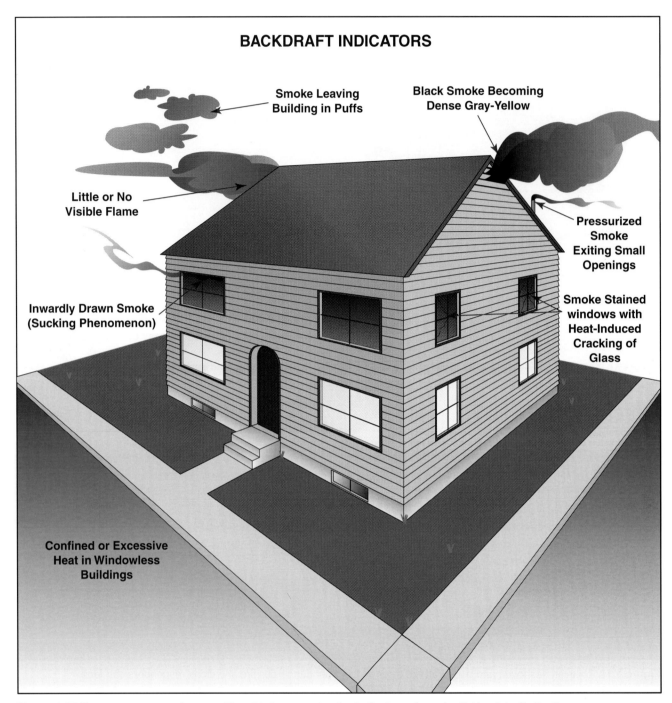

BACKDRAFT INDICATORS

Smoke Leaving Building in Puffs

Black Smoke Becoming Dense Gray-Yellow

Little or No Visible Flame

Pressurized Smoke Exiting Small Openings

Inwardly Drawn Smoke (Sucking Phenomenon)

Smoke Stained windows with Heat-Induced Cracking of Glass

Confined or Excessive Heat in Windowless Buildings

Figure 1.20 Emergency responders must be able to recognize the indicators of a potential backdraft situation.

Smoke

The smoke encountered at most fires consists of a mixture of oxygen, nitrogen, carbon dioxide, carbon monoxide, finely divided carbon particles, and a miscellaneous assortment of products that have been released from the material involved. Most visible smoke is a suspension of small particles that can be in either solid or liquid form. The solid particles provide a location for the condensation of the gaseous products of combustion. However, some combustion products remain as droplets and do not condense on the solid particles.

Toxic products of combustion can enter the body in three ways: (1) inhalation, (2) absorption through the skin, and (3) ingestion into the digestive tract **(Figure 1.21)**. Recall the defense mechanisms of the body that were discussed in the Physiology section earlier. Remember that gases and very small particles have a good chance of reaching the alveoli. With prolonged exposure, the particles and drop-

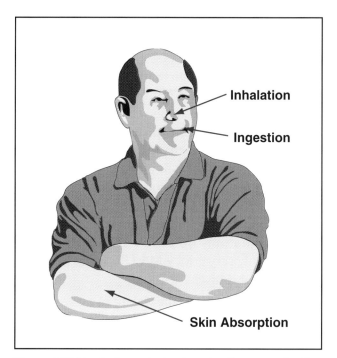

Figure 1.21 The toxic products of combustion can enter the body through inhalation, absorption, and ingestion.

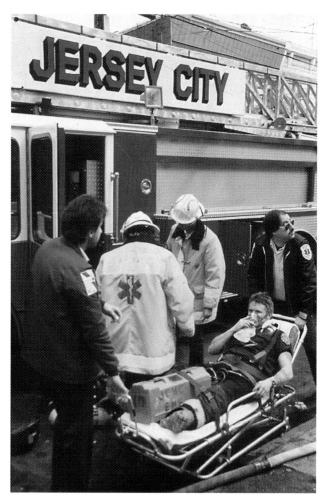

Figure 1.22 Emergency responders who suffer from smoke inhalation should be treated with oxygen, evaluated by a physician, and possibly admitted to a hospital for observation depending on the severity of the exposure. *Courtesy of Ron Jeffers.*

lets overpower the body's defense mechanisms. When enough contaminants reach the alveoli, the gas exchange process stops. In addition to the inhalation and absorption of smaller smoke particles, larger smoke particles can be ingested (swallowed), allowing contaminants to enter the blood from the digestive process. At the very least, swallowing smoke particulates cause nausea, vomiting, and diarrhea.

Tar particles or oil droplets are especially dangerous. Upon entering the alveoli, they may cause intense inflammation. Special cells in the alveoli attempt to remove these particles, but this defense mechanism can soon be overwhelmed. The condition that develops from this inflammation is known as *lipid pneumonia*. Oil droplets can also cause the alveoli to dilate and rupture, thus decreasing the total surface available to exchange oxygen and carbon dioxide. It is recommended that a physician examine emergency responders who have been exposed to heavy, choking smoke for even a few seconds, even if they feel well (**Figure 1.22**). A delay of 1 to 6 hours may occur before symptoms develop.

Toxic Fire Gases

Toxic gases produced by a fire are mixed with smoke. Some gases are colorless and odorless; others are quite irritating. Exposure to one gas is bad enough,

but most toxic gases are present in groups and varying concentrations. When these toxins enter the body, some can cause a *synergistic effect:* a phenomenon that occurs when the combined effect of two or more substances is more toxic or irritating than the total effect would be if each were inhaled separately. Toxic gases can enter the body through the respiratory system in the same manner as smoke particles or absorption through the skin. Therefore, full protective clothing is necessary for protection.

WARNING!

Inhaling toxic gases can cause serious injury or death.

The type and amount of toxic gases released at a fire vary according to the following four factors:

- Physical state of the combustible source
- Rate of heating
- Temperature of the evolved gases
- Oxygen concentration

Parts per Million (ppm) Defined

When discussing amounts of gases in the air, a measurement is given in parts per million (ppm):

$$\frac{\text{level of contaminant}}{1,000,000 \text{ parts air}}$$

Parts per million is actually a very small number. The following analogy helps illustrate how small ppm is: 1 ppm could be compared to 1 cent in $10,000.

Exposure to toxic gases and chemicals is not a new problem. People who work in chemical plants, refineries, or pesticide manufacturing plants have been exposed to toxic chemicals and gases for years. How much exposure is acceptable? Guidelines are established for human exposure to many chemicals such as those given by the American Conference of Governmental Industrial Hygienists (ACGIH), which sets threshold limit values (TLVs), and OSHA, which sets permissible exposure limits (PELs). Additional information is available from NIOSH and the Centers for Disease Control (CDC).

Fires produce large concentrations of toxic gases; these concentrations almost always exceed maximum allowable exposure limits and require the use of protective equipment. **Table 1.2** shows a listing of exposure limits for common fire gases. Two levels are shown: the short-term exposure limit (STEL) and the immediately dangerous to life and health (IDLH) concenetration. The *IDLH concentration* represents an atmospheric concentration of any toxic, corrosive, or asphyxiating substance that poses an immediate threat to life and can cause irreversible or delayed adverse health effects. The *STEL* is a 15-minute, time-weighted average that should not be exceeded at any time during a workday. Exposures at the STEL should not be longer than 15 minutes and should not be repeated more than four times per day with at least 60 minutes between exposures.

Fire fighting operations usually expose firefighters/emergency responders to very high levels of toxic gases. In many cases, the concentrations of these gases are so high that an exposure of only a few minutes can cause injury. The IDLH concentrations listed in the table reflect the maximum concentration levels of exposure a person can be exposed to without injury. Exposure includes skin and eyes as well as the respiratory system. Obviously emergency responders without respiratory protection should never enter an atmosphere containing toxic gases at the IDLH level. Atmospheres containing concentrations up to the STEL level may be tolerated only very briefly. Most fire gases will reach or exceed IDLH levels.

Vapor density (VD) is the weight of a gas or vapor compared to the weight of an equal volume of air. The vapor density of a gas tells whether it is heavier or lighter than air. Air has a value of 1. In a building, gases with a vapor density greater than 1 are found low, near the floor. Gases with a vapor density less than 1 are lighter than air and are found near the ceiling. Knowledge of the vapor densities of fire-released gases tells emergency responders the types of respiratory hazards that will be present during not only the suppression phase but also the loss control and investigation phases of an incident.

Many fire gases are not only toxic but also explosive. Table 1.2 also gives explosive limits for common fire gases. The explosive limits (upper and lower) indicate the percentage of gas that must mix with air in order to cause an explosion; these limits are boundaries of the explosive range. Gases with wide explosive ranges are the most dangerous. Gas concentrations below or above the explosive range are too lean or too rich, respectively, to burn. Flammable fire gases provide fuel for flashover and backdraft conditions.

The term *target organ* refers to the organ or system a toxic gas will affect. A number of these gases affect the eyes and skin. Wearing full facepiece respiratory protection protects the eyes as well as the respiratory system. Since many of these gases are directly absorbed into the skin without the emergency responder's knowledge, full protective clothing should always be worn. In addition to respiratory protection, gloves and hoods give some protection to the skin against these toxic gases during fire fighting operations.

Table 1.2
Chart of Common Fire Gases

Chemical	PEL (ppm)	STEL (ppm)	IDLH (ppm)	Chemical Properties (VD, SG)	Chemical Properties (LEL,UEL)	Traget Organs
Carbon Monoxide (CO)	35	200	1,500	VD: 1.0 SG: GAS	LEL: 12.5% UEL: 74%	Blood, Lungs, Cardiovascular System, Central Nervous System
Carbon Dioxide (CO_2)	5,000	3,000	40,000	VD: 1.5 SG: GAS	Nonflammable	Cardiovascular System, Respiratory System
Hydrogen Chloride (HCl)	5	5	50	VD: 1.3 SG: GAS	Nonflammable	Respiratory System, Skin, Eyes
Hydrogen Cyanide (HCN)	4.7	4.7	50	VD: 0.9 SG: 0.7	LEL: 5.6% UEL: 40%	Liver, Kidney, Central Nervous System, Cardiovascular System
Nitrogen Doxide (NO_2)	5	1	20	VD:1.6 SG: 1.4	Nonflammable	Respiratory System, Eyes, Cardiovascular System
Ammonia (NH_3)	25	35	300	VD: 0.6 SG: --	LEL: 15% UEL: 25%	Respiratory System, Eyes
Phosgene ($COCl_2$)	0.1	--	2	VD: 3.4 SG: GAS	Nonflammable	Respiratory System, Skin, Eyes
Acrolein (CH_2CHCHO)	0.1	0.3	2	VD:1.9 SG: 0.8	LEL: 2.8% UEL: 31%	Heart, Eyes, Skin, Respiratory System
Formaldehyde (HCHO)	0.75	2	20	VD: -- SG:1.1	LEL: 7% UEL: 73%	Respiratory System, Eyes, Skin
Hydrogen Sulfide (H_2S)	10	15	100	VD: 1.2 SG: GAS	LEL: 4.3% UEL: 44%	Respiratory System, Eyes
Benzene (C_6H_6)	1	5	500	VD: 2.7 SG: 0.9	LEL: 1.2% UEL: 7.8%	Blood, Skin, Bone Marrow, Eyes, Respiratory System, Cardiovascular System
Acetic Acid (CH_3COOH)	10	15	50	VD: 2.1 SG: 1.0	LEL: 4.0% UEL: 19.9%	Respiratory System, Skin, Eyes, Teeth
Acetaldehyde (CH_3CHO)	100	150	2,000	VD: 1.5 SG: 0.8	LEL: 4% UEL: 60%	Respiratory System, Skin, Kidneys
Formic Acid (HCOOH)	5	10	30	VD: 1.6 SG: 1.2	LEL: 18% LEL: 57%	Respiratory System, Skin, Kidney, Liver, Eyes

VD: Air = 1   SG: Water = 1

TLV (Threshold Limit Value) — A time-weighted average concentration under which most people can work consistently for 8 hours a day, day after day, with no harmful effects.

PEL (Permissible Exposure Limit) — The maximum time-weighted concentration at which 95 percent of exposed, healthy adults suffer no adverse effects over a 40-hour week — an 8-hour time-weighted average concentration, unless otherwise noted.

STEL (Short-Term Exposure Limit) — A 15-minute time-weighted average that should not be exceeded at any time during a workday. Exposures at the STEL should not be longer than 15 minutes and should not be repeated more than four times per day with at least 60 minutes between exposures.

IDLH (Immediately Dangerous to Life and Health) — Any atmosphere that poses an immediate hazard to life or produces immediate irreversible, debilitating effects on health.

VD (Vapor Density) — The weight of a given volume of pure vapor or gas compared to the weight of an equal volume of dry air at the same temperature and pressure. A figure less than 1 indicates a vapor lighter than air; a figure greater than 1 indicates a vapor heavier than air.

SG (Specific Graphic) — The weight of a substance compared to the weight of an equal volume of water, If the specific gravity is less than 1, the material is lighter than water and will float; if it is greater than 1, the material is heavier than water and will sink.

LEL (Lower Explosive Limit) — Below the flammability range or lower explosive limit, a gas or vapor is too lean to burn (too little fuel and too much oxygen).

UEL (Upper Explosive Limit) — Above the flammability range or upper explosive limit, a gas or vapor is too rich to burn (too much fuel and too little oxygen).

Definitions of Exposure Levels

Threshold Limit Value/Time-Weighted Average

The time-weighted average (TWA) of a substance is the maximum airborne concentration to which an average, healthy person may be exposed repeatedly for 8 hours each day, 40 hours per week without suffering adverse effects. These threshold limit values (TLVs) are based upon current available data and are adjusted on an annual basis. TLVs/TWAs are expressed in parts per million (ppm) and milligrams per cubic meter (mg/m^3). The lower the TLV, the more toxic the substance. At a hazardous materials incident, emergency response personnel should never assume that the concentration is below the TLV/TWA. TLVs/TWAs are primarily used for measuring exposures in the workplace and are not applicable for use in hazardous materials emergencies. However, they are useful during pre-incident planning.

Threshold Limit Value/Short-Term Exposure Limit

The threshold limit value/short-term exposure limit (TLV/STEL) value is the 15-minute, time-weighted average exposure that should not be exceeded at any time or repeated more than four times a day. A 60-minute rest period is required between each TLV/STEL exposure. This short-term exposure can be tolerated without suffering from irritation or chronic or irreversible tissue damage. Also, during this short time, none of the following conditions should occur: narcosis of a sufficient degree to increase the likelihood of accidental injury, impairment of self-rescue, or reduction of worker efficiency. TLVs/STELs are also expressed in ppm and mg/m^3. Under no circumstances is an employee allowed to work in an area with the TLV/STEL value longer than 15 minutes without proper personal protective equipment.

Threshold Limit Value/Ceiling Level

The threshold limit value/ceiling level (TLV-C) is a maximum concentration that should never be exceeded and where exposure protection is mandatory. When working in conditions where the hazardous material concentration is equal to or greater than the TLV-C, appropriate personal protective equipment including respiratory protection must always be used. TLV-C is reported in ppm or mg/m^3.

Permissible Exposure Limit

Permissible exposure limits (PELs) are very similar to TLVs/TWAs. The difference is that a TLV/TWA is determined by the American Conference of Governmental Industrial Hygienists (ACGIH), and PELs are adopted by the Occupational Safety and Health Administration (OSHA) upon recommendation by the ACGIH or the National Institute for Occupational Safety and Health (NIOSH). PELs are the maximum allowable amount of exposure for an eight-hour day. PELs are expressed in terms of ppm and mg/m^3.

Lethal Dose

The lethal dose (LD) of a substance is the minimum amount of solid or liquid that when ingested, absorbed, or injected through the skin will be fatal to 50 percent of all subjects exposed to that dosage. LD is an oral or dermal exposure expressed in milligrams per kilogram (mg/kg). The lower the number, the more toxic the material. Note that this does not mean the other half of the subjects will necessarily be all right. They may be very sick or almost dead, but only half will actually die.

Lethal Concentration

The lethal concentration (LC) of a substance is the minimum concentration of an inhaled substance in the gaseous state that will be fatal to 50 percent of a test group. These values are generally established by testing the effects of exposure on animals under laboratory conditions. As the LC value decreases, it becomes more toxic. LC is expressed in ppm, mg/m^3, and milligrams per liter (mg/L). First responders exposed to hazardous materials should know that exertion, stress, and their individual metabolisms or chemical sensitivities (allergies) may make them more vulnerable to the harmful effects of hazardous materials. The 50 percent of the population not killed may suffer effects ranging from no response to severe injury.

Immediately Dangerous to Life and Health

An immediately dangerous to life and health (IDLH) level is an atmospheric concentration of any toxic, corrosive, or asphyxiating substance that poses an immediate threat to life. It can cause irreversible or delayed adverse health effects and can interfere with an individual's ability to escape from a dangerous atmosphere. IDLHs are expressed in ppm or mg/m^3. At IDLH levels, personal protective equipment and respiratory protection are required.

Determining the concentration of toxic gases in an atmosphere requires specialized equipment and a thoroughly trained, knowledgeable operator (**Figure 1.23**). Generally, this equipment cannot be used during fire fighting operations; therefore, firefighters/emergency responders should be aware of symptoms that result from overexposure to toxic gases. Overexposure may occur during the initial response to the emergency or during postsuppression operations such as loss control and

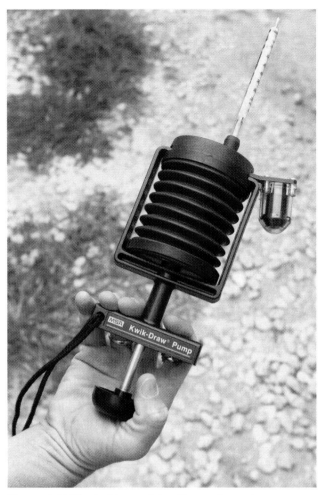

Figure 1.23 The incident safety officer, a hazardous materials officer, or other trained personnel should sample the atmosphere to determine the need for respiratory protection if it is not obvious.

investigation. Symptoms can be classified as *acute* (immediate) and *chronic* (long-term). Acute symptoms may be immediate reactions from overexposure to a toxic substance or symptoms may occur several hours after exposure. Recognizing these symptoms alerts firefighters/emergency responders to the need for proper medical attention. Firefighters/emergency responders should be able to recognize abnormal reactions in themselves as well as others. Chronic symptoms may not be readily detectable without medical testing. Therefore, it is recommended that firefighters/emergency responders receive regular medical examinations by qualified physicians. Such examinations are required for firefighters/emergency responders acting as hazardous material response teams by NFPA 1500, NFPA 1582, *Standard on Medical Requirements for Fire Fighters*, and Title 29 *CFR* 1910, Subpart L, Appendix A (Fire Protection).

The list of toxic gases presented in Table 1.2 is by no means complete. Further information can be obtained by consulting an industrial hygienist. Nonetheless, it should be clear that even an ordinary house contains many products that produce toxic gases during a fire. Because of the injuries these gases can cause, firefighters/emergency responders should never enter a hazardous atmosphere without wearing respiratory protection. The following paragraphs contain descriptions of some toxic gases found in most fire situations and symptoms that may occur with overexposure.

> # WARNING!
> **Do not remove SCBA during the overhaul stage of fire fighting. Levels of toxic fire gases such as carbon monoxide, hydrogen chloride, hydrogen cyanide, phosgene, nitrogen dioxide, acrolein, formaldehyde, hydrogen sulfide, sulfur dioxide, and benzene are extremely high during this stage due to incomplete combustion.**

Carbon monoxide. This colorless, odorless, and tasteless gas is present at all fires. According to the NFPA *Fire Protection Handbook*, carbon monoxide poisoning contributes to more fire deaths than any other toxic product of combustion. The poorer the ventilation and the more inefficient the burning, the greater the quantity of CO formed. A rule of thumb, although subject to much variation, is that the darker the smoke, the higher the CO levels. Black smoke is high in particulate carbon and carbon monoxide because of incomplete combustion. Carbon monoxide levels are extremely high during the overhaul stage of fire fighting due to this incomplete combustion. Do not remove SCBA during this stage of fire fighting. It is essential that CO levels be measured prior to removing respiratory protection equipment (**Figure 1.24**).

Carbon monoxide combines with the blood's hemoglobin much more readily than does oxygen. The most significant characteristic of CO is that it combines with the blood's hemoglobin so readily that the available oxygen is excluded. The blood's

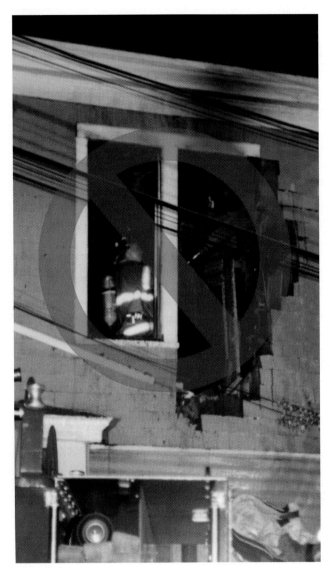

Figure 1.24 Fire and emergency service personnel should continue to wear respiratory protection during overhaul operations unless the atmosphere has been sampled and is determined to be safe. *Courtesy of Ron Jeffers.*

Table 1.3 Effects of Carboxyhemoglobin	
Carboxyhemoglobin (COHb) in Bloodstream (Percent)	Symptoms
0-10	No symptoms
10-20	Shortness of breath during physical exertion, tightness across the forehead
20-30	Headache, shortness of breath
30-50	Confusion, severe headache, dizziness, fatique, collapse from exertion
50-70	Unconsciousness, respiratory failure, and death if exposure continued

hemoglobin combines with and carries oxygen in a loose, chemical combination called *oxyhemoglobin.* The loose combination of oxyhemoglobin becomes a stronger combination called *carboxyhemoglobin (COHb)* when it combines with carbon nonoxide. In fact, CO combines with hemoglobin about 200 times more readily than does oxygen. **Table 1.3** shows the effects of carboxyhemoglobin when carbon monoxide occupies the positions normally taken by oxygen.

Carbon monoxide does not act on the body directly; rather, it crowds oxygen from the blood and leads to eventual hypoxia of the brain and tissues, followed by death if the process is not reversed. Exposure to a 5-percent carbon monoxide atmosphere can cause a 50-percent carbon monoxide level in the blood within 30 to 90 seconds. A room air concentration of 1 percent carbon monoxide causes a 50-percent carbon monoxide blood level in 2½ to 7 minutes. CO exposures are not cumulative, but because it takes the body some time to rid itself of CO, two or three small exposures over a day or two would have the same effect as one large exposure.

Table 1.4 shows the toxic effects of CO. The characteristic cherry red or mottled skin color is not always a reliable indicator of exposure, particularly in cases of long exposures to low concentrations. Other symptoms of exposure include shortness of breath, mild to throbbing headache, irritability, emotional instability, rapid fatigue, weakness, nausea, dizziness, confusion, and collapse. Treatment for exposure to carbon monoxide should include 100 percent oxygen given by mask at high flow rates or as directed by local protocols or regulations. A physician or professional health care provider should evaluate further any firefighter/emergency responder who has any CO exposure (**Figure 1.25**). Heavy exposure can permanently damage the cardiovascular system and/or lead to respiratory arrest. Heavy exposure may require immediate transport to a medical facility equipped with hyperbaric treatment capabilities.

Hydrogen chloride. Hydrogen chloride (HCl) is a colorless gas but can be detected by its pungent odor. It is produced as a by-product of the combustion of plastics, most commonly polyvinyl

Table 1.4
Toxic Effects of Carbon Monoxide

Carbon Monoxide (CO) (ppm)	Carbon Monoxide (CO) in Air (Percent)	Symptoms
100	0.01	No symptoms — no damage
200	0.02	Mild headache; few other symptoms
400	0.04	Headache after 1 to 2 hours
800	0.08	Headache after 45 minutes; nausea, collapse, and unconsciousness after 2 hours
1,000	0.10	Dangerous — unconsciousness after 1 hour
1,600	0.16	Headache, dizziness, nausea after 20 minutes
3,200	0.32	Headache, dizziness, nausea after 5 to 10 minutes; unconsciousness after 30 minutes
6,400	0.64	Headache, dizziness, nausea after 1 to 2 minutes; unconsciousness after 10 to 15 minutes
12,800	1.26	Immediate unconsciousness, danger of death in 1 to 3 minutes

ppm - parts per million

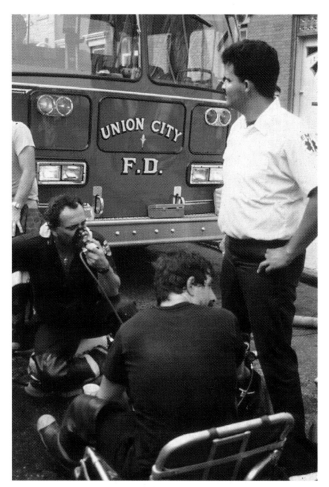

Figure 1.25 Carbon monoxide exposure is treated with oxygen therapy either at the scene or at a medical facility. *Courtesy of Ron Jeffers.*

chloride (PVC). PVC is used in many household furnishings such as wall coverings, upholstery materials, electrical insulation, and furniture laminates. In addition to the usual presence in the home, firefighters/emergency responders can expect to encounter plastics containing PVC in drug, toy, and general merchandise stores. With an increase in the use of plastics, hydrogen chloride is present at practically every fire. The overhaul stage of fire fighting is especially dangerous because breathing apparatus is often removed prematurely, and toxic fumes may linger in a room. For example, heated concrete can remain hot enough to decompose the plastic in telephone or electrical cables, thus releasing more hydrogen chloride. Concentrations of hydrogen chloride as low as 75 to 100 ppm can cause extreme irritation to the upper respiratory tract and to the eyes.

Hydrogen chloride causes irritation of the eyes and respiratory tract. When it is inhaled, it mixes with the moisture in the respiratory tract to form hydrochloric acid. Hydrochloric acid can cause severe burns to the respiratory tract and lungs. These burns can lead to pulmonary edema, shock, and even death. When the burning vapors are first inhaled, the body attempts to protect itself by closing the airway. This protective reaction is known as a *laryngospasm:* a spasm of the laryngeal muscles. Because this spasm reduces the oxygen that can enter the respiratory system, the victim also suffers the effects of oxygen deficiency. Early signs of hydrogen chloride exposure are burning, irritated eyes, nose, and throat. Treatment for hydrogen chloride exposure includes high-flow, high-concentrate oxygen and irrigation of the eyes or as directed by local medical protocols.

Hydrogen cyanide. Hydrogen cyanide (HCN) is a colorless gas but has a faint odor similar to bitter almonds. It is produced by the combustion of nitrogen-bearing substances. These substances include synthetic fibers such as nylon, some plastics (particularly those in aircraft), and natural fibers such as wool. Polyurethane foam, rubber, and paper can also produce HCN.

Hydrogen cyanide interferes with respiration at the cellular and tissue levels. It deactivates certain enzymes, thereby preventing the use of oxygen by the cells. At lower concentrations, HCN can cause an increase in pulse rate, gasping respirations, headache, and confusion. Exposure to higher levels of HCN can lead to respiratory failure and death; however, exposure to even small quantities can be fatal. NFPA reports that the effects of exposure to certain quantities can vary, depending on the amount and length of the exposure. A concentration of 50 ppm can be tolerated for 30 to 60 minutes while an exposure to 100 ppm for the same period can be fatal. An exposure to 130 ppm for 30 minutes can be fatal while 181 ppm for only 10 minutes can have the same effect. For safety sake, a 50-ppm concentration of hydrogen cyanide should be considered an IDLH level. HCN is 25 times more toxic than carbon monoxide.

A person who has been exposed to HCN should receive immediate treatment and transport to a hospital. Immediate treatment requires administering artificial respiration to nonbreathing victims with high-flow 100 percent oxygen as directed by local medical protocols.

Carbon dioxide. Carbon dioxide is a nonflammable, colorless, and odorless gas. Although it is not toxic, CO_2 must be considered dangerous because it is an end product of complete combustion (CO is incomplete) and can be dangerous at high levels. Carbon dioxide is a necessary part of respiration, but at high exposure levels it possesses a dangerous synergistic effect. Free-burning fires generally produce more carbon dioxide than do smoldering fires.

The chief danger of CO_2 exposure is that it causes increased respiratory rates. Recall that the carbon dioxide level in the blood stimulates the breathing center in the brain. When increased carbon dioxide levels are present (20,000 ppm), respirations can be increased by as much as 50 percent. This increased respiratory rate helps increase the amount of smoke and other toxic gases entering the body. **Table 1.5** shows the effects of CO_2. Because it is an asphyx-

Carbon Dioxide (CO_2) (ppm)	Carbon Dioxide (CO_2) in Air (Percent)	Symptoms
5,000	0.5	No symptoms
20,000	2.0	Breathing rate increased by 50 percent
30,000	3.0	Breathing rate increased by 100 percent
50,000	5.0	Vomiting, dizziness, disoriention after 30 minutes
80,000	8.0	Headache, vomiting, dizziness, breathing difficulties after short exposure
100,000	10.0	Death in a few minutes

Table 1.5
Effects of Carbon Dioxide

ppm - parts per million

iant, carbon dioxide in excessive amounts can also create an oxygen-deficient atmosphere that will not support life. Firefighters/emergency responders should anticipate high CO_2 levels when a CO_2 total-flooding system is activated and wear respiratory protection when entering the area. These systems are designed to exclude oxygen from the fire and will also exclude oxygen from firefighters/emergency responders in the process.

Signs of carbon dioxide poisoning include dizziness and difficulty breathing. Because exposure can cause suffocation, victims should be moved to fresh air and given artificial respiration if they are not breathing or oxygen if breathing is difficult.

Phosgene. Phosgene ($COCl_2$) (also known as *carbonyl chloride*) is a colorless, tasteless gas with a musty hay odor. It is produced when refrigerants such as Freon®, plastics containing PVC, or electrical wiring insulation contact flames and extreme temperatures. Phosgene's chief effect is in the lungs: When inhaled, it converts to hydrogen chloride in the alveolar spaces and then into hydrochloric acid and carbon monoxide when it contacts the lungs. The hydrochloric acid produced when phosgene combines with moisture causes pulmonary edema, which prevents the exchange of oxygen in the lungs. The carbon monoxide produced prevents the red blood cells from accepting oxygen and causes cyanosis (skin discoloration from oxygen deficiency in the blood). Phosgene can also be absorbed through the skin, particularly at high concentrations.

Phosgene's odor is perceptible at 6 ppm. The IDLH level of phosgene is 2 ppm (see Table 1.2). By the time the body can tell its presence, the gas is already above the IDLH level. Exposure to a relatively high concentration (10 to 12 ppm) is likely to produce prompt vomiting, followed by a dry throat, pain in the chest, coughing, and shortness of breath. Exposure at the IDLH level produces the cough and irritation after a short exposure but does not cause serious discomfort in the time required to absorb a dangerous or lethal dose. In other words, a lethal dose can be absorbed before the body has time to react. Additional symptoms include severe eye and skin irritation, inability to breathe properly, and cyanosis. Although inhalation exposure damages the respiratory tract, the effects may be delayed for 2 to 24 hours or longer, depending on the length and level of exposure. The victim should be kept under observation during this time.

Treatment of phosgene poisoning requires moving the victim to fresh air and administering artificial respiration to nonbreathing victims with high-flow 100 percent oxygen as directed by local medical protocols. The eyes and any skin contacted should be flushed thoroughly with running water as prescribed by local medical protocols.

Oxides of nitrogen. Two oxides of nitrogen are dangerous: nitrogen dioxide (NO_2) and nitric oxide (NO). Nitrogen dioxide gas has a characteristic reddish brown color and an odor similar to that of household bleach. Nitric oxide is a colorless gas formed by oxidation of nitrogen or ammonia. Nitrogen dioxide is commonly referred to as *silo gas* because it forms under nonfire situations in grain bins and silos. It is most commonly associated with corn but forms during the storage of other crops as well. It is most concentrated within 1 to 3 days after the crop has been placed in the silo, although it may be present for as long as 3 weeks after storage **(Figure 1.26)**. Nitrogen dioxide is also generated when pyroxylin plastics burn. Fires in office supply stores, hobby shops, or hardware stores may create large quantities of nitrogen dioxide.

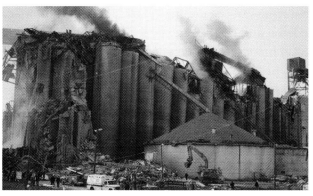

Figure 1.26 Devastating explosions and fires can be caused by the buildup of *silo gas,* also known as nitrogen dioxide. *Courtesy of Chris Mickal.*

Nitrogen dioxide is the more significant of the two because nitric oxide readily converts to nitrogen dioxide in the presence of oxygen and moisture. Nitrogen dioxide can mix with moisture in the air and in the respiratory tract and form nitric and nitrous acids. These acids can then burn the lungs and cause pulmonary edema, which can lead to death. In addition to causing pulmonary edema, nitric and nitrous acids may enter the bloodstream. The body attempts to neutralize these acids and in doing so causes the formation of nitrites and nitrates. These substances chemically attach to the blood and can induce nausea, abdominal pains, vomiting, and cyanosis, which can lead to collapse and coma. Nitrates and nitrites can also cause arterial dilation, variation in blood pressure, headaches, and dizziness. Nitrogen dioxide is especially dangerous because its irritating effects in the nose and throat can be tolerated even though a lethal dose is being inhaled. Therefore, the hazardous effects from its pulmonary irritation action or chemical reaction may not become apparent for several hours. The IDLH level for nitrogen dioxide is 50 ppm.

Treatment of nitrogen dioxide poisoning requires moving the victim to fresh air and administering artificial respiration to nonbreathing victims with high-flow 100 percent oxygen as directed by local medical protocols. Because effects may not be apparent for several hours, the victim should be transported to a hospital and kept under observation.

Acrolein. Acrolein (CH_2CHCHO) is a colorless, highly irritating gas with a piercing, disagreeable odor. It is produced when wood, paper, cotton, plastic materials, and oils and fats burn. Inhaling acrolein can cause nose and throat irritation, nausea, shortness of breath, lung damage, and pulmonary edema and can eventually lead to death. The IDLH level for acrolein is very low (5 ppm). A mild cough may be the only symptom at the time of exposure.

Treatment of acrolein poisoning requires moving the victim to fresh air and administering artificial respiration to nonbreathing victims with high-flow 100 percent oxygen as directed by local medical protocols. The eyes and any skin contacted should be flushed with running water for 15 minutes. The victim should be transported to a hospital and kept under observation as symptoms of edema may be delayed for 5 to 72 hours, depending on the level of exposure.

Formaldehyde. Formaldehyde (HCHO) is a colorless gas that has a characteristic pungent odor. It is produced when wood, cotton, and newspaper burn and is an irritant to the eyes, nose, and throat. At higher concentrations (near 100 ppm), nausea and vomiting can result. Prolonged exposure can result in loss of consciousness. Formaldehyde has an IDLH level of 20 ppm, while inhalation of formaldehyde in a 10–20 ppm concentration causes severe difficulty in breathing, intense lacrimation (tearing of the eyes), and severe cough. Formaldehyde can also be absorbed through the skin and is a known cancer-causing agent or carcinogen of the lung. Emergency treatment requires moving the victim to fresh air and thoroughly flushing the eyes with running water.

Hydrogen sulfide. Hydrogen sulfide (H_2S) is a colorless gas and has a strong rotten-egg odor. It is produced when rubber insulation, tires, and woolen materials burn. It is also commonly produced by the decomposition of sulfur-bearing organic material and is often found in sewers, sewage disposal plants, and oil-drilling operations. Hydrogen sulfide is dangerous because it quickly deactivates the sense of smell. As a result, a person can be exposed to high concentrations without realizing it. The IDLH level for hydrogen sulfide is 100 ppm.

Inhalation of a high concentration of hydrogen sulfide produces sudden asphyxiation — a victim falls, apparently unconscious immediately, and may die without moving again. A complete arrest of respiration occurs, which can often be overcome by prompt application of artificial respiration. In less sudden poisoning, the signs may be nausea, pro-

fuse salivation, diarrhea, belching, cough, headache, dizziness, conjunctivitis of the eyes, and blistering of the lips. Emergency treatment at this level requires moving the victim to fresh air, giving oxygen as directed by local medical protocols, flushing the eyes with running water, and transporting the victim to a hospital for observation.

Sulfur dioxide. Sulfur dioxide (SO_2) is a colorless gas with a highly irritating odor that makes it detectable below its lethal dosage (IDLH level is 100 ppm). It is produced when sulfur-containing materials burn. Inhaled sulfur dioxide acts mainly to irritate the eyes, skin, and mucous membranes to form sulfurous acid. It chiefly affects the upper respiratory tract and bronchi. At the time of exposure, a mild cough may be the only symptom. Later symptoms may include rapid respirations, severe cough, and pulmonary edema. When combined with the moisture in the respiratory tract, sulfur dioxide acts as a corrosive, causing edema of the respiratory tract and lungs and producing respiratory paralysis.

Emergency treatment includes moving the victim to fresh air and administering artificial respiration to nonbreathing victims or oxygen as directed by local medical protocols. The eyes should be thoroughly flushed with running water (**Figure 1.27**).

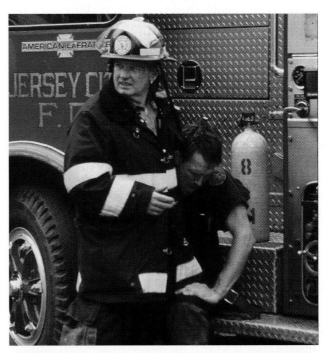

Figure 1.27 Exposure to sulfur dioxide may require oxygen therapy and the flushing of the eyes with water. *Courtesy of Ron Jeffers.*

Benzene. Benzene (C_6H_6), an aromatic hydrocarbon, is a colorless gas with a fairly pleasant aromatic odor. It is produced when PVC plastics and gasoline burn and can be inhaled or absorbed through the skin. A single, heavy exposure may produce a serious acute effect, similar to an anesthetic, with special affinity for the central nervous system. The first sign is usually exhilaration, followed by sleepiness, dizziness, vomiting, tremors, hallucinations, seizures, and unconsciousness. Inhaling high levels of benzene gas can cause unconsciousness and death from respiratory paralysis and cardiovascular collapse. Lesser exposure levels cause irritation to the eyes, nose, and respiratory system as well as headache, nausea, dizziness, weakness, and trembling.

Benzene is particularly dangerous because it is a known carcinogen to blood-forming tissues and has an IDLH level of 100 ppm. NIOSH has identified benzene as an agent that causes leukemia. The main emergency treatment in acute poisonings is to remove the victim to fresh air, administer oxygen, maintain body warmth, and immediately transport to a medical facility.

Respiratory Hazards Not Associated with Fire

[NFPA 1500: 7.9.7, 7.9.8]
[NFPA 1404: 5.1.7 (4) (6) (7), 5.2 (1) (2), 6.6.1, 6.7.2 (2) (3)]

Emergency services personnel respond to many incidents that do not involve fire and may not initially appear to create respiratory hazards. However, the presence of asbestos, polychlorinated biphenyls (PCBs), oxygen-deficient atmospheres, hazardous materials, illegal drug production, and biological/medical pathogens are potential respiratory hazards at most incidents. In addition, the growing threat of weapons of mass destruction (WMD) must be considered as another respiratory hazard to emergency responders.

Asbestos

Asbestos is any of several minerals that separate into long, flexible fibers that were formerly used as fireproof insulating materials. It is not a product of combustion, but emergency responders can be exposed to asbestos fibers during loss control,

overhaul, and fire cause determination. Asbestos can be found in old buildings and on board ships where it was used for insulation. It may be encountered in pipe insulation, floor tiles, and wall and ceiling insulation. Asbestos is classified as a carcinogen to the lungs. When asbestos fibers are inhaled, they travel to the lungs, causing scarring that reduces lung capacity. The effects of asbestos exposure may not appear for many years (**Figure 1.28**).

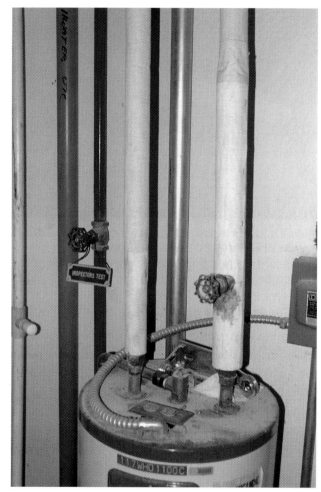

Figure 1.28 Emergency responders should be aware that asbestos might be present in old building especially where heating and plumbing pipes are located.

Polychlorinated Biphenyl

Polychlorinated biphenyl (any of several chemical compounds that are poisonous environmental pollutants; also referred to as PCB) may be found in electrical and mechanical systems manufactured between 1930 and 1976. They were used in fluorescent light ballasts, transformers, and capacitors and as lubricants in compressors and other machinery (**Figure 1.29**). It is still in use today in sealed systems.

PCB can cause skin irritations, effect the nervous system, and is suspected of being a carcinogen. When it burns, it can emit highly toxic and carcinogenic products that can affect the respiratory system. Respiratory protection must be worn when the presence of PCB is suspected.

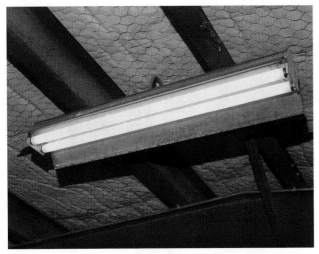

Figure 1.29 Fluorescent light units may contain polychlorinated biphenyls (PCBs) that can escape into the atmosphere when heated and create a respiratory hazard as a carcinogen.

Oxygen-Deficient Atmospheres

Occasionally, an emergency responder may have to enter an oxygen-deficient atmosphere that is not part of a fire fighting operation. This type of entry is usually made for rescue purposes. Entering caves, sewers, storage tanks, cesspools, and other confined spaces requires the use of respiratory protection (**Figure 1.30**). A *confined space* is any space having little or no natural ventilation that can produce dangerous atmospheres. It is impossible to measure oxygen levels in a confined space without a meter, so respiratory protection must be worn. Just having to rescue a person who has lost consciousness in a particular space should be warning enough that the atmosphere of that space does not support life. **Table 1.6** lists concentrations of oxygen in the atmosphere and their various definitions or effects.

Hazardous Materials

The U.S. Department of Transportation (DOT) defines a *hazardous material* as "any substance or material in any form which may pose an unreason-

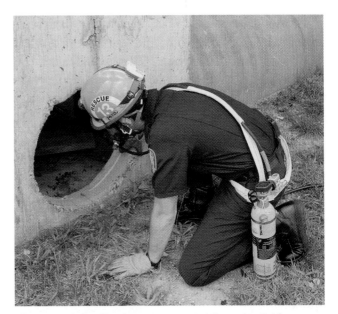

Figure 1.30 Confined spaces present the potential for oxygen-deficient atmospheres that require the use of self-contained breathing apparatus (SCBA) or supplied-air respirator (SAR) units. *Courtesy of Kenneth Baum.*

Table 1.6 Reduced Concentrations of Oxygen	
Concentration of Oxygen (Percent)	**Effect**
21	Usual oxygen content in air
19.5	NFPA/OSHA recommended minimum oxygen content for entry
18	ANSI Z117.1-1977 definition of oxygen-deficient atmosphere
17	Medical problems begin (see Table 1.1)

able risk to health and safety or property when transported in commerce." Because hazardous materials are routinely transported by rail, water, air, and road, every area is a potential site of a hazardous materials incident. Fixed locations such as industrial sites are also likely to present firefighters and emergency services personnel with a variety of hazardous materials situations (**Figure 1.31**).

Hazardous materials can range from chemicals in liquid or gas form to radioactive materials to etiologic (disease-causing) agents. Although these materials can be dangerous in their natural state, they can pose an even greater danger when they

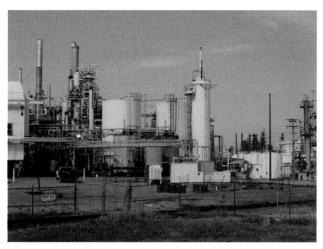

Figure 1.31 Industrial sites including petroleum-processing centers contain numerous hazardous materials that require complete personal protective equipment during an emergency response.

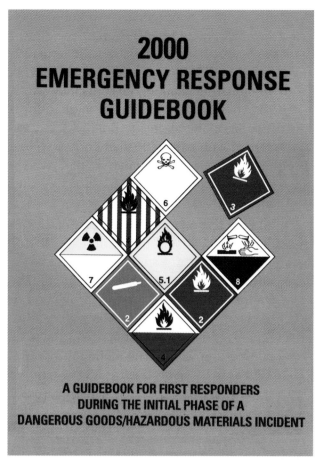

Figure 1.32 The *2000 Emergency Response Guidebook* provides essential information for responses to hazardous materials incidents.

burn. Burning hazardous materials can create an explosion hazard, generate extremely high levels of heat, disperse vapors over wide areas, or combine to create even more toxic gases and vapors. Wearing respiratory protection is mandatory when dealing with hazardous materials — both from a safety standpoint and because its use is required by federal and state/provincial law. Current hazardous materials regulations require extensive training and equipment for responding to a hazardous material incident.

Part of the training involves the ability of emergency services personnel to recognize and understand the *2000 Emergency Response Guidebook (ERG2000)* and the placard system for hazardous materials given in NFPA 704, *Standard System for the Identification of the Hazards of Materials for Emergency Response* (2001 edition) (**Figure 1.32**). The U.S. Department of Transportation, Transport Canada (TC), and the Secretariat of Transport and Communications of Mexico (SCT) jointly developed the *2000 Emergency Response Guidebook* for agencies responsible for hazardous material emergency response. It requires that all vehicles, portable storage tanks, and containers used to transport hazardous materials be clearly marked to indicate the material they contain. NFPA 704 requires that all facilities involved in the manufacture or use of hazardous materials be marked with four-part diamond placards (**Figure 1.33**). This placard informs responders about the substance's fire, life, and reactivity potential as well as special hazards.

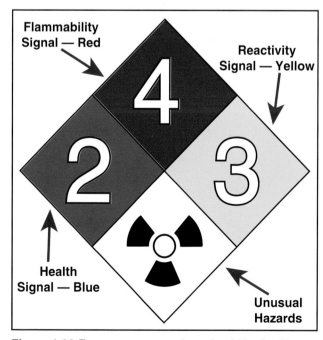

Figure 1.33 Emergency responders should be familiar with the NFPA 704 placard symbols for hazardous materials.

When firefighters/emergency responders see a placard on a vehicle involved in an accident, it serves as a warning that the atmosphere may be toxic and that respiratory protection should be worn. In industrial facilities, placards may also be placed on containers or storage rooms warning of the dangerous materials inside. Buildings may also be placarded with NFPA 704 diamonds. For more information on hazardous materials incidents, see the IFSTA **Hazardous Materials for First Responders** manual.

Emergency responders should not limit the use of respiratory protection to hazardous materials incidents. Common emergency calls such as natural gas leaks or carbon monoxide poisonings may also require the use of respiratory protection. In addition, emergency responders have seen an increase in fires and toxic atmospheres related to the production of the illegal drug methamphetamine (also referred to as *meth*) **(Figure 1.34)**. Meth labs can be found in vehicles, residences, storage buildings, motel rooms, or other structures. Breathing the vapors can be potentially harmful. Responders must treat these incidents as respiratory hazards.

Other common hazards include chemicals such as ammonia and chlorine found around swimming pools, cleaning establishments, or manufacturing plants. Ammonia causes shortness of breath, breathing difficulties, and a burning sensation in the throat. It has a TVL of 25 ppm and an STEL of 35 ppm. Chlorine, which may produce delayed symptoms, causes a burning sensation, labored breathing, nausea, and a sort throat. The TVL is 0.5 ppm, and the STEL is 1 ppm. The IDHL has not been established for either chemical. Attempting rescues in situations involving these chemicals without proper protection rapidly makes the rescuers part of the problem, rather than part of the solution.

Biological/Medical Pathogens

At the beginning of the 21st century, the fire and emergency services are experiencing more responses to emergency medical incidents than to structure fire incidents. Personnel are exposed to an increasing variety of biological and medical hazards. To combat these types of hazards, departments are required by NFPA 1500 to develop, implement, and maintain an infectious disease control program to deal with bloodborne and airborne pathogens. Communicable diseases may be transmitted by bloodborne and airborne pathogens such as viruses, bacteria, and other harmful organisms through exposure to blood, bodily fluids, or exhalation of a contaminated person **(Figure 1.35)**. The pathogens may enter a noninfected person's body by eyes, mouth, or nose or may be absorbed through the skin.

Protection against bloodborne and airborne pathogens consists of full protective clothing, including medical gloves and eye, mouth, and respiratory protection. High-efficiency particulate air (HEPA) filters, SCBA, or approved air-purifying respirators are effective barriers to airborne pathogens **(Figure 1.36)**.

Exposure to Weapons of Mass Destruction

Since the end of World War II, terrorist acts have steadily increased. Nationalism; religious fervor; access to potentially hazardous chemical, radiologi-

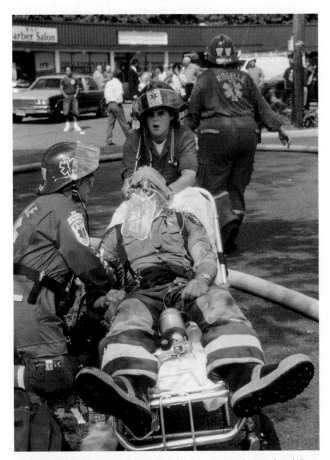

Figure 1.34 Illegal and clandestine methamphetamine labs present a particular hazard to emergency responders who are not protected by respiratory protection equipment. *Courtesy of Bill Tompkins.*

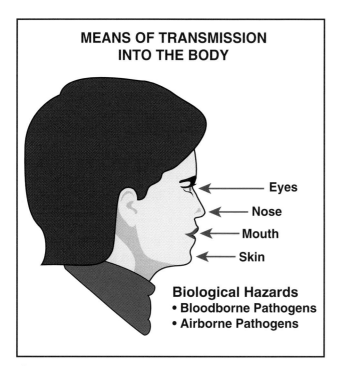

MEANS OF TRANSMISSION INTO THE BODY

← Eyes
← Nose
← Mouth
← Skin

Biological Hazards
• Bloodborne Pathogens
• Airborne Pathogens

Figure 1.35 Bloodborne and airborne pathogens can enter the body through the eyes, mouth, nose, or skin. Full protective clothing including the appropriate level of respiratory protection should be worn.

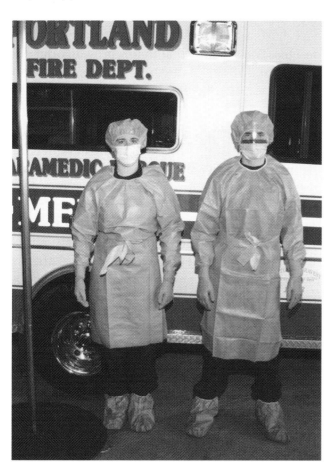

Figure 1.36 Emergency services personnel who respond to medical emergencies should be provided with the appropriate level of personal protection. *Courtesy of Mike Nixon.*

cal, and biological materials; and access to information on the Internet have contributed to this increase. Weapons of mass destruction can take the form of nuclear weapons, hazardous chemicals, explosives, biological weapons, or even commercial airliners. The material can be distributed through a building ventilation system, a municipal water supply, or through the detonation of an explosive device. As the terrorist attack on the New York City World Trade Center in September 2001 proved, targets are no longer military in nature but include symbolic sites such as federal and private office buildings, sites with high population densities such as subways, or sites that can cause great impact on a society such as financial or communications centers (**Figure 1.37**).

Emergency responders must be prepared for the potential that a terrorist attack can have. Primary and secondary releases of hazardous or biological agents may occur as well as attacks using a

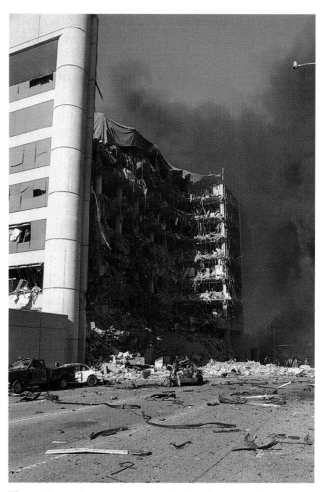

Figure 1.37 Weapons of mass destruction present a particularly terrifying and devastating challenge to emergency responders. *Courtesy of Danny Atchley.*

combination of agents. Respiratory protection resources may be stressed due to the need for reserve equipment and replacement air supplies and the contamination or loss of equipment. Training and the development of protocols based on the recommendations of the federal government should be initiated as part of the organization's standard operating procedures. Respiratory protection will be required not only during the initial response but also during the search and rescue phase and the victim recovery phase. For example, nontoxic particulates released during the collapse of the World Trade Center towers remained in the atmosphere surrounding the site for many days following the initial event.

Short- and Long-Term Effects of Respiratory Hazards

Exposure to respiratory hazards created by both fire and nonfire incidents can result in short- and long-term physical reactions. The effects of respiratory hazards vary depending on the type of hazard and the length of exposure. Short-term effects include but are not limited to dizziness, headache, shortness of breath, nausea, vomiting, loss of muscle coordination, rapid fatigue, and unconsciousness. Long-term effects may include cancer, damage to internal organs, damage to airways and lungs, weakened heart, stroke, mental disorders, or prolonged disease such as meningitis and tuberculosis. Because the potential for long-term illness or disability and death is so high, respiratory protection should always be worn if a respiratory hazard is suspected or known to be present. Respiratory protection can also provide a limited level of splash protection against body fluids and bloodborne pathogens such as human immunodeficiency virus (HIV) and hepatitis.

Types of Respiratory Protection

[NFPA 1404: 5.1.7 (1), 5.2 (2), 6.5.1 (1)]

In general, all respiratory protection equipment requires medical evaluation, training, and physical conditioning. NFPA 1500 and NFPA 1582 establish the medical requirements for all firefighters/emergency responders. Training requirements are defined in NFPA 1500 and NFPA 1404. Physical considerations, which are covered by NFPA 1500, include the following:

- *Physical conditioning* — The wearer must be in sound physical condition in order to maximize the work that can be performed and to stretch the air supply as far as possible.
- *Agility* — Good physical agility helps to overcome the barriers presented by the weight of the SCBA and the restrictions of the harness assembly.
- *Facial features* — The shape and contour of the face affects the wearer's ability to get a good facepiece-to-face seal. Glasses and facial hair can also affect the seal.

To protect fire and emergency service personnel from respiratory hazards that can potentially cause injury, illness, and death, three main classifications of respiratory protection have been developed for use by the fire and emergency services. They are as follows:

- Self-contained breathing apparatus
- Supplied-air respirator
- Air-purifying respirator

Each type is designed for a specific use and to meet a specific type of hazard or hazards. In addition, they each have advantages and disadvantages in their designs. The sections that follow provide brief descriptions of the listed respirators. Detailed information is provided in later chapters of this manual.

Of the three types of respiratory protection systems, only the SCBA and the SAR are designed for use in oxygen-deficient atmospheres. When the oxygen content of the atmosphere is less than 19.5 percent by volume, breathing air must be provided for emergency response personnel. Situations of this type include, but are not limited to, structural fire fighting, confined-space rescue, hazardous materials incidents, and salvage and overhaul operations. All oxygen-deficient atmospheres shall be considered as immediately dangerous to life and health.

Self-Contained Breathing Apparatus

[NFPA 1500: 7.11.1.1]
[NFPA 1404: 6.7.2]

A *self-contained breathing apparatus* is an atmosphere-supplying respirator where the user carries the breathing air supply. The unit consists of a facepiece, pressure regulator, compressed air cylinder, harness assembly, and end-of-service-time indicators (also known as low air supply or low-pressure alarms). SCBA is perhaps the most familiar of the respiratory protection systems in use by the fire and emergency services. Patents for SCBA units date back to the mid-1800s. Practical units finally began appearing in the fire service in the 1950s, and mandatory use began in the 1980s.

All SCBA must be certified for fire fighting and IDLH use by NIOSH and MSHA. The apparatus must meet the design and testing criteria of NFPA in jurisdictions that have adopted the NFPA respiratory standard by law or ordinance. ANSI standards for eye protection apply to the facepiece lens design and testing. Apparatus that is not NIOSH/MSHA certified must not be used. The mixing of components of SCBAs manufactured by various companies is also prohibited. The practice of mixing components may void both the NIOSH approval and the third-party certification required for NFPA compliance. Apparatus are tested and certified as complete systems consisting of facepiece, pressure regulator, harness assembly, air cylinder, and end-of-service-time indicator alarm device(s).

The advantages of using SCBA-type respiratory protection are the independence that is gained from a self-contained system and the maneuverability that it allows the wearer. Disadvantages include the bulkiness of the units, change in profile that may hinder mobility due to the configuration of the harness assembly and location of the air cylinder, limited vision due to facepiece fogging, and limited communications if the facepiece is not equipped with a microphone or speaking diaphragm.

NIOSH classifies SCBA as either *closed-circuit* or *open-circuit*. Three types of SCBA are currently being manufactured in closed- or open-circuit designs: demand, pressure-demand, or positive-pressure. SCBA may also be either high- or low-pressure types.

Closed-Circuit Apparatus
[NFPA 1500: 7.11.1.2, 7.11.1.3]

The closed-circuit type SCBA is also known as a *rebreather* because the exhaled carbon dioxide is removed and the oxygen content is restored by the use of compressed or liquid oxygen or by an oxy-

gen-generating solid. One of the disadvantages of the closed-circuit system is that once the system is turned on, the process cannot be stopped (**Figure 1.38**).

Open-Circuit Apparatus
[NFPA 1500: 7.11.1.1]

The open-circuit type SCBA exhausts the exhaled air into the atmosphere. Replacement breathing air is provided from the compressed breathing air cylinder. Because minute amounts of oil may be present in the valves or regulator that create an explosion hazard when they are mixed with oxygen, the use of compressed oxygen in a system designed for breathing air is prohibited (**Figure 1.39**).

Demand Apparatus

A demand-type breathing apparatus has a regulator that supplies air to the facepiece only when the wearer inhales or when the bypass valve is open.

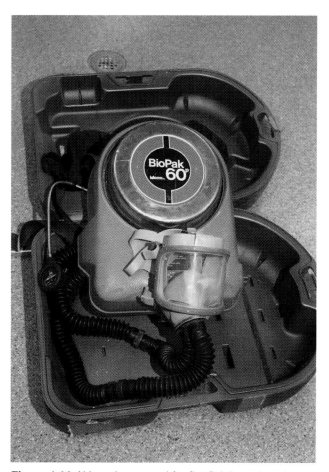

Figure 1.38 Although not used for fire fighting, closed-circuit self-contained breathing apparatus may be found in use by emergency services for long-duration hazardous materials incidents.

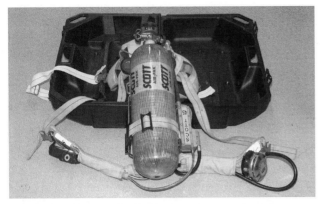

Figure 1.39 Open-circuit self-contained breathing apparatus provide the highest level of respiratory protection and are used primarily for fire fighting situations. *Courtesy of Bob Parker.*

This type of unit is also referred to as a negative-pressure apparatus because the air pressure in the facepiece is less than the surrounding atmosphere, creating a partial vacuum (**Figure 1.40**). This variation in pressure could result in contaminated atmospheres leaking into the facepiece if the seal to the face is not complete. For this reason, demand-type breathing apparatus have not been recommended for use in fire fighting or IDLH atmospheres since 1983, although OSHA still permits their use in other types of emergencies such as mine rescues. Some jurisdictions and nongovernmental organizations still permit the use of demand-type breathing apparatus in fire fighting situations, and some units may still be found in service in states that mandate the use of positive-pressure units. Generally, the continuing reasons for the use of demand-type units are the lack of funds to replace them, the lack of enforcement by jurisdictions, and the lack of education of responders to the fact that this type of unit does not provide adequate protection.

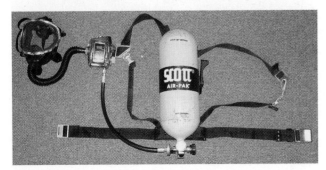

Figure 1.40 Old demand or negative-pressure self-contained breathing apparatus may still be found in use in some areas of North America. *Courtesy of Kenneth Baum.*

Pressure-Demand Apparatus

Pressure-demand apparatus may be operated in either the positive-pressure or negative-pressure (demand) mode. It is designed to provide a positive pressure inside the facepiece during inhalation and exhalation by the wearer. This design addresses the problem of leakage of contaminates into the demand-type apparatus that can occur during inhalation. Pressure-demand type apparatus are still manufactured and may be used in certain instances although most organizations have replaced them with positive-pressure breathing apparatus (see following section) (**Figure 1.41**).

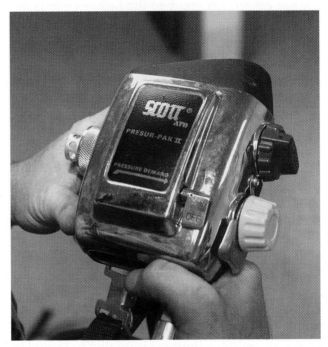

Figure 1.41 Pressure-demand regulators can be recognized by the label and two-position switch.

Positive-Pressure Apparatus

Positive-pressure apparatus provide air to the facepiece under a pressure that is greater than the surrounding atmosphere, approximately $1/27^{th}$ of a psi (0.255 kPa). This apparatus is currently the most common type in use by the fire and emergency services (**Figure 1.42**). Positive-pressure apparatus used in fire fighting and in IDLH atmospheres must be NIOSH approved for those uses. Depending on the model and manufacturer, the units may have facepiece- or belt-mounted regulators, high- or low-pressure breathing air cylinders and first-stage regulators, air-activated personal alert safety systems, or a variety of other accessories.

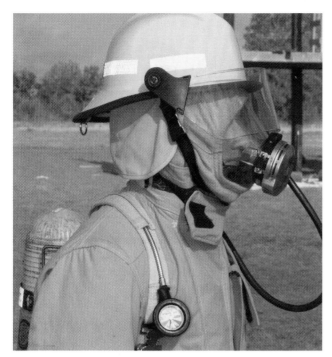

Figure 1.42 The most common self-contained breathing apparatus in the fire and emergency services today is the positive-pressure breathing apparatus. *Courtesy of Bob Parker.*

High- and Low-Pressure Apparatus

SCBA may be either high- or low-pressure-type apparatus. High-pressure apparatus are designed for long duration use from 45 to 60 minutes. The pressures in these types of cylinders range from 3,000 to 5,000 psi (20 684 kPa to 34 474 kPa) and must be reduced to the proper breathing pressure by the regulator. The low-pressure apparatus have cylinder pressure ranges of 1,000 to 2,200 psi (6 895 kPa to 15 169 kPa), which provide from 15 to 30 minutes of operation. The actual operational times of either the high- or low-pressure systems vary and depend on environmental factors, physical fitness, and the user's training and skill level. High-pressure cylinders must not be used with low-pressure regulators (**Figure 1.43**).

WARNING!

Although SCBA has a general appearance to self-contained underwater breathing apparatus (SCUBA), SCBA is not designed for use underwater. Never use SCBA in water rescue or recovery operations.

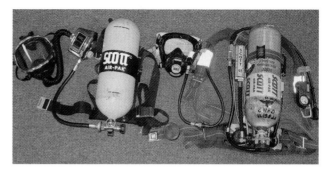

Figure 1.43 Emergency services personnel must be trained to recognize the differences between low-pressure (left) and high-pressure (right) SCBA units. Cylinders may not be interchanged between the units. *Courtesy of Kenneth Baum.*

Supplied-Air Respirator

[NFPA 1500: 7.11.2.1, 7.11.2.2, 7.11.2.3]
[NFPA 1401: 6.8.4]

The supplied-air respirator or airline respirator is an atmosphere-supplying respirator where the user does not carry the breathing air source. The apparatus usually consists of a facepiece, a belt- or facepiece-mounted regulator, a voice communications system, up to 300 feet (90 m) of air supply hose, an emergency escape pack or emergency breathing support system (EBSS), and a breathing air source (either cylinders mounted on a cart or a portable breathing air compressor) (**Figure 1.44**). Due

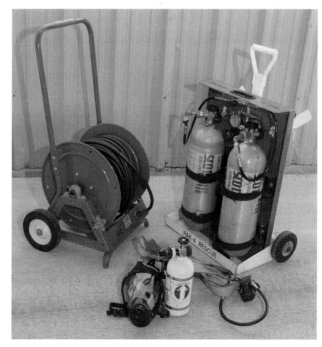

Figure 1.44 A complete supplied-air respirator (SAR) consists of the air supply cart, manifold, air hose, regulator, facepiece, and emergency breathing support system (EBSS).

to the potential for damage to the air supply hose, the EBSS provides enough air, usually 5, 10, or 15 minutes' worth, for the user to escape the hazardous atmosphere. SAR apparatus are not intended or certified for fire fighting operations because of the potential damage to the airline from heat, fire, or debris.

NIOSH classifies SARs as type C respirators. Type C respirators are further divided into two approved types: One type consists of a regulator and facepiece only, while the second consists of a regulator, facepiece, and EBSS. This second type may also be referred to as a supplied-air respirator with egress capabilities. It is used in confined-space environments, IDLH environments, or potential IDLH environments.

SAR apparatus have the advantage of reducing the physical stress to the wearer by removing the weight of the SCBA. However, the air supply line and the limited length of the airline restrict mobility. Other limitations are the same as those for SCBA: restricted vision and communications.

Air-Purifying Respirator

[NFPA 1500: 7.11.3.1, 7.11.3.2, 7.11.3.3]
[NFPA 1404: 6.9.1, 6.9.2 (1) (2) (3)]

Air-purifying respirators have an air-purifying filter, canister, or cartridge that removes specific air contaminants by passing ambient air through the air-purifying element. Respirators with air-purifying filters may have full facepieces that provide a complete seal to the face and protect the eyes, nose, and mouth or half facepieces that provide a complete seal to the face and protect the nose and mouth **(Figure 1.45)**. The disposable filter is mounted on one or both sides of the facepiece. Particle masks, also known as *dust masks,* are also classified as air-purifying filters. They are intended to protect the respiratory system from large-sized particulates and are worn when working with particulate-producing tools such as paint sprayers or sanding equipment. Canister or cartridge respirators pass the air through a filter, sorbent, catalyst, or combination of these items, which removes specific contaminants from the air. The air can enter the system from the external atmosphere through the filter or sorbent or from the user's exhalation combining with a catalyst to provide breathable air.

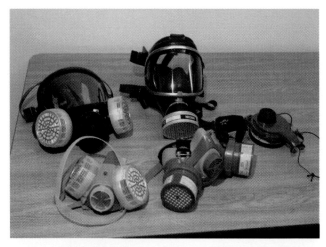

Figure 1.45 Air-purifying respirators (APRs) come in a variety of makes and models and may be full facepiece (top) or half facepiece (bottom) designs.

The latter type dates from World War II when the U.S. Navy developed a rebreather (known as OBA or Chemox™ for use in shipboard fires.

Particulate filters protect the user from particulates in the air, including airborne diseases, and are single-use masks that are disposed of following use. These filters may be used with half facepiece masks, with full facepiece masks, or as particulate (dust) masks. Eye protection must be provided when the full facepiece mask is not worn. Particulate filters are classified by the level of effectiveness and regulated by Title 42 (Public Health) *CFR* 84 (Approval of Respiratory Protection Devices). They are divided into nine classes, three levels of filtration (95, 99, and 99.97 percents), and three categories of filter degradation (N, R, and P). The categories of filter degradation indicate the use limitations of the filter as follows:

- *N*— not resistant to oil
- *R*— resistant to oil
- *P*— used when oil or nonoil lubricants are present

In the fire and emergency services, these filters are used primarily at emergency medical incidents, but they may also be appropriate for investigations or inspections in situations involving body recovery; where bird, bat, or rodent excrement is present; and involving agricultural and industrial incidents among others. HEPA filters used for medical emergencies must be 99.97 percent efficient, while 95 and 99 percent effective filters may be used depending on the health risk hazard **(Figure 1.46)**.

Air-Purifying Items

Catalyst

A *catalyst* is a substance that influences the rate of chemical reaction between other substances. A catalyst used in respirator cartridges and canisters is Hopcalite®, a mixture of porous granules of manganese and copper oxides that speeds the reaction between toxic carbon monoxide and oxygen to form carbon dioxide.

Sorbent

A *sorbent* is a material, compound, or system that holds by adsorption or absorption. Adsorption retains the contaminant molecule on the surface of the sorbent granule by physical attraction. The intensity of the attraction varies with the type of sorbent and contaminant. Adsorption by physical attraction holds the adsorbed molecules weakly. When chemical forces are involved in the process (chemisorption), the bonds holding the molecules to the sorbent granules are much stronger and can be broken only with great dif-

ficulty. An absorbent is a solid or liquid that absorbs other substances. A characteristic common to all adsorbents is a large specific surface area, up to 1,500 m^2/g of sorbent. Activated charcoal is the most common adsorbent and is used primarily to remove organic vapors, although it does have some capacity for adsorbing acid gases.

Filters

Particulate filters are of two types: absolute and nonabsolute. Absolute filters use screening to remove particles from the air; that is, they exclude the particles that are larger than the filter's pores. However, most respirator filters are nonabsolute filters, which means they contain pores that are larger than the particles to be removed. Absolute and nonabsolute filters use combinations of interception capture, sedimentation capture, inertial impaction capture, diffusion capture, and electrostatic capture to remove the particles.

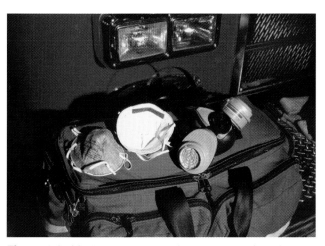

Figure 1.46 Medical response units may be equipped with HEPA-filter masks or particulate masks in addition to air-purifying respirator (APR) units.

Limitations to the APR are the limited life of the filters and canisters, the need for constant monitoring of the contaminated atmosphere, and the need for a normal oxygen content of the atmosphere before use. Usage should be restricted to the unit's certified hazards.

Summary

Fire and emergency services personnel must be aware of the respiratory hazards that may confront them on a daily basis, potential short- and long-term effects of those hazards, and types of respiratory protection available for each type of hazard. It is the responsibility of the fire department or emergency services agency to supply and maintain the proper equipment to meet the potential hazards and to provide training to all personnel in the use of the equipment. It is the responsibility of fire and emergency service responders to learn the operation of the equipment and to use it when the situation demands.

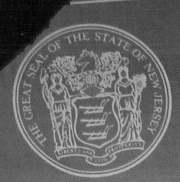

Regulations and Standards

Job Performance Requirements

This chapter provides information that will assist the reader in meeting the following job performance requirements from NFPA 1500, *Standard on Fire Department Occupational Safety and Health Program*, 2002 Edition.

4.8.1 The health and safety officer shall develop, review, and revise rules, regulations, and standard operating procedures pertaining to the fire department occupational safety and health program.

4.8.1.1 Based upon the directives and requirements of applicable laws, codes, and standards, the health and safety officer shall develop procedures that ensure compliance with these laws, codes, and standards.

4.8.1.2 These recommended or revised rules, regulations, or standard operating procedures shall be submitted to the fire chief or the fire chief's designated representative by the health and safety officer.

Reprinted with permission from NFPA 1500, *Standard on Fire Department Occupational Safety and Health Program*, Copyright © 2002, National Fire Protection Association, Quincy, MA 02269. This reprinted material is not the complete and official position of the National Fire Protection Association on the referenced subject, which is represented only by the standard in its entirety.

Chapter 2
Regulations and Standards

[NFPA 1500: 4.8.1, 4.8.1.1, 4.8.1.2]

The requirements that affect respiratory protection in the workplace can be divided into two segments: regulations and standards. *Regulations* are codes, laws, orders, rules, or ordinances that are created through the act of legislation by the authority having jurisdiction (AHJ) and must be obeyed. *Standards* are recommended practices developed by a standards-writing organization within a particular area of concern. Some standards-writing organizations use the consensus method involving volunteer committees and a validation process. However, standards may be enforceable when adopted as law by the authority having jurisdiction.

Regulations and standards are also concerned with design, manufacturing, and testing requirements of respiratory protection equipment and operational use of the equipment. This chapter provides a general overview of the various regulations and standards that effect respiratory protection equipment used by the fire and emergency services in the United States and Canada.

Fire and Emergency Services Standards

In the United States, the National Fire Protection Association (NFPA), the American National Standards Institute (ANSI), the American Society of Mechanical Engineers (ASME), and the Compressed Gas Association (CGA) develop standards that apply to the fire and emergency services. In Canada, standards written by the Canadian Standards Association (CSA), NFPA, ANSI, ASME, and other standards-writing organizations have been adopted or referred to in respiratory protection statutes.

All standards provide minimum levels of protection. Therefore, design, manufacturing, testing, and operational use of respiratory protection equipment must meet or exceed these standards. Some standards do allow for equivalency in the requirements as long as the deviation can be justified by the organization making the change.

Standards are considered good industry practices; however, they are not mandatory unless the authority having jurisdiction adopts them. An incentive for adopting and implementing standards is that they are typically recognized as industry practices in civil legal proceedings even in jurisdictions that have not adopted them as law. The authority adopting the standards may be federal, state/provincial, county/parish, municipal, or tribal governments or private industry. Standards that deal with the design, manufacturing, and testing of respiratory protection equipment are mandatory in the U.S. because they have been adopted as law by the federal government. Areas that are regulated by the U.S. Department of Labor, Occupational Safety and Health Administration (OSHA) or have state-approved OSHA plans must follow NFPA standards. Determining the standards and authorities that apply to the individual emergency organization is an important part of the respiratory protection development process.

Fire and emergency services personnel should be familiar with these various organizations, the authorities the organizations wield, and the impacts they have on the services. The following sections provide a brief introduction of each of the major organizations.

Understanding Codes, Regulations, Standards, Guides, Laws, and the Authority Having Jurisdiction

Understanding the difference between codes, regulations, standards, guides, and laws is extremely important for fire and emergency services personnel in the U.S. and Canada. In the U.S., two general procedures are used in the establishment of respiratory protection laws: the first is through statutes promulgated or made known to the public by legislative action, that is, through the activities of a duly elected body of representatives, and the second is through codes, regulations, and standards promulgated by agencies with rule-making authority such as the Occupational Safety and Health Administration (OSHA). The latter procedure is by far the more common and is more readily responsive to the need for change. Promulgation through either course of action has the same force and effect of law.

By adhering to codes, regulations, standards, guides, and laws, liability to responders and their respective agencies can be more easily mitigated. Although some jurisdictions, either through neglect or outright omission, fail to adopt regulations and/or standards, these jurisdictions can still be held accountable by the judicial system because these standards are considered to be minimum protections within the industry.

Codes

A *code* is a body of law established either by legislative or administrative agencies with rule-making authority. The code is designed to regulate, within the scope of the code, the topic to which it relates. Examples of codes are fire or building codes such as the *Uniform Fire Code* developed by the International Conference of Building Officials, the *Standard Building Code* developed by the Southern Building Code Congress International, Inc., or the *National Building Code of Canada* developed by the National Research Council of Canada.

Regulations

A *regulation* is an authoritative rule dealing with details of procedures or a rule or order having the force of law issued by an executive authority of government. Regulations usually provide specific applications to acts of legislation. An example of a regulation is the *Code of Federal Regulations (CFR)*, Title 29 (Labor) 1910.134 (Respiratory Protection).

Standards

A *standard* is any rule, principle, or measure established by an authority on the specific topic. For example, the term *occupational safety and health*

standard under the Occupational Safety and Health Act of 1970 means "a standard which requires conditions, or adoption or use of one or more practices, means, methods, operations, or processes, reasonably necessary or appropriate to provide safe or healthful employment and places of employment." Perhaps the most commonly known standards in the fire and emergency services are those developed by the National Fire Protection Association (NFPA). These standards are developed through the consensus process and are considered the industry standard. (Note that not all standards are developed through the consensus process.) If the authority having jurisdiction adopts the standard, the standard then has the force of law within the jurisdiction (see Authority Having Jurisdiction section).

Guides

A *guide* is an instrument that provides direction or guiding information. Although such guides do not have the force of law, they may be considered as part of what is "reasonable" in a negligence case when determining the standard of care. A guide is a useful reference source to understanding what is involved in establishing and maintaining a program or process such as a respiratory protection program or the recommended procedure for cleaning and maintaining respiratory protection equipment. A guide provides guidance but does not prescribe requirements.

Laws

Laws can be divided into two categories: statutory and case. *Statutory laws* pertain to civil and criminal matters. Due to the nature of these laws, they may not take effect for many years. These laws regulate such things as water and air pollution through the Clean Water and Air Act, hazardous waste site cleanup through the Superfund Amendments and Reauthorization Act of 1986, and pollution by petroleum products through the Oil Pollution Act of 1990.

Case law is usually the result of a legal precedent or a judicial decision. These decisions serve as rules for future determinations in similar cases. The impact of these decisions affects emergency responders almost immediately because there is usually no implementation period. Case law, if heard at the federal level, can have nationwide effect. Some case law decisions can impact emergency responders even though the individual case did not involve emergency response personnel. An example of a case law decision is *Whirlpool Corporation v. Marshall*, which determined that an employer could not terminate the employment of a worker who refuses to perform an unsafe act that he or she considers unacceptably risky. However, case law is always subject to change and can provide precedence to both sides of an issue.

Authority Having Jurisdiction

The phrase *authority having jurisdiction* is defined as "the organization, office, or individual responsible for approving equipment, an installation, or a procedure." The NFPA uses this phrase in its documents in a broad manner because jurisdiction and approval agencies vary, as do their responsibilities. When local, municipal, or county/parish ordinance adopt standards such as those developed by the NFPA, the authority having jurisdiction has discretion in interpreting and enforcing the consensus standards and can provide equivalent codes as long as the intent of the standard is met. Failure to adopt standards or codes can make the authority having jurisdiction liable for court action.

Where public safety is primary, the authority having jurisdiction may be an agency or an individual. Some examples include the following:

- Federal department or agency
- State/provincial department or agency
- Local and regional departments or agencies
- Fire chief
- Fire marshal
- Board of fire commissioners/engineers
- Board of directors
- Chief of the fire prevention bureau, labor department, or health department
- Building official
- Electrical inspector
- Any others having statutory authority

For insurance purposes, the AHJ may include the insurance inspection department, rating bureau, and any other insurance company representative. These last three groups tend to work more for the benefit of insurance companies than for the creation of safety guidelines.

In many circumstances, the property owner or designated agent assumes the role of authority having jurisdiction. In government installations, the commanding officer or department official may be the authority having jurisdiction.

In Canada, the authority for provincial/territorial authorities to make regulations is provided through the Canadian Constitution Act and British North American (BNA) Act. These acts identify that certain responsibilities such as safety are the responsibility of provincial/territorial governments. Provincial/territorial governments pass acts that regulate assigned responsibilities or place certain responsibilities under the authority of municipalities. Municipal authorities may then pass bylaws to regulate/administrate the responsibility assigned.

An act in Canada is similar to statutory law in the U.S. The act or statute assigns powers, duties, responsibilities, and authorities to a person or entity. They may also assign quasi-criminal offenses for not fulfilling duties or for violating a requirement of the act.

While the NFPA definition for the *authority having jurisdiction* is valid in Canada, an authority having jurisdiction is also the legal authority responsible for the administration of legislation (act/statute, regulation, or bylaw/ordinance). An authority having jurisdiction may be authorized to pass regulations or bylaws (if a municipal authority). The regulations may be adopted or developed locally by the authority but are normally adopted from standards-writing agencies.

In Canada, the terms *code, guide, recommended practice,* and *standard* have no legal standing unless they are adopted as a regulation or within a regulation by an authority having jurisdiction. While the National Research Council of Canada writes the *National Fire Code* and *National Building Code,* these codes have no legal standing unless adopted by an authority having jurisdiction as a regulation or bylaw. An authority having jurisdiction may adopt a variety of documents as regulations, and thus it is not unusual in Canada to see NFPA codes, standards, guides, and recommended practices adopted as regulations.

National Fire Protection Association

Most firefighters are familiar with the National Fire Protection Association and its multitude of standards that relate to fire safety. Since the NFPA was organized in 1896, it has developed close to 300 standards that deal with everything from building construction to protective clothing for firefighters.

NFPA committees composed of representatives from the fire service, product manufacturers, government agencies, labor organizations, testing laboratories, and the general public develop the standards. The NFPA standards are developed and voted on by a technical committee, then voted on by a correlating committee prior to review and comment by the public. The technical committee answers public comments, and the process is repeated. The implementation date is established at the beginning of the cycle (**Figure 2.1**). Design, manufacturing, and testing standards that are concerned with respiratory protection are as follows:

● NFPA 1971, *Standard on Protective Ensemble for Structural Fire Fighting* — Provides requirements for the interface between the self-contained breathing apparatus (SCBA) and the coat, helmet, and flashover hood of the structural fire fighting ensemble

● NFPA 1976, *Standard on Protective Ensemble for Proximity Fire Fighting* — Provides the requirements for the interface between the SCBA facepiece and the proximity fire fighting ensemble

● NFPA 1981, *Standard on Open-Circuit Self-Contained Breathing Apparatus for the Fire Service* — Standard specifically concerned with the design, manufacture, and testing of SCBAs

● NFPA 1982, *Standard on Personal Alert Safety Systems (PASS)* — Standard specifically concerned with the design, manufacture, and testing of PASS devices; provides information on the integration of the PASS device with the SCBA unit

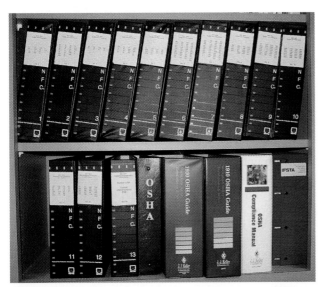

Figure 2.1 National Fire Protection Association standards provide fire and emergency services organizations with accepted industry standards upon which to base respiratory protection programs. Other regulatory requirements may be found in government documents such as the OSHA portions of the *Code of Federal Regulations (CFR)*. *Courtesy of Kenneth Baum.*

● NFPA 1991, *Standard on Vapor-Protective Ensembles for Hazardous Materials Emergencies* — Provides information on the interface between the SCBA facepiece and the vapor-protective ensemble

● NFPA 1999, *Standard on Protective Clothing for Emergency Medical Operations* — Provides the design, manufacture, and testing criteria for protective clothing worn during emergency medical operations

Design, manufacture, and testing requirements for supplied-air respirators (SARs) and air-purifying respirators (APRs) may be included in future revisions of the NFPA standards. NFPA currently does not have standards that concern the design, manufacture, or testing of types of respiratory protection other than self-contained breathing apparatus.

Self-contained breathing apparatus that is manufactured to NFPA standards must be tested and certified by a third-party testing laboratory such as Underwriters Laboratories Inc (UL) or Factory Mutual (FM). SCBAs are submitted and tested as a single unit consisting of facepiece, air hoses, regulator, PASS device (if integrated with the system), harness, and cylinder. If the end user substitutes parts or components from another system or manufacturer or the unit is used in a situation for which it was not designed or certified, the certification is voided. Currently, all SCBA sold in the United States for use by fire and emergency services must meet NFPA design, manufacturing, and testing standards. Some noncertified SCBA are manufactured and sold in the United States for use in industrial applications. Canadian readers should refer to the Canadian Requirements section later in this chapter.

Operational standards for respiratory protection are covered in the following NFPA standards:

● NFPA 472, *Standard on Professional Competence of Responders to Hazardous Materials Incidents,* 2002 edition — Provides guidelines for respiratory protection during hazardous materials incidents

● NFPA 600, *Standard on Industrial Fire Brigades* — Provides guidelines for the organizing, operating, training, and equipping of industrial (private) fire brigades

- NFPA 1404, *Standard for Fire Service Respiratory Protection Training,* 2002 edition — Provides the guidelines for developing an NFPA-compliant respiratory protection training program within a fire department

- NFPA 1500, *Standard on Fire Department Occupational Safety and Health Program,* 2002 edition — Establishes the requirements for a respiratory protection program within a fire department

- NFPA 1521, *Standard for Fire Department Safety Officer* — Establishes the authority for a health and safety officer in relation to a respiratory protection program

- NFPA 1581, *Standard on Fire Department Infection Control Program* — Establishes the requirements for infection control protection for emergency medical service (EMS) providers

- NFPA 1582, *Standard on Medical Requirements for Fire Fighters* — Establishes the requirements for minimum medical standards for firefighters, including medical testing and records keeping

- NFPA 1852, *Standard on Selection, Care, and Maintenance of Open-Circuit Self-Contained Breathing Apparatus,* 2002 edition — Establishes guidelines for selecting, cleaning, and repairing SCBA

- NFPA 1977, *Standard on Protective Clothing and Equipment for Wildland Fire Fighting* — Provides limited guidelines for respiratory protection during wildland fire incidents

American National Standards Institute

The American National Standards Institute was established in 1918 as a private, nonprofit membership organization. Its primary goal was to make the U.S. economy more competitive in the world market. The organization coordinates the private sector voluntary standardization system through ANSI-accredited member organizations. ANSI does not itself develop the standards. Instead, it facilitates development through the consensus process. The organization also oversees the creation of conformity assessment or testing systems; that is, ANSI sets the testing criteria for respiratory protection equipment to ensure that it meets the NFPA design criteria. The following ANSI standards located in the Z88 series affect respiratory breathing equipment. Additional requirements for respiratory protection during confined-space operations are located in ANSI Z117.1-1995, Safety Requirements for Confined Spaces.

- ANSI Z88.2-1992, Practices for Respiratory Protection

- ANSI Z88.5-1981, Practices for Respiratory Protection for the Fire Service

- ANSI Z88.6-1984, For Respiratory Protection — Respirator Use — Physical Qualifications for Personnel

- ANSI Z88.7-2001, Color Coding of APR Canisters, Cartridges, and Filters

- ANSI Z88.8-2001, Performance Criteria and Test Methods for APRs

- ANSI Z88.10-2001, Fit Testing Methods

American Society of Mechanical Engineers

The American Society of Mechanical Engineers is a worldwide, nonprofit educational and technical organization that was originally founded in 1880. The organization is primarily concerned with the development of technical standards through the consensus committee process. Many of the ASME standards such as the Boiler Code have been incorporated into U.S. and Canadian laws. ASME has developed standards that apply to the design and construction of compressed air cylinders and storage containers used with respiratory protection equipment (**Figure 2.2**).

American Society for Testing and Materials

The American Society for Testing and Materials (ASTM) was established in 1898 and is a consensus standards organization that establishes testing procedures and minimum quality levels for manufacturing materials. Such standards apply to the materials used in the manufacture of respiratory protection equipment.

Compressed Gas Association

The Compressed Gas Association established in 1913 is a private sector organization that develops and promotes safety standards and safe practices for the industrial gas industry. Technical and safety standards for the storage, use, and handling of compressed gases are developed through the consensus

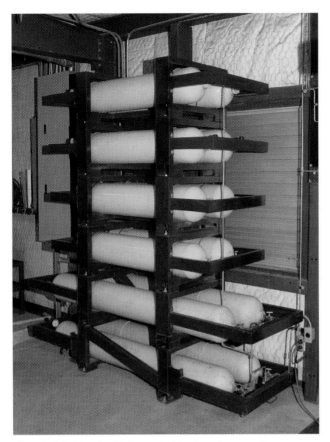

Figure 2.2 Standards that regulate the storage of compressed gases, including large-capacity breathing air cylinders such as these, are developed by organizations such as the American Society of Mechanical Engineers and the Compressed Gas Association.

committee system. Additionally, CGA develops training programs and educational material to promote safety in the workplace. The organization works closely with government agencies at all levels in formulating regulations regarding compressed and liquefied gases. CGA standards that apply to respiratory protection involve the design and testing of storage cylinders and the transportation of compressed air cylinders.

Examples of CGA standards that apply to the fire and emergency services are as follows:

- C-1, Methods for Hydrostatic Testing of Compressed Gas Cylinders

- C-6, Standards for Visual Inspection of Steel Compressed Gas Cylinders

- C-6.1, Standards for Visual Inspection of High Pressure Aluminum Compressed Gas Cylinders

- C-6.2, Guidelines for Visual Inspection and Requalification of Fiber Reinforced High Pressure Cylinders

- C-6.3, Guidelines for Visual Inspection and Requalification of Low Pressure Aluminum Compressed Gas Cylinders

- C-7, Guide to Preparation of Precautionary Labeling and Marking of Compressed Gas Containers

- C-8, Standard for Requalification of DOT-3HT, CTC-3HT, and TC-3HTM Seamless Steel Cylinders

- C-9, Standard Color Marking of Compressed Gas Containers Intended for Medical Use

- C-15, Procedures for Cylinder Design Proof and Service Performance Tests

- C-16, CGA Registration Program for Cylinder Owner Symbols

- C-19 FRP-3, Guidelines for Filament-Wound Composite Cylinders with Nonloadsharing Liners

U.S. Government Requirements

Numerous departments of the U.S. federal government enforce regulations concerning respiratory protection. They include the Department of Labor (DOL), Department of Transportation (DOT), Department of Health and Human Services (DHHS), Department of Defense (DOD), Department of the Interior (DOI), Department of Agriculture (USDA), and the Nuclear Regulatory Agency (NRC).

Department of Labor

Within the Department of Labor, two administrations have authority over respiratory protection: The Occupational Safety and Health Administration (OSHA) and the Mine Safety and Health Administration (MSHA). The act that created OSHA also provided guidelines and authority for each state to develop and implement similar federally approved safety and health plans.

Occupational Safety and Health Administration

In December 1970, President Richard Nixon signed into law the Occupational Safety and Health (OSH) Act of 1970 (Public Law [PL] 91-596). This law is commonly referred to as the Williams-Steiger Occupational Safety and Health Act, named after the two legislators who were the primary authors and sponsors. The act instructed the Secretary of the U.S. Department of Labor to promulgate mandatory occupational safety and health standards among other requirements. The creation of the Occupational Safety and Health Administration under the existing U.S. Department of Labor was a result of this act.

Prior to the initiation of OSHA, there were few national safety and health requirements for employee safety in North America. Numerous states had safety and health regulations that varied in quality and enforcement from excellent to poor. Under the OSHA regulations, the employers covered by the law were required to do the following things:

- Furnish each employee a place of employment free from recognized hazards that would cause or likely cause death or serious physical harm.

- Comply with occupational safety and health standards included in PL 91-596. In addition, Section 5 (b) of the Williams-Steiger Act required all employees to comply with the "standards, rules, regulations, and orders issued pursuant to this Act."

Although primarily concerned with safety in the private sector, sections of this law were found applicable to the public sector as a whole. The fire service was required to comply with all applicable OSHA regulations published in Title 29 (Labor) of the *Code of Federal Regulations* (*CFR*) or equivalent regulations issued by state governments that elected to assume responsibility for the development of standards and enforcement as allowed by Section 18, State Jurisdiction and State Plans, of the OSH Act. Although Title 29 (Labor) *CFR* 1910, Subpart L (Fire Protection) did not apply directly to municipal fire departments or fire protection districts, it contained applicable requirements for the fire service. This standard or regulation contained requirements for personal protective equipment, training, respiratory protection, and the use of fire fighting equipment (**Figure 2.3**). In addition, Title 29 *CFR* 1910.134 (Respiratory Protection Requirements), Title 29 *CFR* 1910.120 (Hazardous Waste Operations and Emergency Response Requirements), Title 29 *CFR* 1910.1000 (Air Contaminants), and Title 29 *CFR* 1910.1200 (Hazard Communication) were particular concerns to the fire service. Fire departments were covered by numerous other applicable regulations of the general industry stan-

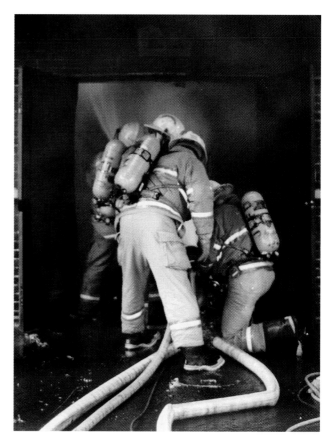

Figure 2.3 Personal protective equipment including respiratory protection equipment is required by OSHA for all structural fire fighting. *Courtesy of Chris Mickal.*

dards (Title 29 *CFR* 1910, Occupational Safety and Health Administration, Department of Labor) and parts of the construction standards (Title 29 *CFR* 1926, Safety and Health Regulations for Construction), in particular Title 29 *CFR* 1926, Subpart P (Excavations). Basically, Title 29 *CFR* 1910 was the fire service's introduction to mandated safety and health requirements.

In the years since the adoption of Title 29 *CFR* 1910, these requirements have increased with mandates for the following areas:

- Hazardous materials mitigation
- Confined-space entry
- Increased respiratory protection
- Incident management
- Occupational safety and health
- Health and safety officer
- Infection control, identification, and notification

NOTE: Because federal OSHA regulations do not apply to all states, it is important for fire service personnel to check with individual state departments of labor concerning the applicable safety and health regulations.

State Occupational Safety and Health Plans

Section 18 of the Occupational Safety and Health Act of 1970 encourages states to develop and operate their own job safety and health programs. These state plans are approved and monitored by OSHA. Currently, the following states and territories have OSHA-approved state plans:

Alaska	New Mexico
Arizona	New York
California	North Carolina
Connecticut	Oregon
Hawaii	Puerto Rico
Indiana	South Carolina
Iowa	Tennessee
Kentucky	Utah
Maryland	Vermont
Michigan	Virgin Islands
Minnesota	Virginia
Nevada	Washington
New Jersey	Wyoming

NOTE: The Connecticut, New York, and New Jersey plans cover public sector (state and local government) employment only. Addresses of state OSHA offices are included in Appendix A, Federal OSHA Office Directory, which includes the Directory of States with Approved Occupational Safety and Health Plans.

Mine Safety and Health Administration

The Mine Safety and Health Administration was created in 1978 when all federal mine safety programs were transferred from the Department of the Interior to the Department of Labor. Prior to 1978, the mine safety agency was referred to as the Bureau of Mines, after which it became the Mine Environmental Safety Agency (MESA). MSHA governs safety in the mining industry where respiratory protection is intended to reduce or eliminate the effects of airborne particulates and oxygen-deficient atmospheres. MSHA respiratory protection testing, certification, and use requirements are compiled in Title 42 (Public Health) *CFR* Part 84 (Approval of Respiratory Protection Devices).

Department of Agriculture

The Department of Agriculture regulates wildland and forestry fire fighting on federal government land through the Forest Service. OSHA regulations apply to these organizations also **(Figure 2.4)**.

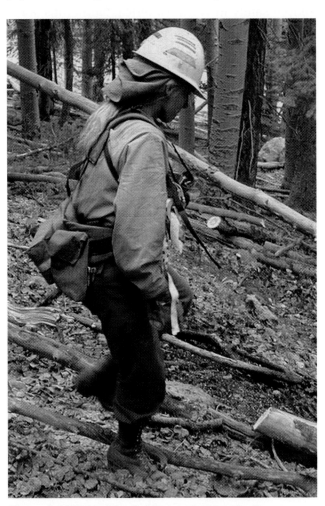

Figure 2.4 Wildland fire fighting personal protective equipment is regulated by federal, state, and provincial requirements. *Courtesy of Federal Emergency Management Agency (U.S.).*

Department of the Interior

The Department of the Interior is responsible for safety and risk management within the Bureau of Indian Affairs (BIA). The BIA administers OSHA regulations on Native American lands and works with the individual Native American Nations to provide respiratory protection to firefighters and emergency responders assigned to those lands.

Department of Transportation

The Department of Transportation regulates the transportation and storage of compressed gases. These regulations include the design, manufacture, and certification testing of the containers and also the filling, marking, and periodic service testing of them. Since breathing air used in SCBAs and supplied-air respirators is classified as a compressed gas, DOT-approved cylinders must be used for storage **(Figure 2.5)**. All SCBA cylinders are regulated by the DOT and must meet ASME, ANSI, and CGA standards.

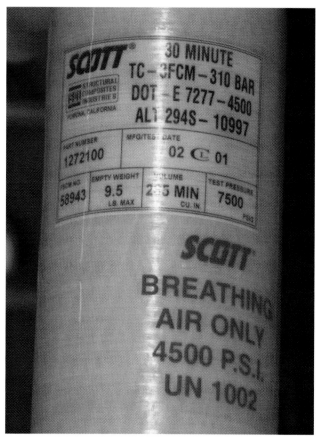

Figure 2.5 All breathing air cylinders used in the United States must have Department of Transportation (DOT) labels applied to them. *Courtesy of Bob Parker.*

Nuclear Regulatory Commission

The Nuclear Regulatory Commission defines the type of respiratory protection necessary to protect workers from airborne radioactive particles. The regulations concern respiratory protection in nuclear laboratories, nuclear power stations, and nuclear waste dumps. It is important to understand these regulations because larger quantities of nuclear waste are transported from controlled sites to dumps around the country. Respiratory protection requirements covered by the NRC are found in Title 10 (Energy) *CFR* 20.1703 (Standards for Protection Against Radiation, Use of Individual Respiratory Protection Equipment).

Department of Health and Human Services

The Department of Health and Human Services is responsible for educating the public on safety hazards. Through the collection of data by the National Institute for Occupational Safety and Health (NIOSH), the DHHS compiles injury, illness, and fatality information. This information is analyzed, and safety violations are noted. Recommendations are then made to reduce the safety hazards, and NIOSH bulletins are issued to the general public. NIOSH also issues product warnings when a particular piece of equipment is the cause of injuries or fatalities **(Figure 2.6)**.

In addition, NIOSH is responsible for establishing testing procedures for respiratory protection equipment. NFPA refers to NIOSH-required testing within its own standards. All manufacturers of SCBAs and respiratory protection equipment must submit their units to NIOSH for testing as required by OSHA Title 42 *CFR* 84. Units that pass the test are certified for use. All approved SCBA in the United States must bear the NIOSH/MSHA certification labels. Voiding of the certification through alteration or misuse of an SCBA also voids the third-party certification for NFPA compliance as well as potentially violating any applicable OSHA regulations.

NIOSH guidelines are published in the following publications:

- NIOSH 87-116, Guide to Industrial Respiratory Protection

- NIOSH 87-108, Respiratory Decision Logic

Department of Defense

Military facilities are operated and governed by the Department of Defense. OSHA regulations and NFPA standards apply to respiratory protection within these sites. Military personnel, a civilian vendor under contract, or mutual aid resources may provide fire and emergency services.

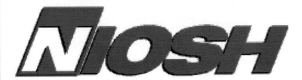

Respirator Users' Notice

January 15, 1982

NIOSH Emergency Information Bulletin on the Use of Self-Contained Breathing Apparatus in Low Temperatures

Extreme caution should be exercised by all persons using open circuit self-contained breathing apparatus (SCBA) in hazardous environments during sub-freezing weather. SCBAs are widely used by fire fighters combatting winter fires. All users who wear SCBAs in cold temperatures should take particular note of the following important precautions:

1. Moisture in the air cylinders must be kept at an absolute minimum since small amounts of moisture in the air supply may freeze and result in failure of the breathing apparatus.

2. Always use a nosecup in the SCBA facepiece when temperatures are below freezing. Failure to use a nosecup under such circumstances can result in facepiece fogging and severely impaired vision. Chemical anti-fog agents may not perform adequately in low temperatures.

3. Carefully read the approval label on the respirator to determine if it is necessary to install special accessories prior to use of the SCBA in sub-freezing weather. Certain older U.S. Bureau of Mines approved SCBAs require such low temperature accessories (SCBAs approved prior to March 25,1972).

4. When leaving an extremely hot environment, such as a fire scene, and entering cold air (below or near freezing), always place the SCBA facepiece in your turnout coat to keep it warm if it is to be quickly reused. SCBAs when not being actively breathed can freeze-up very quickly.

5. Use special care after washing SCBA facepieces and breathing tubes to remove all moisture to prevent water drainage and freeze-up of the regulator.

6. SCBA alarms can fail in low temperatures; therefore, visual checks of remaining service time should be made when SCBAs are used in sub-freezing conditions.

7. Be familiar with procedures on how to cope with exhalation valves which can freeze open or closed in low temperatures. (Contact the manufacturer or the State Fire Training Officer for specific instructions.)

8. SCBAs are NIOSH laboratory approved for use in temperatures down to -25° F. Therefore, if SCBAs are to be used in temperatures below -25° F, extreme caution should be used.

9. Also observe the following general precautions:
a. Use G-7.1, Type I, Grade D air or air of equivalent specification.
b. Follow all information listed on the NIOSH/MSHA or BOM approval label for the specific SCBA in use.
c. Follow the manufacturer's recommendations included in their instruction and maintenance manual accompanying the SCBA.
d. Follow all applicable Federal, State, and Local regulations concerned with the use of SCBAs.
e. Keep SCBAs in a warm location between uses.

Figure 2.6 The National Institute for Occupational Safety and Health Internet website provides a source for respiratory protection equipment warnings and fatality/injury reports.

Canadian Requirements

In Canada, the provincial and territorial governments regulate health and safety within their own jurisdictions. Although the Canadian federal government does have an occupational health and safety (OH&S) agency, it only regulates the activities of some federal government employees. Federal regulations may be found in the *Canada Labour Code.* Other federal employees are regulated by the OH&S regulations of the province/territory in which they are located. For instance, the Royal Canadian Mounted Police (RCMP) is a federal agency but is required to comply with the provincial/territorial OH&S regulations in the particular province/territory in which it operates. However, prison guards, who are also federal law enforcement officers, must comply with the federal OH&S regulations and not the local province/territory regulations.

The titles of the provincial/territorial agencies responsible for administration of OH&S regulations vary. Some of the agencies are the Worker's Compensation Board (WCB), Workplace Safety and Insurance Board (WSIB), Worker's Health and Safety Centre, and Atomic Energy Commission of Canada (AECC) among others. The provincial/territorial agency may be a government agency, a "Crown" corporation, or a government board.

Just as the titles of agencies vary from province to province, the OH&S regulations also vary. Regulations only apply in the province/territory enacting them and do not have authority in any other province/territory. Some regulations cover specific fire service subjects such as respiratory protection or protective clothing requirements **(Figure 2.7)**. Others cover general safety issues for all workers, portions of which also apply to firefighters and emergency responders.

Provincial/territorial OH&S regulations typically adopt standards or parts of standards within the regulations. Once a standard has been adopted as part of a regulation, the standard must be followed. As in the case of the United States, standards are only enforceable when they are adopted by the appropriate legislation. The responsibility for enforcement is retained by the provincial/territorial government and not granted by the standards-writing agency. This means that

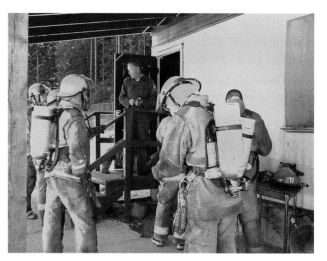

Figure 2.7 Canadian respiratory protection requirements usually vary from province to province. *Courtesy of Lloyd Lees.*

Manitoba (the legal adopting jurisdiction) and not the Canadian Standards Association (the standards-writing organization) would enforce CSA standards adopted in Manitoba. NFPA standards are also in use in some Canadian provinces/territories.

Standards may also be listed as reference documents within the OH&S regulations. As a reference document, the cited standard is considered a *recommended practice* that meets the requirements of the OH&S regulation. It is not unusual for provincial/territorial OH&S regulations to adopt or reference NFPA standards.

The Standards Council of Canada (SCC) is the verification agency for standards-writing agencies. This organization is similar to ANSI in the United States. ANSI is also a recognized verification agency in Canada. The National Research Council of Canada also establishes standards. Standards developed by NFPA and NIOSH may be adopted in a province/territory because they carry ANSI approval. Canadian standards-writing agencies include Canadian Standards Association, Underwriters Laboratories of Canada (ULC), Canadian General Standards Board (CGSB), and Bureau de normalisation du Quebec (BNQ). However, Canadian regulations may adopt standards from any recognized standards-writing agency such as NFPA, ANSI, and ASME. Underwriters Laboratories Inc is accredited by the Standards Council of Canada as a testing and certification agency for Canadian standards.

The following standards may be applicable in provinces/territories in relation to respiratory protection. Fire and emergency service personnel in Canada are urged to consult their provincial OH&S agency to determine the appropriate requirements.

- CAN/CSA Z180.1-00, Compressed Breathing Air Systems
- CAN/CSA Z94.4-93, Selection, Use, and Care of Respirators
- CAN/CSA B339-96, Cylinders, Spheres and Tubes for the Transportation of Dangerous Goods

International Requirements

Respiratory protection requirements internationally relate to the design, manufacture, and testing of respiratory protection equipment. Operational requirements are national and not international concerns. United States federal government OSHA or Canadian OH&S agency regulations govern overseas U.S. and Canadian government facilities. These regulations apply to fire protection services provided on facilities staffed by foreign nationals.

Some of the more prominent international regulations include those by the International Organization for Standardization (ISO), the European Norm (EN), and the Deutsches Institut fur Normung (DIN). The ISO and DIN standards have been in place for many years while the EN has developed as a result of the creation of the European Union (formerly known as the European Economic Community). The European Union is an attempt by the nations of Europe to create a strong economic, political, and military alliance to counter the factionalism that has marked the history of Europe.

International Organization for Standardization

In Europe, Australia, and New Zealand, respiratory protection equipment must meet International Organization for Standardization (ISO) 9000 quality control standards. Current components include ISO 9000, 9001, and 9004 sections. The ISO system is intended to ensure that equipment is constructed and tested to similar standards (**Figures 2.8 a and b**). U.S. and Canadian firms doing business in Europe must have an ISO rating and meet the ISO

standards. Some products manufactured overseas and imported into the U.S. and Canada must also meet these standards.

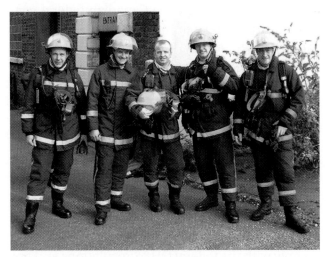

Figure 2.8a Firefighters in Great Britain wear personal protective equipment that is similar to apparel/equipment worn in North America. Design requirements are based on ISO standards that are similar to NFPA standards that are applied in the U.S. *Courtesy of Neil Constantine.*

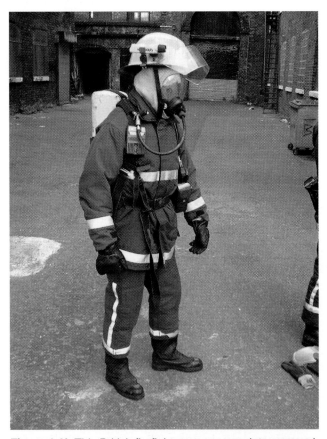

Figure 2.8b This British firefighter wears complete personal protective clothing and respiratory protection equipment. Compare this photo to other images of U.S. firefighters and note both the similarities and differences in the clothing and equipment. *Courtesy of Neil Constantine.*

European Norm

A quality standard that has been established in the European Union is the European Norm (EN). Some of the EN standards are based on ISO requirements while others are based on NFPA standards. The EN standards are intended to provide greater standardization of manufacturing, the equalization of trade opportunities between the member nations, and a stronger economic balance to U.S. trade. There is currently an effort to combine the various standards and conform to one EN standard for respiratory protection equipment.

Deutsches Institut fur Normung

Similar to ANSI, the Deutsches Institut fur Normung (DIN) has been active in Germany and Europe for many years. The DIN is a nongovernmental organization established to promote the development of standardization and related activities in Germany and related markets. The organization has worked to develop over 12,000 standards through the consensus process that ensures quality and conformity of materials, testing, and processes. The DIN is currently active in the European Union to represent the interests of German business in the development of European standards that will be critical to completion of a single European market.

Other International Areas

Other areas of the world, including South America, Asia, and Africa, have their own standards and regulations, although they are not necessarily as strict as the United States, Canada, Australia, New Zealand, and the European Union. These standards and regulations are only of concern in the United States and Canada when considering respiratory protection equipment manufactured in those areas and imported into the U.S. and Canada. This equipment must meet or exceed NFPA standards and be NIOSH/MSHA tested and certified.

State/Provincial/Territorial, Local, and Tribal Laws and Ordinances

Government authorities at the state, province, territory, county/parish, municipal, or tribal level may have their own regulations regarding personal safety and respiratory protection. These regulations are intended to protect not only the employee but also the authority having jurisdiction. Usually based on nationally recognized standards, the regulations provide the employee with a minimum level of protection and safety. At the same time, the existence of the nationally recognized standard as part of the law lessens the jurisdiction's legal liability and protects it from lawsuits based on negligence.

Various agencies or departments within the individual authorities administer the regulations governing respiratory protection. Fire and emergency personnel should research the appropriate laws to determine the relevant authority and how it applies to the fire and emergency services. An overview of the various governmental jurisdictions is as follows:

● *State/Provincial/Territorial* — Respiratory protection regulations are usually administered by the state/provincial/territorial Department of Labor. Agencies that manage wildland and forestry fire fighting such as the California Forestry Department also regulate respiratory protection. State laws usually govern rural fire protection districts.

● *Local* — Local government (county/parish, city, township, or village) may adopt consensus standards as part of local laws or ordinances to regulate the jurisdiction's fire protection. Appropriate departments such as personnel, safety, and human services or emergency medical authorities or fire commissioner's offices would administer these regulations.

● *Tribal* — Many states, provinces, and territories in the United States and Canada have semiautonomous areas referred to as *tribal lands* or *reservations.* The particular Native American Nation's elected government (such as Cherokee, Sac and Fox, and Pawnee Nations) governs these lands. These governments provide police and fire protection and other governmental services to residents of the tribal lands. Consensus standards may be used to form the basis for fire protection ordinances and laws within the tribal area of authority. The U.S. Federal government's Department of the Interior, Bureau of Indian Affairs, may also regulate fire protection in reservation lands that do not have an organized tribal government. The BIA applies OSHA safety regulations where applicable (**Figure 2.9**).

Fire and emergency agencies must determine the various jurisdictions they operate within, the types of hazards they respond to, and the respiratory protection regulations that govern those jurisdictions and hazards. Overlapping jurisdictions can create multiple levels of jurisdiction for these emergency agencies. For instance, a municipal fire department operating in the county/parish jurisdiction to protect a federal government facility through a mutual aid agreement can be faced with increased operational regulations (**Figure 2.10**). The possibility of such a situation occurring should be considered during the planning of the respiratory protection program, during the development of mutual aid agreements, and when purchasing new equipment.

Summary

Determining the regulations that govern respiratory protection for a specific fire or emergency organization may seem challenging. However, most regulations already exist within the laws and ordinances that created the organization. If respiratory protection is not defined or regulated for the fire or emergency services department, then the department should consider proposing such laws to the authority having jurisdiction. A strong case should be made for the benefits to both the employees and the liability imposed on the jurisdiction by the lack of respiratory protection regulations.

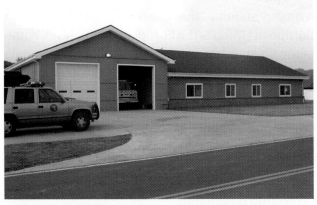

Figure 2.9 The Bureau of Indian Affairs regulates fire fighting activities on Native American land (such as at this Pawnee Tribal Fire Station) through the application of OSHA regulations. *Courtesy of Nathan Traurnicht.*

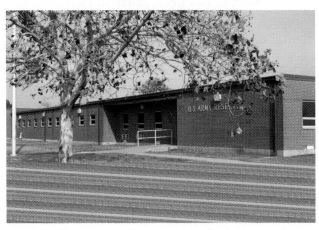

Figure 2.10 Many jurisdictions include federally owned facilities such as this U.S. Army Reserve facility that depends on the local fire department for protection.

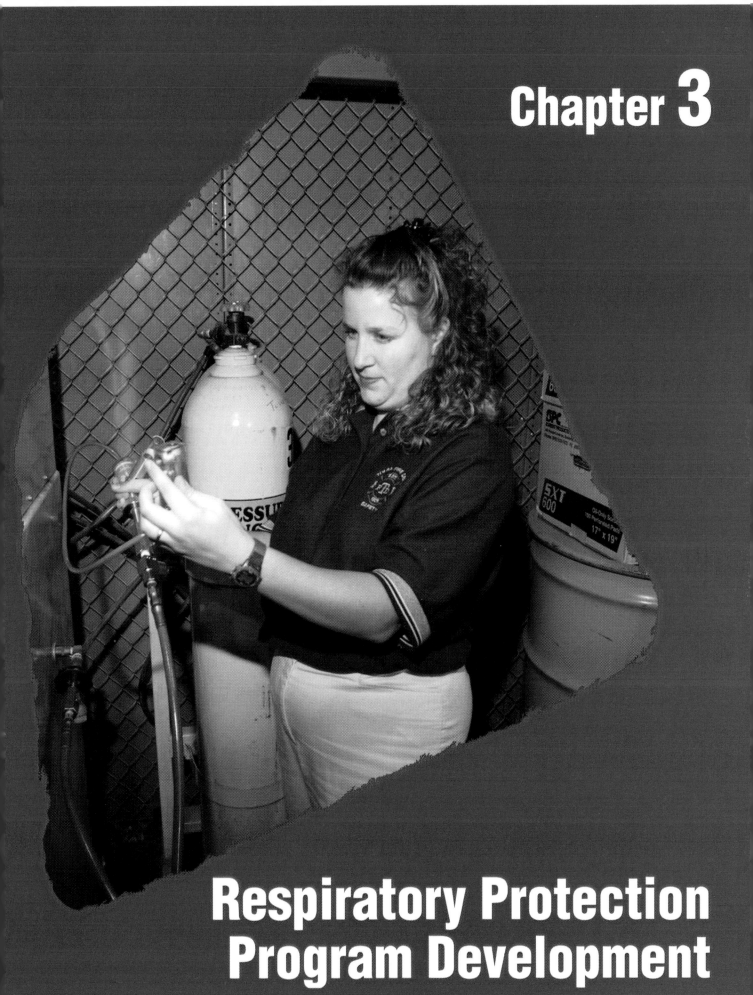

Respiratory Protection Program Development

This chapter provides information that will assist the reader in meeting the following job performance requirements from NFPA 1404, *Standard for Fire Service Respiratory Protection Training*, 2002 Edition, and NFPA 1500, *Standard on Fire Department Occupational Safety and Health Program*, 2002 Edition.

NFPA 1500

4.5.1 An occupational safety and health committee shall be established and shall serve in an advisory capacity to the fire chief.

4.5.1.1 The committee shall include the following members:

(1) The designated fire department health and safety officer

(2) Representatives of fire department management

(3) Individual members or representatives of member organizations

4.5.1.2 The committee shall also be permitted to include other persons.

4.5.1.3 Representatives of member organizations shall be selected by their respective organizations, but other committee members shall be appointed to the committee by the fire chief.

4.8.1 The health and safety officer shall develop, review, and revise rules, regulations, and standard operating procedures pertaining to the fire department occupational safety and health program.

4.8.1.1 Based upon the directives and requirements of applicable laws, codes, and standards, the health and safety officer shall develop procedures that ensure compliance with these laws, codes, and standards.

4.8.1.2 These recommended or revised rules, regulations, or standard operating procedures shall be submitted to the fire chief or the fire chief's designated representative by the health and safety officer.

4.8.2 The health and safety officer shall periodically report to the fire chief or the fire chief's designated representative on the adequacy of, effectiveness of, and compliance with the rules, regulations, and standard operating procedures specified in 4.8.1 and 4.8.1.1 of this section.

7.9.1 The fire department shall adopt and maintain a respiratory protection program that addresses the selection, care, maintenance, and safe use of respiratory protection equipment, training in its use, and the assurance of air quality.

7.9.2 The fire department shall develop and maintain standard operating procedures that are compliant with this standard and that address the safe use of respiratory protection.

7.9.3 Members shall be tested and certified at least annually in the safe and proper use of respiratory protection equipment that they are authorized to use.

NFPA 1404

5.1.1 The authority having jurisdiction shall adopt and maintain a respiratory protection program that meets the requirements of Section 7.9 of NFPA 1500, *Standard on Fire Department Occupational Safety and Health Program*.

5.1.2 The authority having jurisdiction shall conduct ongoing respiratory protection training that meets the requirements of this standard.

Chapter 3
Respiratory Protection Program Development

[NFPA 1500: 7.9.1, 7.9.2]
[NFPA 1404: 5.1.1]

The increase in the chemical and biological toxins associated with chemical manufacturing and transportation prompted the U.S. government to issue requirements for respiratory protection in Title 29 (Labor) *CFR* 1910.134 (Respiratory Protection Requirements) to provide work practices and a safe work environment for all employees. This regulation from the U.S. Department of Labor (DOL), Occupational and Safety Health Administration (OSHA), and the recognition by the fire and emergency services that respiratory protection was necessary for the protection of their members during emergency responses led to the creation of respiratory protection requirements in NFPA 1500, *Standard on Fire Department Occupational Safety and Health Program*. As mentioned in Chapter 2, Regulations and Standards, the DOL/OSHA regulation carries the force of law where applicable, while the NFPA standard recommends the establishment of a comprehensive respiratory protection program within the fire department/emergency response organization. As a minimum, a respiratory protection program consists of the following items:

- Written standard operating procedures for the safe use of respiratory protection equipment in a hazardous atmosphere

- Written standard operating procedures on the selection, care, storage, and maintenance of the respiratory protection equipment

- Initial and periodic training requirements in the proper use of the respiratory protection equipment

- Procedures for annual testing and recertification of members in the use of the respiratory protection equipment

- Annual medical evaluations of members who are assigned to use respiratory protection equipment

- Periodic air-quality testing program for breathing air from the charging air source for air-supplied respirators (required by OSHA and recommended by NFPA 1500, Section 7.10)

For the program to be successful, there must be complete support by the administration and members of the department/organization. This chapter discusses how to develop a written respiratory protection program that meets safety and regulatory requirements. The formation of a respiratory protection committee and guidelines for limited-resource emergency organizations are also discussed.

Administrative Commitment

[NFPA 1500: 4.5.1, 4.8.1, 4.8.1.1, 4.8.1.2, 4.8.2, 7.9.1, 7.9.2]

For a respiratory protection program or any other type of program to be successful, it must be supported completely by the organization's administration. The administration can show this support by obtaining the necessary resources and equipment and being involved in the program compliance. Support must be consistent and the mandate for compliance must be communicated to all members of the organization. Management's commitment and support to the success of the respiratory protection program and its policies assist program acceptance, program implementation, and users' acceptance of responsibility for the equipment.

One way of providing support and ensuring member compliance is through participatory management and decision-making policies. The administration must include all levels of the organization in writing the respiratory protection program, which can be accomplished by establishing a respiratory protection program committee or assigning the task to the safety and health program committee (**Figure 3.1**). The committee must be provided with specific guidelines, deadlines, and expectations based on the standards and regulations to be met.

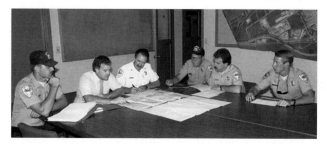

Figure 3.1 The organization's safety and health program committee can provide the nucleus for the development of a respiratory protection program.

The committee or developing body must also factor in the perceptions of the population that the organization serves. An excellent way to educate the public and other involved parties is to present a cost/benefit risk analysis. To do this analysis, the administration has to demonstrate a cost benefit and risk benefit from the respiratory protection program. This demonstration involves educating government officials, citizens, and the organization's membership about the scope of the hazards faced by fire and emergency service personnel. An analysis of the hazards and a correlation between them and potential injuries, illnesses, and fatalities and the medical and liability costs to the authority should then be generated. This data is then compared to the cost of implementing a respiratory protection program. The intangible benefits to employee quality of life, health, and life expectancy should also be emphasized.

Once the respiratory protection program is established and implemented, it must be monitored. A specific administrative position must be assigned the task of monitoring the program. This administrative position may be the health and safety officer, a training officer, or a senior staff officer (**Figure 3.2**). The person who monitors the program must report directly to the fire chief/director and have the authority to act in his or her behalf. Data on the effectiveness of the program must be continually collected and analyzed by the person responsible for the program and the respiratory protection program committee. This data includes postincident analyses, injury reports, training records, and respiratory protection equipment maintenance costs. Periodically, the administration must review the data and determine if changes to the program are needed.

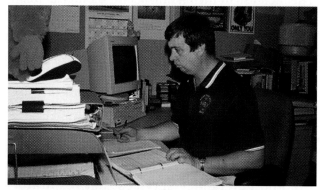

Figure 3.2 The health and safety officer is a principle member of the safety and health program committee and can be assigned the responsibility for the respiratory protection program.

Committee Representation

[NFPA 1500: 4.5.1.1, 4.5.1.2, 4.5.1.3]

To gain complete support of the organization's membership for the program, the respiratory protection program committee (or safety and health program committee) must include members from all levels of the organization. Representation should include but is not limited to the following people:

- Senior management officials
- Health and safety officer
- Training personnel
- Operational personnel
- Respiratory protection equipment maintenance technician
- Emergency services organization physician
- Representatives of employee organization

Each representative brings to the committee specific concerns and viewpoints. The senior management representative brings administrative concerns such as budgetary constraints, concerns of elected officials, and implementation and enforcement concerns. The health and safety officer, required by NFPA 1500 and NFPA 1521, *Standard for Fire Department Safety Officer,* provides the technical expertise in health and safety regulations and concerns. Training personnel provide the limitations and needs for respiratory protection training based on the requirements found in NFPA 1403, *Standard on Live Fire Training Evolutions,* and NFPA 1404, *Standard for Fire Service Respiratory Protection Training.* The operational personnel bring the view of the people who have to wear the equipment on active duty. The emergency services organization physician has the medical background and provides the medical testing information. Finally, the employee representatives bring the concerns of the membership as a whole to the meetings.

An effective respiratory protection program committee should not be larger than 12 members. Additional personnel with special skills or knowledge can be invited to provide information as needed. These additional personnel are listed in Chapter 5, Respiratory Protection Equipment Selection and Procurement, as part of the respiratory protection equipment selection committee. Leadership of the respiratory protection program committee must be assigned to one person, usually the health and safety officer. The committee must establish its goals and objectives, meeting schedule, and program development process within the mandate of the administration. A committee secretary must be appointed to take accurate notes and maintain the group's records.

Safety and Regulatory Requirements

When developing a respiratory protection program, the primary responsibilities should always be addressing personal safety and meeting or exceeding regulatory requirements. Regulatory requirements, which were covered in depth in Chapter 2, Regulations and Standards, depend on the local, state/provincial, and federal laws that govern the fire and emergency services in that jurisdiction. Safety re-

quirements are based on the types of hazards faced by an organization. These hazards are determined by a hazard or risk assessment of the tasks performed by the organization and potential hazards found in the area the organization serves. For instance, an emergency services organization that provides only basic or advanced life support for a residential community may only require a program that includes respiratory protection against airborne pathogens. If that organization does not provide hazardous materials protection to the area, it may not need supplied-air-type respiratory protection. In any event, the hazard or risk assessment must be thorough and accurate, listing all potential hazards and tasks.

Limited-Resource Organizations

It must be recognized that some organizations lack the resources necessary for a comprehensive respiratory protection program. Organizations with limited resources must develop a program that has attainable goals and deadlines and falls within the scope and ability of the organization. A program that is too large can overstress resources such as time, finances, and personnel (**Figure 3.3**). This stress will result in failure by the organization to fully implement the basic requirements of the program and a loss of credibility among the employees, governing body, and community. Time required for

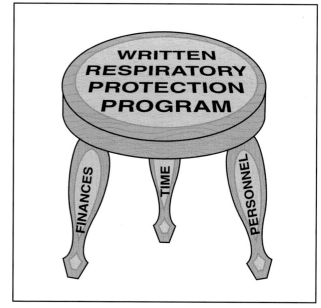

Figure 3.3 The respiratory protection program requires a commitment of time, finances, and personnel.

training, equipment maintenance, and reevaluation of the program and the financial commitment of the following items must be considered:

- Initial purchase
- Parts and maintenance
- Replacement costs
- Training costs
- Medical evaluation costs
- Facepiece fit-testing costs

Data collection and analysis costs must be fully understood by the organization, government, and community. The scope of the organization is usually found in the charter that created the organization or the organization's mission statement. By attempting to meet only the mandated tasks of the organization, the respiratory protection program committee can use its time better and remain close to or within the financial constraints of the budget (**Figure 3.4**).

To implement a respiratory protection program, the committee may have to go beyond its traditional funding source for support. The committee should research the availability of funding in order to recommend funding sources to the administration. Other sources include but are not confined to the following:

- Federal grants
- State/provincial grants
- Capital bond issues
- Special sales taxes
- Private grants
- Insurance funds

The committee should also be aware of other government agencies that can provide equipment, training, or support of a respiratory protection program. Equipment may be acquired through state/provincial or federal donations or low-cost purchases. For many years the U.S. Department of the Interior has provided rural departments with wildland fire fighting equipment through the Forestry Department. Rural fire protection districts established by the individual states or provinces also help to fund or equip volunteer emergency services organizations. State/provincial and national training programs can help reduce local training costs through state/provincial academies or regional training programs. Universities may also provide training programs and even training facilities for an organization's use (**Figure 3.5**). The committee should make every attempt to locate potential government support from the appropriate agencies. Research may be done through the National Fire Academy, through the local library system, or on the Internet. In addition, state/provincial fire commission or fire marshal offices and insurance offices may have information on available grants and programs.

RESPIRATORY PROTECTION PROGRAM

COSTS	FUNDING SOURCE
Initial Purchase	Federal Grants
Parts and Maintenance	State/Provincial Grants
Replacement Costs	Capital Bonds
Training Costs	Special Sales Tax
Medical Evaluation Costs	Private Grants
Fit Testing Costs	Other Sources
Data Collection and Analysis Costs	

Figure 3.4 Multiple costs are associated with the respiratory protection program.

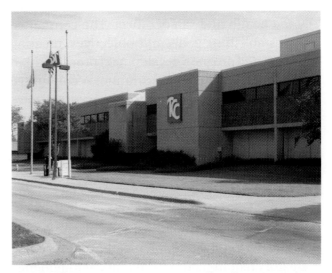

Figure 3.5 Fire protection programs offered at community colleges such as this one can be valuable sources for developing and implementing a respiratory protection program.

Written Policies and Procedures

[NFPA 1500: 7.9.1, 7.9.2, 7.9.3]
[NFPA 1404: 5.1.2]

The respiratory protection program must be in written form and always accessible to members of the organization. Small departments may choose to provide copies to all members while larger organizations may place single copies in stations and other facilities. As regulations, standards, and federal guidelines change, the respiratory protection program must continuously adapt. An example of a written respiratory protection program may be found in Appendix B, Respiratory Protection Program Sample.

Basic to a written policies and procedures manual is the hazard assessment for the organization. This assessment is the justification for the level of protection outlined in the respiratory protection program. It defines each hazard that an organization is likely to encounter and the type of respiratory protection required to protect employees.

The basic components of the program are equipment/use criteria, medical requirements, facepiece fit testing, training requirements, inspection/maintenance, cylinder air specifications, and program support/evaluation. They should be well organized and easily accessed within the program document.

Equipment/Use Criteria

Included in the program manual is a list of the types of equipment in use by the organization and the criteria for their use. This list would include all self-contained breathing apparatus (SCBA), supplied-air respirators (SARs), air-purifying respirators (APRs), and particle masks and the specific hazards they are designed to address. A hypothetical example of a use criteria based on NFPA 1500 might be as follows:

> Respiratory protection shall be worn when personnel might encounter atmospheres that are immediately dangerous to life or health (IDLH), when atmospheres are unknown, or when atmospheres are likely to be oxygen deficient.

More specifically, the criteria may include requirements for wearing respiratory protection when involved in salvage and overhaul operations, confined-space operations, or medical emergencies.

Medical Requirements

Medical requirements for personnel using respiratory protection must also be included in the written policy. NFPA and OSHA both require that all personnel who use respirators must have a medical evaluation. General guidelines for these evaluations can be found in NFPA 1582, *Standard on Medical Requirements for Fire Fighters*. The initial medical evaluation, which usually takes place when an individual is hired, provides a baseline for all future evaluations (**Figure 3.6**). Thereafter, annual evaluations are performed on each employee. It must be remembered that an employee's medical records are confidential, and the organization's physician may only release a pass/fail result of the pulmonary test.

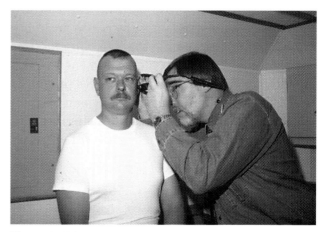

Figure 3.6 Fire and emergency services personnel must undergo both initial and periodic medical evaluations and examinations to participate in the respiratory protection program.

Facepiece Fit Testing

In order to ensure a proper seal for the respirator facepiece, fit testing of each wearer must take place (**Figure 3.7**). The written policy and procedures manual must contain the facepiece fit-testing procedures used by the organization and the requirements for periodic retesting. Restrictions on the wearing of facial hair (long sideburns, bushy mustaches, or beards) and the conditions for

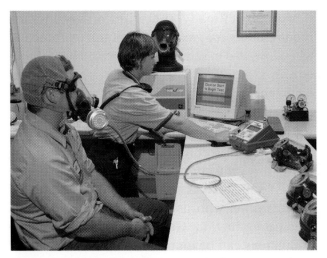

Figure 3.7 All personnel who are required to wear respiratory protection must be fit tested for each type of facepiece used by the organization.

wearing eyeglasses with the facepiece must be included in the policy. Proper fit testing is an essential part of the respiratory protection program and must be emphasized in the manual.

Training Requirements

The program must also outline the training requirements for respiratory protection, including training in the care, storage, inspection, maintenance, and use of the equipment. Training should include classroom theory, skills training in donning and doffing and inspecting and cleaning the equipment, and live operational fire training evolutions. A schedule for recertification should also be defined (**Figure 3.8**).

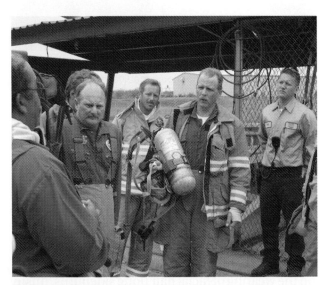

Figure 3.8 Respiratory protection equipment training includes both classroom theory and skills training.

Inspection/Maintenance

Criteria for respirator equipment inspection must also be established in the written policy and procedures manual. Inspections by company personnel should occur daily and after each use of the equipment. Annual inspections by qualified personnel must also be defined. The manual should include the inspection procedures, cleaning procedures, and criteria for placing a unit out of service.

Maintenance procedures must also be part of the manual. Company personnel should be provided with guidelines for the type of maintenance that they may perform on a unit based on the manufacturer's recommendations. Qualified personnel must perform all other maintenance. The manufacturer or vendor for a specific respiratory system usually provides certification for respiratory protection equipment maintenance technicians. The certification is tied to manufacturer-provided training programs (**Figure 3.9**).

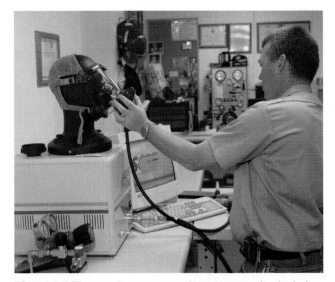

Figure 3.9 The respiratory protection program also includes the requirement for a maintenance program based on the manufacturer's recommendations. Factory-trained and certified technicians repair and test the organization's respiratory protection equipment.

Cylinder Air Specifications

The organization's respiratory protection program should include specifications for cylinder air quality, air testing, air storage, air-transfer protocol, and air transportation. The air source may be an organization-owned breathing air compressor or cascade system, in which case operating procedures and responsibility for the system must be clearly

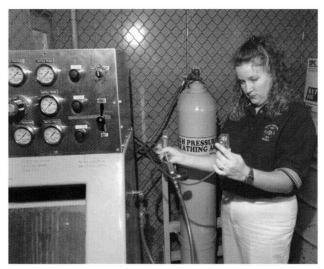

Figure 3.10 All breathing air, purchased from a vendor or produced by the organization, must be tested for purity by an independent laboratory. The health and safety officer is responsible for taking the test samples and submitting them to the lab for analysis.

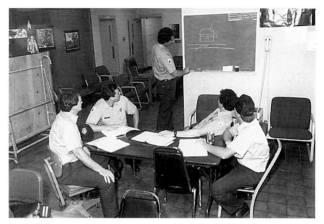

Figure 3.11 Periodic evaluation of the respiratory protection program can be the result of postincident critiques and analyses.

defined. An alternate source for breathing air may be an outside contractor or other governmental agency. Procedures for replenishing air cylinders must be provided. This section of the manual also describes how to fill individual air cylinders, regardless of the source of the breathing air. Finally, the air-quality testing procedures must be provided, including the time schedule, who is responsible for drawing the air samples, and who performs the testing (**Figure 3.10**).

Program Support/Evaluation

The procedures necessary for supporting the program must be well documented. This documentation includes the source and method for replacing the breathing air, replacement cartridges, or canisters and the process for replacing single-use masks and filters. In addition, disposal of contaminated masks, filters, cartridges, and canisters should also be defined. The criteria for end-of-service life for capital items such as SCBA and SAR units should also be included in the manual. The purchasing department of the authority having jurisdiction may mandate disposal of these types of capital items. The potential for liability for product failure of the units must also be taken into consideration when the units are sold or donated to other users.

The respiratory protection program must be able to conform to the changing needs of the organization. Therefore, the program must be evaluated periodically. The evaluation can be done monthly through a quality assurance evaluation performed by the administration. It can also occur during postincident critiques following a major incident or an incident where deficiencies in the program become apparent (**Figure 3.11**). In no case should the program operate longer than 1 year without an evaluation.

Summary

The elements of a respiratory protection program are essential in preventing immediate or chronic injuries to emergency services personnel. Furthermore, they allow emergency responders to be more effective in the performance of their duties. On the other hand, failure of the respiratory protection program can have tragic and long-lasting consequences to both the victims of incidents and emergency responders.

Safety and Risk Management

This chapter provides information that will assist the reader in meeting the following job performance requirements from NFPA 1404, *Standard for Fire Service Respiratory Protection Training*, 2002 Edition; NFPA 1852, *Standard on Selection, Care, and Maintenance of Open-Circuit Self-Contained Breathing Apparatus*, 2002 Edition; and NFPA 1500, *Standard on Fire Department Occupational Safety and Health Program*, 2002 Edition.

NFPA 1500

3.3.38   Incident Safety Officer. An individual appointed to respond or assigned at an incident scene by the incident commander to perform the duties and responsibilities of that position as part of the command staff.

4.2.1   The fire department shall develop and adopt a comprehensive written risk management plan.

4.2.2   The risk management plan shall at least cover the risks associated with the following:

(1) Administration

(2) Facilities

(3) Training

(4) Vehicle operations, both emergency and non-emergency

(5) Protective clothing and equipment

(6) Operations at emergency incidents

(7) Operations at non-emergency incidents

(8) Other related activities

4.2.3   The risk management plan shall include at least the following components:

(1) *Risk Identification.* Actual and potential hazards

(2) *Risk Evaluation.* Likelihood of occurrence of a given hazard and severity of its consequences

(3) *Risk Control Techniques.* Solutions for elimination or mitigation of potential hazards; implementation of best solution

(4) *Risk Management Monitoring.* Evaluation of effectiveness of risk control techniques

4.5.1   An occupational safety and health committee shall be established and shall serve in an advisory capacity to the fire chief.

4.5.1.1   The committee shall include the following members:

(1) The designated fire department health and safety officer

(2) Representatives of fire department management

(3) Individual members or representatives of member organizations

4.5.1.2   The committee shall also be permitted to include other persons.

4.5.1.3   Representatives of member organizations shall be selected by their respective organizations, but other committee members shall be appointed to the committee by the fire chief.

4.6.4   The fire department shall maintain training records for each member indicating dates, subjects covered, satisfactory completion, and, if any, certifications achieved.

4.7.2   The health and safety officer shall be involved in the development, implementation, and management of the written risk management plan.

4.7.3   The health and safety officer shall communicate the health and safety aspects of the risk management plan to all members through training and education.

4.7.4   The health and safety officer shall make available the written risk management plan to all fire department members.

4.7.5   The health and safety officer shall monitor the effectiveness of the risk management plan and shall ensure the risk management plan is revised annually as it relates to fire fighter health and safety.

4.7.6   The health and safety officer shall develop an incident risk management plan that is implemented into the fire department's incident management system for incident scene operations as required in Section 8.2 of this standard.

4.9.3   The health and safety officer shall cause safety supervision to be provided for training activities, including all live burn exercises.

4.9.4   All structural live burn exercises shall be conducted in accordance with NFPA 1403, *Standard on Live Fire Training Evolutions*.

4.9.5   The health and safety officer or qualified designee shall be personally involved in pre-burn inspections of any acquired structures to be utilized for live fire training.

4.11.2   The health and safety officer shall investigate, or cause to be investigated, all occupational injuries, illnesses, exposures, and fatalities, or other potentially hazardous conditions involving fire department members and all accidents involving fire department vehicles, fire apparatus, equipment, or fire department facilities.

4.11.3   The health and safety officer shall develop corrective recommendations that result from accident investigations.

4.11.4   The health and safety officer shall submit such corrective recommendations to the fire chief or the fire chief's designated representative.

4.11.5   The health and safety officer shall develop accident and injury reporting and investigation procedures and shall periodically review these procedures for revision.

4.11.5.1 These accident and injury reporting procedures shall comply with all local, state, and federal requirements.

4.11.6 The health and safety officer shall review the procedures employed during any unusually hazardous operation. Wherever it is determined that incorrect or questionable procedures were employed, the health and safety officer shall submit corrective recommendations to the fire chief or the fire chief's designated representative.

4.12.3 The health and safety officer shall identify and analyze safety and health hazards and shall develop corrective actions to deal with these hazards.

4.12.4 The health and safety officer shall ensure that records on the following are maintained as specified in 4.4.5:

(1) Fire department safety and health standard operating procedures

(2) Periodic inspection and service testing of apparatus and equipment

(3) Periodic inspection and service testing of personal safety equipment

(4) Periodic inspection of fire department facilities

4.12.5 The health and safety officer shall maintain records of all recommendations made and actions taken to implement or correct safety and health hazards or unsafe practices.

4.12.6 The health and safety officer shall maintain records of all measures taken to implement safety and health procedures and accident prevention methods.

4.20.1 The health and safety officer shall develop procedures to ensure that safety and health issues are addressed during postincident analysis.

4.20.4 The health and safety officer shall include information about issues relating to the use of protective clothing and equipment, personnel accountability system, rehabilitation operations, and other issues affecting the safety and welfare of personnel at the incident scene.

7.9.1 The fire department shall adopt and maintain a respiratory protection program that addresses the selection, care, maintenance, and safe use of respiratory protection equipment, training in its use, and the assurance of air quality.

7.9.2 The fire department shall develop and maintain standard operating procedures that are compliant with this standard and that address the safe use of respiratory protection.

7.9.3 Members shall be tested and certified at least annually in the safe and proper use of respiratory protection equipment that they are authorized to use.

7.10.3 When a fire department compresses its own breathing air, the fire department shall be required to provide documentation that a sample of the breathing air obtained directly from the point of transfer from the filling system to the SCBA cylinder has been tested at least quarterly and that it is compliant with the requirements of 7.10.1 of this section.

7.10.4 When a fire department obtains compressed breathing air from a supplier and transfers it to other storage cylinders, cascade system cylinders, storage receivers, and other such storage equipment used for filling SCBA, the supplier shall be required to provide documentation that a sample of the breathing air obtained directly at the point of transfer from the filling system to the storage cylinders, cascade system cylinders, storage receivers, and other such storage equipment has been tested at least quarterly and that it is compliant with the requirements of 7.10.1 of this section.

7.10.5 The fire department shall obtain documentation that a sample of the breathing air obtained directly from the point of transfer from the storage cylinders, cascade system cylinders, storage receivers, and other such storage equipment to the SCBA cylinder has been tested at least quarterly and that it is compliant with the requirements of 7.10.1 of this section.

7.12.7 Nothing shall be allowed to enter or pass through the area where the respiratory protection facepiece is designed to seal with the face, regardless of the specific fitting test measurement that can be obtained.

7.12.8 Members who have a beard or facial hair at any point where the facepiece is designed to seal with the face or whose hair that could interfere with the operation of the unit shall not be permitted to use respiratory protection at emergency incidents or in hazardous or potentially hazardous atmospheres.

7.12.8.1 These restrictions shall apply regardless of the specific fitting test measurement that can be obtained under test conditions.

7.12.9 When a member must wear spectacles while using a full facepiece respiratory protection, the facepiece shall be fitted with spectacles in such a manner that it shall not interfere with the facepiece-to-face seal.

7.12.10 Spectacles with any strap or temple bars that pass through the facepiece-to-face seal area shall be prohibited.

7.12.11 Use of contact lenses shall be permitted during full facepiece respiratory protection use, provided that the member has previously demonstrated successful long-term contact lens use.

7.12.12 Any head covering that passes between the sealing surface of the respiratory protection facepiece and the member's face shall be prohibited.

7.12.13 The respiratory protection facepiece and head harness with straps shall be worn under the protective hoods.

7.12.14 The respiratory protection facepiece and head harness with straps shall be worn under the head protection of any hazardous chemical-protective clothing.

7.12.15 Helmets shall not interfere with the respiratory protection facepiece-to-face seal.

7.14.1 PASS devices shall meet the requirements of NFPA 1982, *Standard on Personal Alert Safety Systems (PASS)*.

7.14.2 Each member shall be provided with, use, and activate their PASS device in all of the following situations:

(1) Fire suppression

(2) Rescue

(3) Other hazardous duty

7.14.3 Each PASS device shall be tested at least weekly and prior to each use, and shall be maintained in accordance with the manufacturer's instructions.

8.1.6 As incidents escalate in size and complexity, the incident commander shall divide the incident into tactical-level management components and assign an incident safety officer to assess the incident scene for hazards or potential hazards.

8.1.9 The fire department shall establish and ensure the maintenance of a fire dispatch and incident communications system that meets the requirements of NFPA 1561, *Standard on Emergency Services Incident Management System*, and NFPA 1221, *Standard for the Installation, Maintenance, and Use of Emergency Services Communications Systems*.

8.1.10 The fire department standard operating procedures shall provide direction in the use of clear text radio messages for emergency incidents.

8.3.1 The fire department shall establish written standard operating procedures for a personnel accountability system that is in accordance with NFPA 1561, *Standard on Emergency Services Incident Management System*.

8.3.2 The fire department shall consider local conditions and characteristics in establishing the requirements of the personnel accountability system.

8.3.3 It shall be the responsibility of all members operating at an emergency incident to actively participate in the personnel accountability system.

8.3.4 The incident commander shall maintain an awareness of the location and function of all companies or crews at the scene of the incident.

8.3.5 Officers assigned the responsibility for a specific tactical level management component at an incident shall directly supervise and account for the companies and/or crews operating in their specific area of responsibility.

8.3.6 Company officers shall maintain an ongoing awareness of the location and condition of all company members.

8.3.7 Where assigned as a company, members shall be responsible to remain under the supervision of their assigned company officer.

8.3.8 Members shall be responsible for following personnel accountability system procedures.

8.3.9 The personnel accountability system shall be used at all incidents.

8.4.21 When members are performing special operations, the highest available level of emergency medical care shall be standing by at the scene with medical equipment and transportation capabilities. Basic life support shall be the minimum level of emergency medical care.

8.4.22 Emergency medical care and medical monitoring at hazardous materials incidents shall be provided by or supervised by personnel who meet the minimum requirements of NFPA 473, *Standard for Competencies for EMS Personnel Responding to Hazardous Materials Incidents*.

8.4.23 At all other emergency operations, the incident commander shall evaluate the risk to the members operating at the scene and, if necessary, request that at least basic life support personnel and patient transportation be available.

8.5.1 The fire department shall provide personnel for the rescue of members operating at emergency incidents.

8.5.2 A rapid intervention crew/company shall consist of at least two members and shall be available for rescue of a member or a crew.

8.5.2.1 Rapid intervention crews/company shall be fully equipped with the appropriate protective clothing, protective equipment, SCBA, and any specialized rescue equipment that could be needed given the specifics of the operation underway.

8.5.3 The composition and structure of a rapid intervention crew/company shall be permitted to be flexible based on the type of incident and the size and complexity of operations.

8.5.4 The incident commander shall evaluate the situation and the risks to operating crews and shall provide one or more rapid intervention crew/company commensurate with the needs of the situation.

8.5.5 In the early stages of an incident, which includes the deployment of a fire department's initial attack assignment, the rapid intervention crew/company shall be in compliance with 8.4.11 and 8.4.12 and be either one of the following:

(1) On-scene members designated and dedicated as rapid intervention crew/company

(2) On-scene members performing other functions but ready to re-deploy to perform rapid intervention crew/company functions

The assignment of any personnel shall not be permitted as members of the rapid intervention crew/company if abandoning their critical task(s) to perform rescue clearly jeopardizes the safety and health of any member operating at the incident.

8.5.6 As the incident expands in size or complexity, which includes an incident commander's requests for additional resources beyond a fire department's initial attack assignment, the dedicated rapid intervention crew/company shall upon arrival of these additional resources be either one of the following:

(1) On-scene members designated and dedicated as rapid intervention crew/company

(2) On-scene crew/company or crews/companies located for rapid deployment and dedicated as rapid intervention crews

During fire fighter rescue operations, each crew/company shall remain intact.

8.5.7 At least one dedicated rapid intervention crew/company shall be standing by with equipment to provide for the rescue of members that are performing special operations or for members that are in positions that present an immediate danger of injury in the event of equipment failure or collapse.

8.6.1 The fire department shall develop standard operating procedures that outline a systematic approach for the rehabilitation of members operating at incidents.

8.6.2 The incident commander shall consider the circumstances of each incident and initiate rest and rehabilitation in accordance with the standard operating procedures and with NFPA 1561, *Standard on Emergency Services Incident Management System.*

8.6.3 Such on-scene rehabilitation shall include at least basic life support care.

NFPA 1404

6.1.2 Records of all respiratory protection training shall be maintained, including training of personnel involved in maintenance of such equipment, in accordance with Section 4.3 of NFPA 1852 *Standard on Selection, Care, and Maintenance of Open-Circuit Self-Contained Breathing Apparatus.*

6.6.2 Fire department members shall be trained to handle problems related to the following situations that can be encountered during the use of respiratory protection equipment:

(1) Low temperatures

(2) High temperatures

(3) Rapid temperature changes

(4) Communications

(5) Confined spaces

(6) Vision

(7) Facepiece-to-face sealing problems

(8) Absorption through or irritation of the skin

(9) Effects of ionizing radiation on the skin and the entire body

(10) Punctured or ruptured eardrums

(11) Use near water

(12) Overhaul

6.8.1 Understanding the Components of a SAR. The training program of the authority having jurisdiction shall evaluate the ability of members to perform the following skills:

(1) Describe the air source, air hose limitations, and NIOSH-approved inlet pressure gauge range

(2) Identify the components of facepieces, regulators, harnesses, manifold system, and cylinders or compressors used by the authority having jurisdiction

(3) Describe the operation of the SAR used by the authority having jurisdiction

(4) Describe the limitations of the escape cylinder

(5) Describe the potential incompatibility of different makes and models of SAR units

(6) Describe proper procedures for inspection, cleaning, and storage of SAR units

6.8.2 Understanding the Safety Features and Limitations of a SAR. The training program of the authority having jurisdiction shall evaluate the ability of members to perform the following skills:

(1) Describe the operational principles of an emergency escape cylinder required on a SAR when used in IDLH atmospheres

(2) Identify the limitations of the SAR used by the authority having jurisdiction

(3) Describe the limitations of the SAR's ability to protect the body from absorption of toxins through the skin

(4) Describe the possible means of communications when wearing a SAR

(5) Describe the prohibition in using compressed oxygen with a SAR system

(6) Describe how to recognize medical signs and symptoms that could prevent the effective use of a SAR

7.2.1 Inspection, maintenance, and repair records shall be maintained for SAR units used in training as required in Chapter 4 of this standard.

7.3.1 Inspection, maintenance, and repair records for FFAPR use in training shall be maintained as required in Chapter 6 of this standard.

NFPA 1852

4.4.1 The organization shall create a written procedure to manage the record-keeping system.

4.4.2 The record-keeping system shall accommodate the documents listed in 4.4.8 and all additional documents that are needed after considering the following factors:

(1) The need for the record, report, or document

(2) How the record, report, or document will contribute to realizing the organization's goals within the selection, care, and maintenance program component

(3) The number of copies needed

(4) The person(s) responsible for producing the record, report, or document

(5) The format and substance of the record, report, or document

(6) The person(s) who will receive, forward, review, process, and use the record, report, or document

(7) The disposition of the record, report, or document after it has been completely developed

4.4.3 The organization shall consult with legal counsel concerning specific laws that determine the length of time records, reports, and documents shall be retained. Additionally, legal counsel shall advise the organization about the form, written or electronic, that is permitted and under what circumstances original or copied documents are needed for various purposes.

4.4.4 The organization shall determine how required records, reports, and documents will be created, processed, maintained, and stored. Regardless of the method selected, the organization shall take measures to prevent loss and damage.

4.4.5 The record-keeping system shall be managed by a person who is trained and qualified to ensure that information is obtained, collected, communicated, retrieved, used, and stored according to the plan. The record-keeping manager shall also consider how to reduce waste, redundancy, and cost in the system.

4.4.6 The manager of the record-keeping system shall educate and train personnel within the organization in completing, filing, and using various components of the record-keeping system. The manager shall be assisted by sufficient staff to fulfill his duties.

4.4.7 The manager of the record-keeping system shall conduct an annual inventory and audit of records, reports, and documents. Following the inventory and audit, the manager shall recommend changes in the record-keeping system as needed.

4.4.8 The organization shall create, maintain, and disseminate the following as required:

(1) Written instructions for care, maintenance, and repair that correspond to those provided by the manufacturer

(2) Written instructions for checks while donning SCBA

(3) Written instructions for inspection, including procedures to be followed if defects are found

(4) Forms to document the findings during inspection

(5) Forms to record and to report defects, found during inspection, and to track the SCBA or cylinder as it is repaired

(6) Forms to document inspections, tests, and repairs by SCBA users and technicians that shall include the following:
   a. SCBA make, model, and serial number and other information to identify components
   b. Documentation of the date, result of the inspection or test, and all actions taken as well as who acted

(7) Written instructions for filling and for testing cylinders

(8) Written policy and procedure concerning training and authorization of SCBA technicians as well as documentation of that training and authorization

(9) Written procedures for the inspection of cylinders by technicians

(10) Written procedures for recording information about the inspection and repair of cylinders

(11) Stickers, tags, or other similarly effective means to alert users and technicians to defects, to document inspections, and to certify that tests, repairs, and other actions have been completed

(12) Written procedures for periodic tests and comprehensive inspections that comply with the SCBA manufacturer's instructions

(13) Documentation of the tests to verify SCBA performance

(14) Schedule for retention, disposition, and disposal of each report, record, and document

(15) Methods of identifying all SCBAs, cylinders, parts, and components so that these can be identified and tracked from initial receipt by the organization until removed from the possession and control of the organization

(16) Documentation when a defective or obsolete SCBA or component part is removed from service in accordance with the following:
   a. Until retirement and disposal of a defective or obsolete SCBA or component as specified in 4.6.3, a tag shall be conspicuously placed on the SCBA or component.
   b. The tag shall indicate the date and time the SCBA or component was removed from service, by whom, and for what reason.
   c. SCBA and components that are removed from service shall be stored separately from other SCBA and components and secured, as necessary.
   d. Access to tagged SCBA and components shall be limited, and only authorized persons shall remove tags after repair or service.

(17) Records for maintenance of each individual SCBA regulator, reducer, harness, cylinder including valve assembly, and facepiece including the following information:
   a. The manufacturer's serial number or other unique identifier
   b. Date of manufacture, receipt, service, inspection, test, maintenance, and repair
   c. Inspections, service, repairs, and tests
   d. Who performed the work
   e. Other comments

(18) Records of training provided to each user showing date(s) and subject(s) covered

(19) Such other reports, records, and documents including forms, tags, stickers, and other means necessary to effectuate the purposes of record keeping and the intent of this standard.

4.5.1 When issuing new SCBA, the organization shall provide users with the instructions provided by the manufacturer on the care, use, and maintenance of their SCBA, including any warnings provided by the manufacturer.

4.5.2 Where the manufacturer's instructions regarding the care, use, and maintenance of their SCBA differ from the requirements in this standard, the manufacturer's instructions shall be followed.

Reprinted with permission from NFPA 1404, *Standard for Fire Service Respiratory Protection Training;* NFPA 1852, *Standard on Selection, Care, and Maintenance of Open-Circuit Self-Contained Breathing Apparatus;* and NFPA 1500, *Standard on Fire Department Occupational Safety and Health Program,* Copyright © 2002, National Fire Protection Association, Quincy, MA 02269. This reprinted material is not the complete and official position of the National Fire Protection Association on the referenced subject, which is represented only by the standard in its entirety.

Chapter 4
Safety and Risk Management

The primary concern of the respiratory protection program that is required by NFPA 1500, *Standard on Fire Department Occupational Safety and Health Program*, is to ensure a safe working environment for firefighters/emergency responders. The program addresses the selection, inspection, safe use, maintenance, and training in the use of all respiratory protection equipment. It further requires air-quality testing for the breathing air used by the department/emergency organization. To attain the NFPA recommended level of safety, the fire and emergency services provider must be aware of general safety issues, product warnings, and common safety problems associated with the use of respiratory protection equipment. The use of the risk management model is an effective, efficient, and thorough approach to defining the problems and selecting the appropriate solutions for them. This chapter looks at some of the safety issues related to respiratory protection, reviews the risk management model and its implementation, and outlines the incident safety officer's responsibilities in the respiratory protection process during emergency scene use.

Respiratory Protection Safety Issues

To understand the general safety issues that face a fire and emergency services provider, the officer or committee responsible for the respiratory protection program must know the hazards the organization deals with on a daily basis during emergency operations and in training exercises. This section addresses various concerns such as selecting a respirator based on the type of hazard, safety during training exercises, manufacturers' and government safety warnings, common respirator equipment problems, and emergency scene safety.

Respirator Choice Based on Hazard

Hazards can be determined through a hazards or risk analysis based on the duties that are assigned to the department/organization. The duties and hazards or risks that a fire and emergency services provider usually encounters may include the following:

- Structural fire fighting (**Figure 4.1**)
  — Oxygen-deficient atmospheres
  — Carbon monoxide
  — Unburned products of combustion
  — Toxic gases

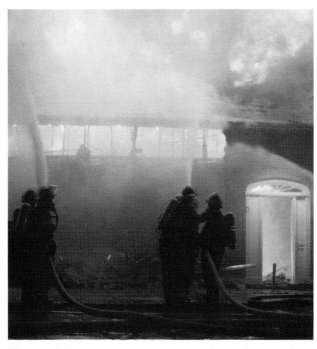

Figure 4.1 Fires in structures create respiratory hazards that include carbon monoxide, unburned products of combustion, toxic gases, and potentially oxygen-deficient atmospheres as well as extreme levels of heat. *Courtesy of Chris Mickal.*

- Medical responses (**Figure 4.2**)
  — Bloodborne and airborne pathogens
  — Hepatitis
  — Tuberculosis
  — Viral diseases
- Hazardous materials operations (**Figure 4.3**)
  — Toxic gases
  — Oxygen-deficient atmospheres
  — Radioactive materials
  — Airborne pathogens
  — Chemical vapors or smoke
- Confined-space operations and structural collapse (**Figure 4.4**)
  — Oxygen-deficient atmospheres
  — Toxic gases
  — Carbon monoxide
  — Airborne particulates
- Trench collapse and excavation operations
  — Oxygen deficiency
  — Toxic organic gases

When the hazards or risk analysis is complete, the department/organization can then determine the type and level of respiratory protection required to protect personnel. It should be recognized that

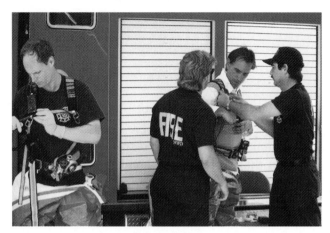

Figure 4.3 Before entering the hot zone, hazardous materials responders must fully inspect respiratory and personal protective equipment. *Courtesy of Chris Mickal.*

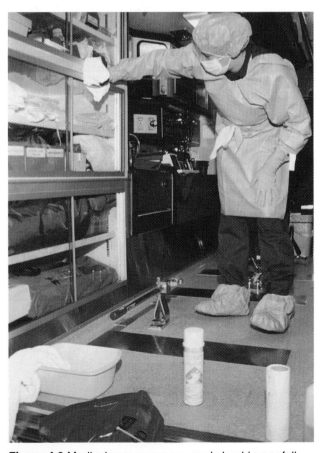

Figure 4.2 Medical response personnel should wear full protective clothing including respiratory protection while decontaminating apparatus and equipment. *Courtesy of Mike Nixon.*

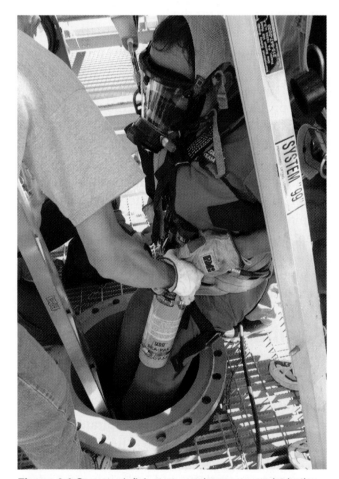

Figure 4.4 Oxygen-deficient atmospheres may exist both above and below ground levels. Fire and emergency services personnel must wear supplied-air apparatus (SAR) equipped with emergency breathing support systems (EBSSs) when entering such spaces.

while one type may provide protection against all the hazards, its use may be inappropriate in certain situations. For instance, self-contained breathing apparatus (SCBA) provides the maximum protection in all cases. Confined-space operations may require the use of a supplied-air regulator (SAR) instead of an SCBA due to the restricted nature of the workspace. Therefore, the department/organization has to investigate the various types of equipment available and the risks they are certified to protect against.

One model that may be of use is the *NIOSH Respirator Decision Logic* publication. This document walks the reader through the steps necessary to determine the appropriate type of protection based on the hazard that is encountered. It is available from the National Institute for Occupational Safety and Health (NIOSH) or Centers for Disease Control (CDC). An example of the NIOSH process is provided in flow-chart form in Appendix C, NIOSH Decision Logic Flow Chart.

Training Safety

[NFPA 1500: 4.9.3, 4.9.4, 4.9.5]

In order to prepare fire and emergency services personnel for the duties they will be performing and the hazards and risks they will face, training must be as realistic as possible. Requirements for respiratory protection training are given in NFPA 1404, *Standard for Fire Service Respiratory Protection Training*, and include the following topics:

• Respiratory protection program understanding

• Responsibilities of the user and provider

• Respiratory protection hazard recognition

• Appropriate respiratory protection selection

• Use, care, and maintenance of the respiratory protection equipment **(Figure 4.5)**

• Training evolutions that involve live fires, simulated hazardous materials incidents, confined-space operations, and emergency medical service (EMS) operations

Repetition in the use of respiratory protection equipment increases proficiency and develops muscle memory that ensures the safe use of the equipment. However, training in the use of respiratory protection equipment must also be accomplished with safety in mind. NFPA 1403, *Standard on Live Fire Training Evolutions,* and NFPA 1500 require that the health and safety officer or an incident safety officer be present during all live fire training **(Figure 4.6)**. The presence of a safety officer ensures that safe procedures are followed during the training activities.

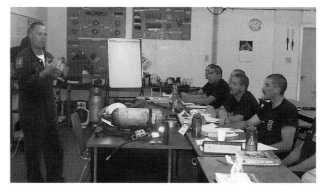

Figure 4.5 An essential part of the respiratory protection program is training personnel in the proper care, cleaning, maintenance, and use of respiratory protection equipment. *Courtesy of Lloyd Lees.*

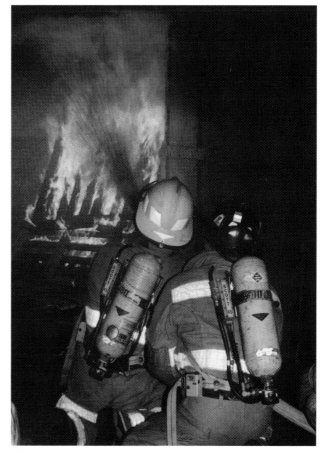

Figure 4.6 Respiratory protection hazards even exist during training exercises. The presence of a safety officer during live-fire training is a requirement of NFPA 1500 and NFPA 1403. *Courtesy of Joe Marino.*

Safety Warnings

[NFPA 1852: 4.5.1, 4.5.2]

The respiratory protection program should include a process for gathering, analyzing, and disseminating product warnings. Two sources for product warnings are NIOSH and the manufacturer of the respiratory protection product.

NIOSH Warnings

As mentioned in Chapter 2, Regulations and Standards, NIOSH is responsible for collecting, analyzing, and publishing information about injuries, illnesses, and fatalities in the workplace. NIOSH investigates an incident, determines the cause of the injury or illness or fatality, specifies any safety violations, and then recommends alterations in procedures or changes in equipment. The review of the incident is published with the NIOSH recommendations. If an incident is due to the malfunction of a specific piece of equipment, the manufacturer is notified. A warning is issued relating to the potential safety hazard posed by the specific piece of equipment. See Appendix D, NIOSH Incident Report and Product Warning, for an example. Warnings are also posted on the NIOSH Internet website at www.cdc.gov/niosh.

Manufacturers' Warnings

Because of the potential for legal actions due to equipment malfunction, manufacturers are particularly sensitive to incidents involving their equipment. The respiratory protection equipment manufacturer may become aware of potential safety problems through NIOSH investigations, user complaints, or internal quality control testing. Once aware of a potential safety problem, a manufacturer issues a safety warning or a product recall. Depending on the severity of the problem, the safety warning may require that the product be restricted in its use, removed from service, or tested to determine if a similar problem exists with the specific unit. Because of the strict testing and certification process by NIOSH and the Mine Safety and Health Administration (MSHA), total respiratory protection system recalls (particularly SCBA units) are rare. However, the fire and emergency services must be prepared for such an occurrence when dealing with any form of respiratory protection and understand that manufacturers' warnings must be complied with. Appendix E, Sample Manufacturer's Warning, contains a sample of a manufacturer's product warning.

Common Respiratory Equipment Safety Concerns

Specific safety concerns for each type of respiratory protection equipment used by the fire and emergency services include procurement, usage, maintenance, storage, cleaning, and disposal. These concerns are addressed in detail later in this manual. Common respiratory protection equipment concerns include facepiece seal and interface, SCBA and personal protective equipment (PPE) interface, supplied-air respirator requirements, and other general equipment concerns.

Facepiece Seal and Interface

[NFPA 1500: 7.12.7, 7.12.8, 7.12.8.1, 7.12.9, 7.12.10, 7.12.11]

In order to provide complete respiratory protection, the breathing air atmosphere must be pure and free of toxins. To provide this level of protection, the facepiece seal to the face must be complete and tight. Design, specification, fit testing, education, and training can ensure that the facepiece seals properly and interfaces with the rest of the ensemble. Any obstructions, including facial hair and eyeglasses, that prevent a complete seal and allow leakage must be eliminated (**Figure 4.7**).

Facial hair. NFPA 1500 expressly prohibits beards, long sideburns, or other facial hair that would interfere with the facepiece seal or the operation of the unit. This restriction is based on a 1990 ruling by the Occupational Safety and Health Administration (OSHA), which stated that anything that interferes with the facepiece seal is in violation of Title 29 (Labor) *CFR* 1910.134 (Respiratory Protection) (g)(1)(i) (Facepiece seal protection) (**Figure 4.8**).

Eyeglasses and contact lenses. The use of eyeglasses while wearing a facepiece is prohibited unless the glasses are specifically designed to mount inside the facepiece without the use of ear temple bars or straps that might break the seal. NFPA 1500, OSHA 29 *CFR* 1910.134, and various state depart-

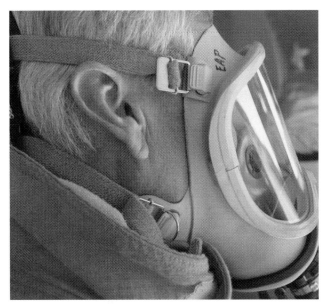

Figure 4.7 A complete seal between the face and facepiece ensures that leakage of toxins or smoke into the respiratory system will not occur.

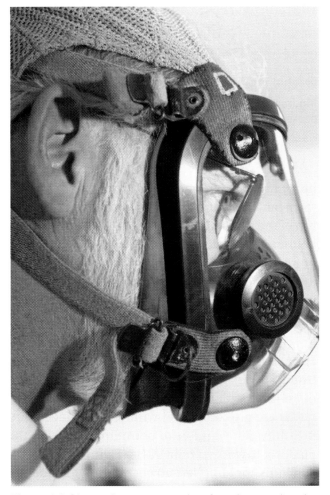

Figure 4.8 Obstructions to a complete facepiece seal such as facial hair and eyeglass frames are prohibited by both NFPA standards and OSHA regulations. *Courtesy of Maura Casey.*

ments of labor permit the wearing of contact lenses with the facepiece as long as the wearer has demonstrated that the lenses can be safely worn for long periods of time (**Figure 4.9**).

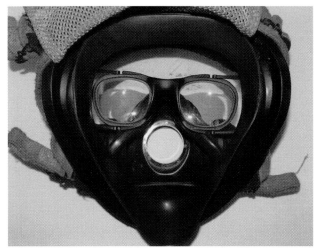

Figure 4.9 Easily installed eyeglass frame kits are provided by respiratory protection facepiece manufacturers. *Courtesy of Kenneth Baum.*

SCBA/PPE Interface
[NFPA 1500: 7.12.12, 7.12.13, 7.12.14, 7.12.15]

Respiratory protection equipment is used as part of the total personal protective ensemble including the protective hood, coat, pants, boots, gloves, and helmet. Alterations to any of this equipment, including the attachment of tools, removal of required labels, or unauthorized repairs, are prohibited. Parts of the personal protective clothing ensemble may also interfere with the facepiece and its seal.

Protective hood interface. NFPA 1500 stipulates that facepiece and head harness straps be worn in direct contact with the head to ensure a proper fit. If a protective hood is worn, it must be worn over the head harness and dressed over the facepiece seal. The interface between the protective hood and facepiece must be complete to prevent exposure of unprotected skin. If a protective hood has a loose face opening due to wear, it should be replaced (**Figure 4.10**).

PPE clothing interface. Self-contained breathing apparatus and supplied-air respirators interface with the personal protective clothing in other parts of the ensemble also. Backpacks, shoulder harnesses, and waist belts create

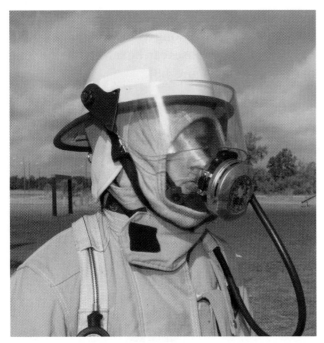

Figure 4.10 The protective hood is worn outside the facepiece seal and is tucked into the coat collar to provide complete protection to the face, head, and neck of the wearer. *Courtesy of Bob Parker.*

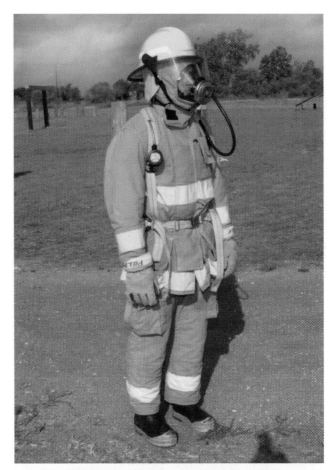

Figure 4.11 To prevent movement of the air cylinder backpack, the shoulder straps must be pulled snug to the shoulders and the waist strap fastened in place. *Courtesy of Bob Parker.*

compression points in the turnout coat that reduce its thermal protection and can contribute to injuries. This effect must be taken into consideration when specifying both protective clothing and respiratory protection units. Additionally, the waist strap of the SCBA must be secured when in use (**Figure 4.11**). Respiratory protection training and education must emphasize the importance of securing the waist belt and pulling the shoulder harness tight. However, it may be necessary to specify longer waist straps for personnel who are larger-than-average sizes.

Helmet interface. The helmet and facepiece interface is another point that may create problems. Due to the variety of facepiece and helmet designs, it is unlikely that the two will fit together properly. Some manufacturers are building helmets and SCBA units that are designed to work together. The majority, however, do not. Two points of difficulty are the forehead area and the back of the head. When wearing the facepiece, it is often necessary to have the helmet pushed back on the head at a slight angle. The helmet will not have a tight fit and give the intended protection from falling debris. The helmet may also be prone to being knocked off a wearer's head. Therefore, the helmet chin strap must

be secured under the wearer's chin. At the back of the head, the rear bill of the helmet may strike the top of the air cylinder, which may also dislodge the helmet. The wearer must be aware of these two points of contact and prepared to deal with them during emergency operations (**Figure 4.12**).

Supplied-Air Respirator Requirements
[NFPA 1404: 6.8.1, 6.8.2]

Supplied-air respirators are generally used for confined-space rescue operations and hazardous materials operations. However, some elevating platforms are also equipped with SARs connected to breathing air cylinders to permit personnel in the platform to work without SCBA (**Figure 4.13**). Safety concerns for supplied-air respirators include the same facepiece problems mentioned earlier plus additional requirements for hose length and protection, number of fittings/couplings, and emergency escape packs.

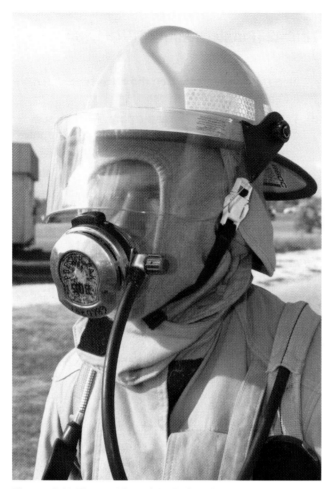

Figure 4.12 The position of the helmet has to be adjusted to properly cover the head while not affecting the facepiece seal. Earflaps and helmet shields are worn in the down position, and the chin strap is tightened under the facepiece. *Courtesy of Bob Parker.*

Hose length/protection. NIOSH specifies the maximum length of air-supply hose for SAR units based on the type of respirator. See sidebar on page 84 for descriptions of SAR types. The maximum hose lengths for three types are listed as follows:

- Type A supplied-air respirator: 300 feet (90 m)
- Type B supplied-air respirator: 75 feet (23 m)
- Type C supplied-air respirator: 300 feet (90 m)

Use of hose in excess of the specified length may result in injury to the user and nullify NIOSH/MSHA certification. Air-supply hoses must also be protected from mechanical, thermal, and chemical damage while in use. Protective sleeves made of Tyvek® high-density polyethylene material or PBI/Kevlar® polybenzimidazole/aramid fibers may be purchased from the manufacturer to protect the hose against damage. Personnel should be trained

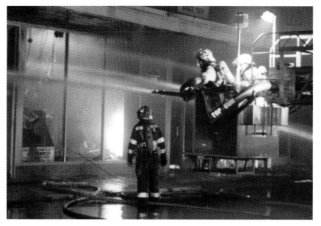

Figure 4.13 Respiratory protection equipment must be supplied to all personnel operating on aerial devices. Some elevating platforms are designed to provide air connections for supplied-air respirator (SAR) units or for quick filling of SCBA cylinders. *Courtesy of Bill Tompkins.*

in the proper procedures to follow in the event the air-supply hose becomes snagged or damaged (**Figure 4.14**).

Number of fittings/couplings. Follow the manufacturer's instructions regarding not only the length of air-supply hose but also the number of fittings or couplings in the hose. The number of fittings is restricted by the manufacturer because of the effect fittings have on airflow. The quantity of air at adequate pressure can be reduced by increased hose length and an excessive number of fittings. Refer to the manufacturer's instructions for the specific SAR brand and model.

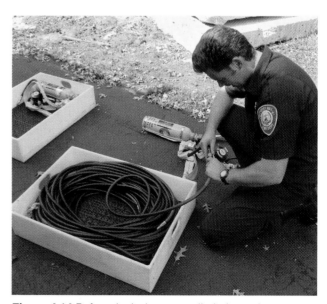

Figure 4.14 Before deploying a supplied-air respirator system, all hose, fittings, and connections must be inspected for damage or wear. *Courtesy of Kenneth Baum.*

Supplied-Air Respirator Descriptions from Title 42 (Public Health) *CFR* 84.130, Subpart J

Supplied-air respirators, including all completely assembled respirators designed for use as respiratory protection during entry into and escape from atmospheres not immediately dangerous to life or health, are described as follows:

(a) Type A supplied-air respirators. A hose mask respirator, for entry into and escape from atmospheres not immediately dangerous to life or health, consisting of a motor-driven or hand-operated blower that permits the free entrance of air when the blower is not operating, a strong large-diameter hose having a low resistance to airflow, a harness to which the hose and the lifeline are attached, and a tight-fitting facepiece

(b) Type AE supplied-air respirators. A Type A supplied-air respirator equipped with additional devices designed to protect the wearer's head and neck against impact and abrasion from rebounding abrasive material and with shielding material such as plastic, glass, woven wire, sheet metal, or other suitable material to protect the window(s) of facepieces, hoods, and helmets that do not unduly interfere with the wearer's vision and permit easy access to the external surface of such window(s) for cleaning

(c) Type B supplied-air respirators. A hose mask respirator for entry into and escape from atmospheres not immediately dangerous to life or health, consisting of a strong large-diameter hose with low resistance to airflow through which the user draws inspired air by means of the lungs alone, a harness to which the hose is attached, and a tight-fitting facepiece

(d) Type BE supplied-air respirators. A type B supplied-air respirator equipped with additional devices designed to protect the wearer's head and neck against impact and abrasion from rebounding abrasive material and with shielding material such as plastic, glass, woven wire, sheet metal, or other suitable material to protect the window(s) of facepieces, hoods, and helmets that do not unduly interfere with the wearer's vision and permit easy access to the external surface of such window(s) for cleaning

(e) Type C supplied-air respirators. An airline respirator for entry into and escape from atmospheres not immediately dangerous to life or health, consisting of a source of respirable breathing air, a hose, a detachable coupling, a control valve, orifice, a demand valve or pressure demand valve, an arrangement for attaching the hose to the wearer, and a facepiece, hood, or helmet

(f) Type CE supplied-air respirators. A type C supplied-air respirator equipped with additional devices designed to protect the wearer's head and neck against impact and abrasion from rebounding abrasive material and with shielding material such as plastic, glass, woven wire, sheet metal, or other suitable material to protect the window(s) of facepieces, hoods, and helmets that do not unduly interfere with the wearer's vision and permit easy access to the external surface of such window(s) for cleaning

Emergency escape packs. OSHA regulations require the wearing of an emergency escape pack or emergency breathing support system (EBSS) with the SAR. The emergency escape packs provide between 3 and 60 minutes of air, depending on the design. These units provide a measure of safety in the event that the air supply is interrupted. The respiratory protection policy/program must include guidelines for use of escape packs and the proper escape procedures. Combination SCBA/SAR units are available that provide the benefits of both types of units (**Figure 4.15**). It must be remembered that air under pressure increases in temperature. Some SARs are provided with accessories for reducing the temperature of the breathing air at the regulator.

Other Respiratory Protection Equipment Safety Concerns

[NFPA 1404: 6.6.2]

Other areas of concern include the limitations of the respiratory protection equipment, exposure limits, escape times, and temperature extremes. These concerns should be taken into consideration when developing a respiratory protection program and when selecting types of respiratory protection for the organization. The limitations may be addressed in the selection process, through policy implementation, and through training.

Equipment limitations. Limitations inherent with respiratory protection equipment are as follows:

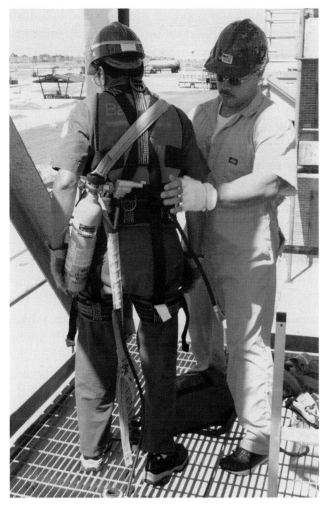

Figure 4.15 An emergency breathing support system (EBSS) is a small-capacity, lightweight air cylinder that provides a limited breathing air supply in the event that the SAR air supply is interrupted.

- *Limited visibility* — A facepiece reduces peripheral vision. Forward vision may be restricted by the design of some facepiece-mounted regulators. These issues can only be corrected by selecting a facepiece that provides a wide unobstructed area of vision and is made of nondistorting material. Other visibility factors are as follows:

  — Mechanical damage of the lens and dirt, filth, and grime on the lens can reduce overall vision. A maintenance policy and proper training in the care and cleaning of facepieces will correct this problem.

  — Fogging of the facepiece lens may also impair vision. Fogging is caused by the difference in temperatures between the inside and the outside of the facepiece. External fogging occurs when the outside air is moist, while internal fogging is caused by exhaled moist air in the facepiece. External fogging can be controlled by physically wiping the moisture off with the hand. Internal fogging can be controlled with the use of a properly fitted nose cup that deflects exhalation away from the lens or an antifogging chemical that is applied to the inside of the lens. The use of any antifogging material or device must follow the manufacturer's recommendations.

- *Decreased ability to communicate verbally* — The facepiece restricts the ability of the wearer to communicate verbally. This problem can be overcome with hand signals and physical touch when wearers are in close proximity. Bone microphones that contact the user's head, throat microphones that press against the side of the throat, or facepiece-mounted microphones can improve radio communications. These types of communications devices may not work to the satisfaction of the individual or organization. Voice amplification and radio interface devices that attach directly to the facepiece are also available (**Figure 4.16**). The respiratory protection equipment manufacturer can provide NIOSH-compliant devices for a specific facepiece. If none of these methods are available, personnel should be trained in the effective use of handheld radios while wearing facepieces.

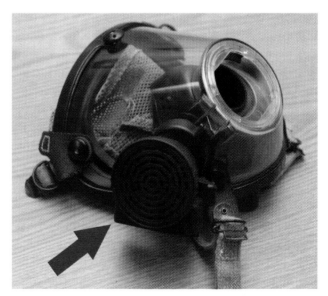

Figure 4.16 Voice amplification systems are provided for facepieces to improve communications while wearing respiratory protection equipment

- *Decreased mobility*—The weight of an SCBA and the splinting effect of the shoulder harness reduce user mobility. The facepiece can also restrict side-to-side and up-and-down head movement.

- *Increased weight* — An SCBA can add up to 35 pounds (16 kg) of additional weight to the firefighter/emergency responder and may increase the workload as much as 20 percent while also increasing the respiratory breathing and cardiovascular rates. The weight of the various types of units should be considered during the selection process. A physical fitness training program can improve the user's respiratory and cardiovascular systems and provide greater stamina while using respiratory protection equipment.

- *Air hose restrictions* — An SAR air-supply hose restricts the user's ability to move through mazelike areas. Wearers have to retrace their original paths when leaving the work area. The distance from the air source to the work area is also restricted to a maximum of 300 feet (90 m). Training helps to overcome some of the effects created by air-supply hoses.

Exposure limits. Fire and emergency services personnel should be aware of the exposure limits of hazardous materials, airborne diseases, and products of combustion. Exposure limits are the maximum lengths of time an individual can be exposed to an airborne substance before injury, illness, or death occurs. Through testing and research, NIOSH and OSHA have established specific permissible exposure limits for hazardous materials, biological diseases, and other substances. Permissible exposure limits (PELs) and materials and diseases that are immediately dangerous to life and health (IDLH) for which no PEL has been determined are addressed in detail in Chapter 1, Introduction to Respiratory Protection. In addition, the American Conference of Governmental Industrial Hygienists (ACGIH) has established threshold limit values (TLVs) that are published in *Threshold Limit Value and Biological Exposure Indices*.

Escape times. Escape time is based on the maximum exposure to a hazardous material, biological hazard, or oxygen-deficient atmosphere that an individual can experience without sustaining adverse effects to his or her health. Personnel who are working in an IDLH atmosphere must have a sufficient breathing air supply to escape the contaminated

area without endangering themselves. Maximum escape time has been set by NIOSH as 30 minutes. NIOSH requires that escape packs certified for use with SAR systems have a minimum operating capacity of 5 minutes. SCBAs must have an end-of-service alarm that activates when the air supply reaches 25 percent of the maximum-rated cylinder pressure. The escape time and minimum air supply required to meet that time are determined by the hazard that the wearer is exposed to.

Temperature extremes. Ambient temperatures can also have an effect on respiratory protection equipment. As indicated earlier, facepieces can fog when the outside temperature is lower than the air temperature inside the mask. Likewise, cold temperatures can cause the moisture inside the regulator of SCBA and SAR units to freeze, which causes the regulator to cease functioning. Respiratory protection equipment must be stored on the apparatus in such a way that moisture is not allowed to collect or form within the system (**Figure 4.17**).

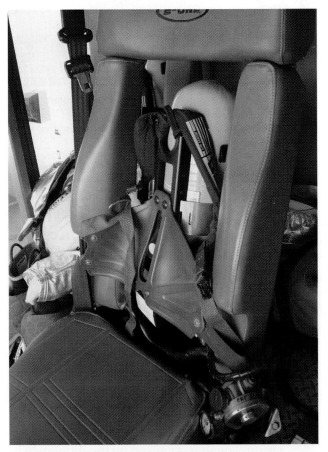

Figure 4.17 To prevent damage and exposure to the elements, SCBA must be properly stored on the apparatus. At the same time, the harness assembly must be easily accessible to provide rapid donning of the unit.

Emergency Scene Safety

During an incident, the incident commander (IC) has the ultimate responsibility for safety-related issues, one of which is respiratory protection. At a large incident, the safety function may be given to another chief officer, a trained company officer, the health and safety officer, another member of the safety office, a staff officer trained to perform this function, or a combination of these individuals (**Figure 4.18**). In small departments/organizations, the incident commander may find that he or she has to perform this function along with other duties. Beside the general role of the incident safety officer, some of the respiratory protection related functions include accountability, personal alert safety system device use, incident scene communications, rehabilitation, and rapid intervention crew supervision.

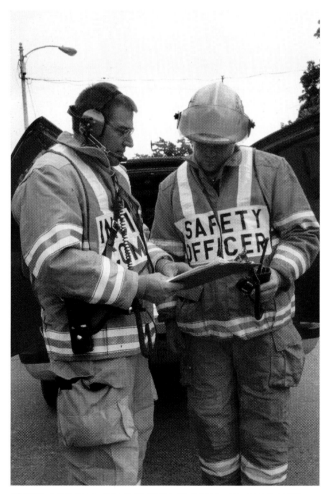

Figure 4.18 As a member of the incident command staff, the incident safety officer provides the incident commander with information on potential safety hazards that might affect responders.

Role of Incident Safety Officer
[NFPA 1500: 3.3.38, 8.1.6]

Regardless of the type of incident, the role of the incident safety officer must be defined in the fire and emergency services organization's written standard operating procedures (SOPs). NFPA 1521, *Standard for Fire Department Safety Officer*, outlines the role of the incident safety officer and is a good starting point for developing SOPs. Due to the increasing responsibilities of the health and safety officer, NFPA 1521 has separated the duties of the health and safety officer and the incident safety officer. While the health and safety officer is a permanent position responsible for the organization's safety and health program, the incident safety officer is only responsible for safety issues that arise during specific emergency scene operations. The separation of duties gives the administrations of fire departments/emergency services organizations the ability to assign this second function to other qualified personnel.

Statistics published in the November/December 1999 issue of the *NFPA Journal* indicate that more firefighters are killed and injured at incident scenes than during any other activity. Using an incident safety officer provides a means of focusing specifically on emergency scene safety while monitoring conditions, activities, and operations to determine whether appropriate risk management procedures are being followed. Through continual risk assessment, the incident safety officer evaluates and suggests effective tactics that provide a successful outcome of the incident while ensuring the safety of the members operating at the incident. Other duties of the incident safety officer are outlined in NFPA 1521, and the IFSTA **Fire Department Safety Officer** manual gives additional information on the duties and authorities of the incident safety officer and the health and safety officer.

Accountability
[NFPA 1500: 8.3.1, 8.3.2, 8.3.3, 8.3.4, 8.3.5, 8.3.6, 8.3.7, 8.3.8, 8.3.9]

The accountability system that tracks all personnel at the incident scene is essential to personnel safety. The IC or incident safety officer (when appointed) is responsible for ensuring that the system is in place and that all members comply with it. The

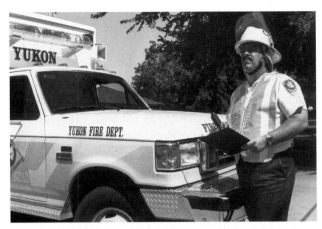

Figure 4.19 The incident safety officer may be assigned the duty of monitoring the accountability function at an incident.

incident safety officer must have the authority to enforce the use of the system and correct any violations. This authority may include altering tactical operations until all personnel are accounted for, but the incident safety officer always works through the IC when making any alterations (**Figure 4.19**).

Personal Alert Safety System Device Use

[NFPA 1500: 7.14.1, 7.14.2, 7.14.3]

The incident safety officer is responsible for ensuring that all personnel operating within the designated hot zone at an emergency incident scene are properly protected with personal protective equipment. The hot zone is part of the control system of barriers surrounding designated areas at emergency incident scenes that are intended to limit the number of persons exposed to the hazard and to facilitate mitigation. At a major incident, three zones are established: restricted (hot), limited access (warm), and support (cold). Protection in the hot zone includes the use and activation of personal alert safety system (PASS) devices. PASS devices must be activated anytime the wearer is working in an IDLH situation, including confined-space rescue and wildland operations (**Figure 4.20**).

Incident Scene Communications

[NFPA 1500: 8.1.9, 8.1.10]

Communications at an incident scene take many forms. The incident safety officer must be prepared to use the radio system and the approved clear-text message system. The incident safety officer is responsible for monitoring all radio traffic during the

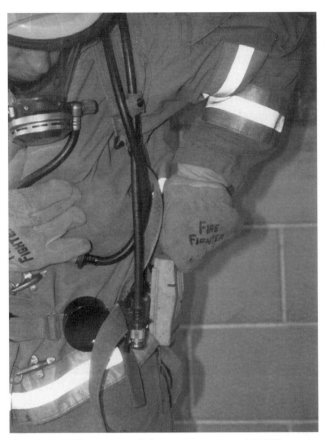

Figure 4.20 The personal alert safety system (PASS) must be tested and activated before entering the hot zone at any incident.

incident to listen for signs of duress and/or other significant information from members committed to the hot zone. When possible, face-to-face communication is the most effective because it reduces the possibility for misunderstandings, produces immediate responses, and adds the benefits of non-verbal aspects of communications: facial expressions, gestures, etc.

The incident safety officer provides both feedback and reports to the incident commander. Feedback occurs when questions are asked and responses are given. Feedback works best in face-to-face situations such as safety briefings but may also occur over the telecommunications system. Reports give assessments of the situation from other parts of the scene. They include the results of the incident safety officer's reconnaissance or 360-degree walk around the site, information on deployment of or need for additional resources, and lists of potential risks or hazards that may be encountered (**Figure 4.21**). This information must be precise and to the point.

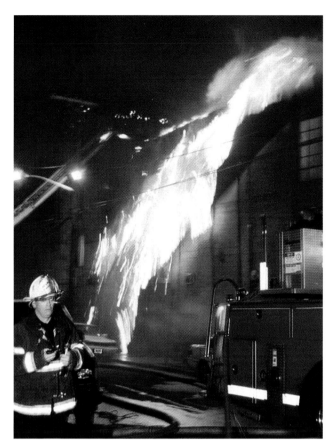

Figure 4.21 The incident safety officer must survey the perimeter of the incident and provide the incident commander with an accurate assessment of the developing situation. *Courtesy of Bill Tompkins.*

Rehabilitation

[NFPA 1500: 8.4.21, 8.4.22, 8.4.23, 8.6.1, 8.6.2, 8.6.3]

Emergency incident scene rehabilitation is just as important at a small incident as it is at a large one. The incident safety officer is responsible for monitoring the condition of all personnel at an incident and ensuring that they receive the level of rehabilitation necessary to protect their health. At a small incident, this rehabilitation may simply mean the replacement of fluids and a brief rest. At long-duration incidents, the incident safety officer may need to establish a rehabilitation section within the Incident management System (IMS) structure.

A rehabilitation site may include an ambulance and crew, apparatus equipped for rehabilitation, and area protected from the environment (wind, rain, or temperature extremes). Physiological monitoring of emergency personnel may be performed by the incident safety officer, health and safety officer, or trained emergency medical technicians

(**Figure 4.22**). Monitoring can include recording body temperatures, heart rates, or breathing rates. Some departments/organizations use the capacity time of one SCBA cylinder to determine the point when rehabilitation should occur. The incident safety officer shall ensure that personnel are certified to return to duty after rehabilitation. Personnel who cannot be certified for return to duty should be transported to the appropriate medical facility for further monitoring and evaluation. See the IFSTA/Brady *Emergency Incident Rehabilitation* book for more information.

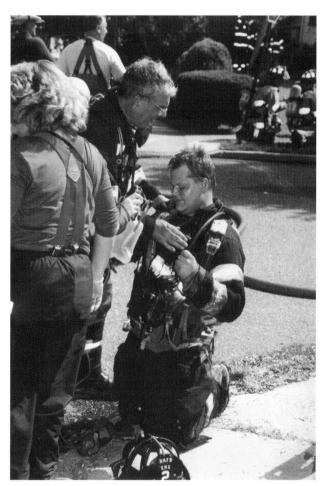

Figure 4.22 Emergency medical technicians monitor the conditions of emergency responders and provide the incident safety officer with evaluations of personnel at the rehabilitation site. *Courtesy of Bill Tompkins.*

Rapid Intervention Crew/Two-In Two-Out

[NFPA 1500: 8.5.1, 8.5.2, 8.5.2.1, 8.5.3, 8.5.4, 8.5.5, 8.5.6, 8.5.7]

The concept known as *two-in two-out* is found in Title 29 *CFR* 1910.134 (g)(4)(i), Procedures for Interior Structural Firefighting. The regulation requires personnel engaged in interior structural fire fighting to operate in teams of at least two people. This attack or search and rescue team must be equipped with respiratory protection, and members must remain in visual or voice contact with each other at all times. A second team composed of at least two people, referred to as a *rapid intervention crew (RIC)*, must be fully equipped with respiratory protection and complete personal protective clothing and ready to assist in rescue if the interior crew requires assistance. OSHA allows one member of the exterior RIC team to perform other functions such as serving as incident commander. The incident safety officer is responsible for ensuring that the two-in two-out rule is followed and that an RIC team is established during interior structural fire fighting operations and IDLH incidents (**Figure 4.23**).

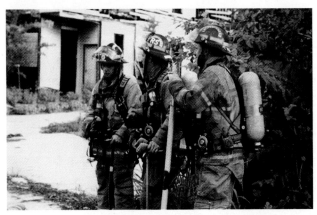

Figure 4.23 The rapid intervention crew (RIC) is fully equipped and ready to respond in the event an interior attack crew requires assistance or rescue. *Courtesy of Chris Mickal.*

Risk Management

The risk management model adopted in NFPA 1500 has been successfully used by general industry for decades. The safety and health components of risk management were incorporated into NFPA 1500 during the 1992 revision process. In the 1997 edition of the standard, they are outlined in Chapter 2 and applied to emergency operations in Chapter 6. With the 2002 edition, the safety and health components moved to Chapter 4, respiratory protection equipment requirements are included in Chapter 7, and emergency operations are moved to Chapter 8. Because the risk management model can be applied to all phases of emergency services operations, the following sections provide a general

overview of the fire and emergency services risk management plan, respiratory protection program responsibilities, safety and health program committee, and implementation procedures as they relate to respiratory protection.

Fire and Emergency Services Risk Management Plan

[NFPA 1500: 4.2.1, 4.2.2, 4.2.3, 4.7.2, 4.7.3, 4.7.4, 4.7.5, 4.7.6]

The risk management plan described in NFPA 1500 is a process that incorporates several components that can be applied to the operations of any fire and emergency services organization. This plan is not a stagnant document that is developed, described in a printed document, placed in a manual on a shelf, and used occasionally. Essentially, a risk management plan serves as documentation that risks have been identified and evaluated and that a reasonable control plan has been implemented and is being followed. An effective risk management program has a positive impact on the department/organization from the operational, safety, financial, and liability standpoints.

The fire chief/director or authority having jurisdiction (AHJ) has the ultimate responsibility for the risk management plan but may delegate it to the health and safety officer. This risk management plan must be reviewed and revised annually if necessary. Responsibility for the review and revision may be assigned to the health and safety officer, the safety and health program committee, or retained by the fire chief/director or AHJ (**Figure 4.24**). The plan may be part of the overall community/ jurisdiction plan and may be the responsibility of that organization's risk manager such as the community health and safety manager or loss control manager.

In the appropriate chapter of NFPA 1500, the requirements of the risk management plan are simply stated. The fire and emergency services organization shall adopt an official written risk management plan that covers administration, facilities, training, vehicle operations, respiratory protection, protective clothing and equipment (including respiratory protection equipment), operations at emergency incidents, operations at nonemergency incidents, and other related activities. At a minimum, the plan

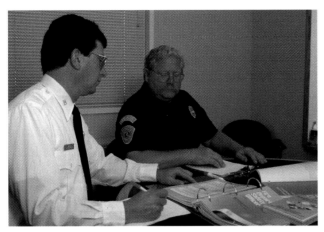

Figure 4.24 The organization's health and safety officer may be asked to assist the head of the organization in developing a comprehensive risk management plan.

shall include risk identification, risk evaluation, risk control techniques, and risk monitoring. However, in this chapter we are going to add an additional step in the process called *risk prioritization*. A sample plan can be found in Appendix A.4.2.2 (6) of the 2002 edition of NFPA 1500.

Risk Identification

To identify the risks, the health and safety officer compiles a list of all emergency and nonemergency operations and duties in which the organization participates. Ideally, the health and safety officer should take into consideration the worst possible conditions or potential events, including major disasters and multiple events. Many sources are available to assist with this identification process. The first and possibly the most effective is the organization's loss prevention data, which consists of annual fire loss reports by occupancy type, loss value, frequency, etc. (**Figure 4.25**). Although most departments/organizations are too small to rely on

---

Steps in the Development of a Risk Management Plan from NFPA 1500

1. **Risk identification.** List potential problems for every aspect of the operation of the fire department/emergency services organization at the facility or station. The following are examples of sources of information that may be useful in the process:
   - List of the risks to which members are or may be exposed
   - Records of previous accidents, illnesses, and injuries (both locally and nationally)
   - Facility and apparatus survey/inspection results

2. **Risk evaluation.** Evaluate each item listed in the risk identification process using the following two questions:
   - What is the potential frequency of occurrence?
   - What are the potential severity and expense of its occurrence?

   Use this information to set priorities in the control plan (needs assessment). Some sources of information include the following:
   - Safety audits and inspection reports
   - Prior accident, illness, and injury statistics
   - Application of national data to local circumstances
   - Professional judgment in evaluating risks unique to the jurisdiction

3. **Risk control.** Once the risks are identified and evaluated, determine which control should be implemented and documented. The two primary methods of controlling risk, in order of preference, are the following:
   - Wherever possible, totally eliminate/avoid the risk or the activity that presents the risk. For example, if the risk is falling on ice, do not allow members to go outside when icy conditions are present.
   - Where it is not possible or practical to avoid or eliminate the risk, take steps to control it. In the previous example, methods of control would be applying sand/salt or wearing proper footwear. Also consider the specific development of safety programs, standard operating procedures, training, and inspections as control methods.

4. **Risk management monitoring and follow-up.** Periodically evaluate the selected controls to determine whether they are working satisfactorily. If not, identify and implement new control measures.

Adapted from Section A.4.2.3 of NFPA 1500, *Standard on Fire Department Occupational Safety and Health Program*, 2002 edition, National Fire Protection Association, Quincy, MA 02269. The 1997 edition of NFPA 1500 also contains these steps.

their own databases for a statistically valid trend, national averages and trends are available from NFPA and the National Fire Academy. It is important to note that national data is not always complete or accurate due to collection inconsistencies and that a time lag of 1 to 2 years is required to collect, analyze, and publish it.

The health and safety officer should also seek input and ideas from organization personnel, trade journals, professional associations, and other service providers to identify the potential risks. When using information provided by other fire departments or emergency services organizations, the health and safety officer should consider local circumstances when formulating the list of all emergency and nonemergency operations and duties. Other risk identification sources include risk management plans developed by local industry and hazardous substance sites, vulnerability analyses, and Environmental Protection Agency (EPA) plans among others.

Risk Evaluation

Once the health and safety officer identifies the risks, they can be evaluated from both frequency and severity standpoints. Frequency, referred to by OSHA as *incidence rate*, addresses the likelihood of occurrence. Typically, if a particular type of incident such as injuries related to respiratory protection has occurred repeatedly, it will continue to occur until a job hazard or task analysis has been performed to identify the root causes and effective control measures have been implemented. In this example, the health and safety officer or safety and health program committee must develop and implement guidelines that outline proper respiratory protection techniques, the correct equipment to use, and physical fitness requirements that may mitigate the problem.

Severity addresses the degree of seriousness of the incident and can be measured in a variety of ways such as lost time away from work, cost of damage, cost of and time for repair or replacement of equipment, disruption of service, or legal costs. Refer to Appendix F, Risk Management Formulas, for the formulas for calculating frequency of occurrence and severity of incidents. Incidents of high frequency and high severity must have the highest priority in the risk analysis while those of low frequency and low severity receive the lowest priority. The method for calculating the risk may vary from organization to organization (**Figure 4.26**).

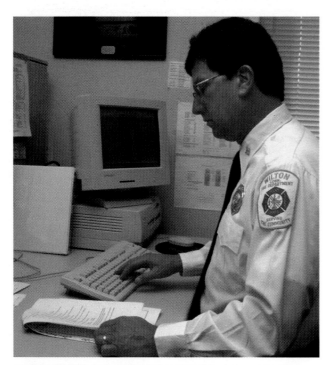

Figure 4.25 To help identify the possible risks related to respiratory protection that face the organization, the health and safety officer must collect information regarding the history of respiratory protection use, respiratory injuries, and the types of hazards protected.

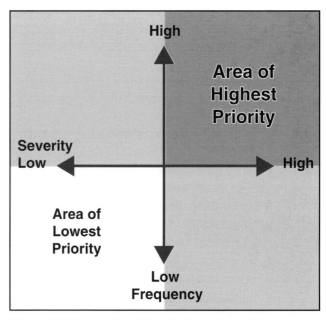

Figure 4.26 To prioritize risks, the frequency of occurrence of the risk must be weighed against the severity of the risk. The risks that occur the most frequently with the greatest severity must be addressed first.

Risk Prioritization

Taken in combination, the results of the frequency and severity determinations help to establish priorities for determining action. Any risk having a high probability of occurrence and serious consequences deserves immediate action and is considered a high-priority item. Low-severity incidents with a low likelihood of occurrence are a lower priority and can be placed near the bottom of the "action-required" list.

Risk Control Techniques

Once the health and safety officer prioritizes the risks, it is now time to apply risk control measures. Several approaches can be taken toward risk control, including risk avoidance, risk transfer, and implementation of control measures.

Risk avoidance. In any situation, the best risk control choice is risk avoidance. Simply put, personnel should avoid the activity that creates the risk. In a fire and emergency services organization, this approach frequently is impractical. Entering an oxygen-deficient area to perform a rescue creates a risk to rescuers, but personnel cannot avoid this risk and provide effective service. Therefore, training must be provided in the use of respiratory protection equipment and search and rescue techniques. However, risk avoidance could include a policy prohibiting other risks such as smoking by fire and emergency services organization candidates when they are hired, thereby reducing the potential for lung cancer among members. Mandatory use of respiratory protection in oxygen-deficient or toxic atmospheres is another example of risk avoidance.

Risk transfer. Risk transfer can be accomplished in one of two primary ways: (1) by physically transferring the risk to someone else and (2) through the purchase of insurance. For a fire and emergency services organization, the transfer of risk may be difficult if not impossible. However, an example of risk transfer would be contracting the cleanup and disposal of hazardous waste to an outside source. The risks associated with those activities would then transfer to a private contractor who accepts the liability. However, this approach does not address the need to protect emergency responders from the hazardous materials before cleanup. The purchase of insurance transfers financial risk only. In addition, insurance coverage does nothing to affect the likelihood of occurrence. Buying fire insurance for a station/facility — while highly recommended for protecting the assets of a department/organization — does nothing to prevent the station/facility from burning. Therefore, fire insurance is no substitute for an effective fire control measure such as an automatic sprinkler system.

Control measures. The most common method used for the management of risk is the adoption of effective control measures (risk reduction). While control measures will not eliminate the risk, they can reduce the likelihood of occurrence or mitigate the severity. Some typical control measures instituted to control incident scene injuries include accountability systems, full-protective clothing, mandatory respiratory protection programs, ongoing training and education programs, health and wellness programs, and well-defined SOPs. These control measures coupled together make an effective program that promotes safe emergency-incident operations (**Figure 4.27**). A classic example

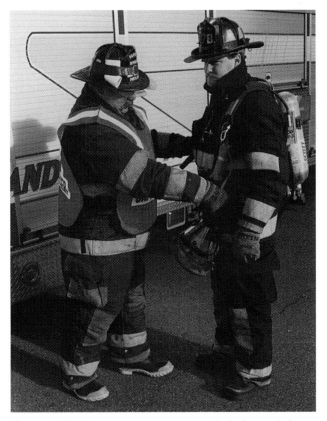

Figure 4.27 Risk control measures may include regulations regarding the wearing of full protective gear within the hot zone and the authority of the incident safety officer to prevent improperly equipped personnel from entering that area. *Courtesy of Mike Nixon.*

of a control measure is the mandatory use of respiratory protection equipment in situations that are immediately dangerous to life and health. This requirement was the result of high rates of emergency responder injury and death due to concentrations of toxic atmospheres.

Risk Monitoring

Once control measures have been implemented, they need to be evaluated to measure their effectiveness. The last step in the process is risk management monitoring. This step ensures that the system is dynamic and facilitates periodic reviews of the entire program. Any problems that occur in the process have to be revised or modified.

The intent of the risk management plan is to develop a strategy for reducing the inherent risks associated with fire and emergency service operations. Regardless of its size or type, every organization should operate within the parameters of a risk management plan. The operation of this plan is a dynamic and aggressive process that the health and safety officer must monitor and revise at least annually or as needed.

Respiratory Protection Program Responsibilities

[NFPA 1500: 7.9.1, 7.9.2, 7.9.3]

The fire or emergency services administration is required by NFPA 1500 to establish a respiratory protection program. The chief or director has ultimate authority over the program and the application of the risk management model to it. The health and safety officer is usually given responsibility for developing and administering the program based on the results of the risk management model. The operational personnel are responsible for applying the program policy and adhering to it during emergency operations. Because these three groups or positions are intimately involved in the program, they must be represented on the department's safety and health program committee (**Figure 4.28**).

Safety and Health Program Committee

[NFPA 1500: 4.5.1, 4.5.1.1, 4.5.1.2, 4.5.1.3]

Instrumental and valuable components of a fire and emergency service organization's safety and health program are the development, implementation,

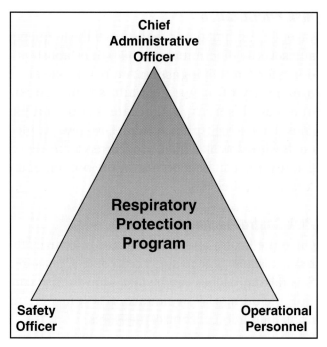

Figure 4.28 The head of the organization, health and safety officer, and operational personnel of the organization share responsibility for the respiratory protection program.

and operation of a safety and health program committee. This committee is a centralized group within a fire or emergency services organization that functions as a clearinghouse for activities, problems, and issues relating to firefighter/emergency responder safety and health.

The issues that confront this committee are unlimited. Ensuring firefighter/emergency responder safety and health are constantly changing processes based upon the needs of the organization and its commitment to safety. Other factors that can impact the successful operation of this committee are the level of activity of the committee and the examination and management of current safety and health issues within the organization. The goals of the safety and health program committee are to develop and recommend solutions to resolve conflicts. One issue that is *not* an objective of this committee is disciplinary action. The activities and issues that are addressed must be within the scope of the committee. NFPA 1500 defines the criteria for establishing and using a safety and health program committee. The requirements are as follows:

• The fire and emergency services organization needs to establish a safety and health program committee that serves in an advisory capacity to the fire chief/director.

- The intent of the safety and health program committee is to conduct research, develop recommendations, and study and review matters pertaining to occupational safety and health within the fire and emergency services organization. This function relates directly to the development of a respiratory protection program (**Figure 4.29**).

- The safety and health program committee must hold regularly scheduled meetings and special meetings as deemed necessary. Regular meetings must be held at least once every 6 months. Written minutes of each meeting must be maintained and distributed to all members of the fire and emergency services organization.

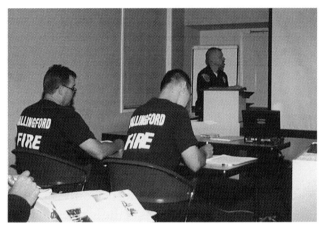

Figure 4.29 The health and safety officer and safety and health program committee members review safety regulations and concerns of the organization and recommend changes as necessary.

The health and safety officer is responsible for directing the operations of the safety and health program committee; however, other members of the committee vary from organization to organization depending on its size and type. The authority having jurisdiction establishes membership on the safety and health program committee based on recommendations of NFPA 1500. An effective safety and health program committee usually consists of three members from management, three members from the member organization, and the health and safety officer as a nonvoting member. Additional members may be appointed, including the organization's physician. Committees consisting of more than 12 members can become unwieldy

and ineffective. The safety and health program committee is slightly different from the respiratory protection program committee because the respiratory protection program committee contains some additional personnel.

Regardless of the size and type of the fire and emergency services organization, every organization should employ a safety and health program committee. For example, a career fire department can use members from each shift, each battalion, each division, or other combinations depending on the size of the department plus representatives from the member department. As with any organization, the key for the success of the organization's safety and health program committee is time management. With training mandates as well as other time requirements, the key to participation is efficiency and effectiveness. An organization must emphasize the importance of good time management to make the process work.

Implementation Procedures

The health and safety officer, respiratory protection officer, or safety and health program committee must ensure that the respiratory protection program is properly implemented and that procedures are followed. This overview is part of the monitoring step of the risk management model. It includes incident investigation, postincident analysis, case study reviews, and record keeping.

Incident Investigation
[NFPA 1500: 4.11.2, 4.11.3, 4.11.4, 4.11.5, 4.11.5.1, 4.11.6]

When an incident occurs that results in an injury or death of an employee, the incident safety officer or health and safety officer must make a thorough investigation of the event. The objective of the incident investigation is to determine the factors that contributed to firefighter/emergency responder fatality or injury or damage to departmental/organizational property. Investigations are fact-finding rather than faultfinding procedures (**Figure 4.30**). The health and safety officer or incident safety officer must determine whether an unsafe act or negligence was a part of the incident. The purposes of this type of investigation include the following:

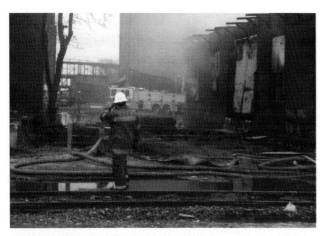

Figure 4.30 One of the responsibilities of the health and safety officer is to make a postincident investigation and provide recommendations for improving incident safety including any respiratory protection concerns.

- Avoid future loss of human resources and equipment.

- Ensure better cost-effectiveness in the use of personnel and equipment.

- Improve the morale of both fire and emergency services' personnel and members of the community.

- Determine the change or deviation that caused an incident.

- Determine hazardous conditions to which fire and emergency services personnel may be exposed.

- Direct the attention of management or officers to the causes of incidents.

- Examine facts as though they have a legal impact on incident cases.

During the investigation phase of the incident, the health and safety officer collects information from many sources such as the following:

- Dispatch records

- Interviews with participants

- Emergency incident reports

- Incident action plan

- Incident safety plan

- Police reports

- Photographs and videotapes of the scene or incident

- Site diagrams

- Physical property involved in the incident

- Laboratory analysis of evidence relating to the incident

- Testimony from experts

- Incident safety officer report

This information provides the health and safety officer with a fairly accurate description of the incident. A written report is then compiled on the incident relating to health and safety issues. This report is the basis for the postincident analysis and any corrective actions that need to be taken by the organization.

Personal protective clothing and equipment and respiratory protection equipment directly involved in the incident must be confiscated and held as evidence or for testing. NIOSH and the manufacturer of the equipment involved must be notified as soon as possible.

Postincident Analysis

[NFPA 1500:4.12.3, 4.20.1, 4.20.4]

The postincident analysis lists the cause of the incident, the organization's actions in bringing the incident under control, and the effects of the incident. The health and safety officer is concerned with the health and safety aspects of the incident on personnel. He or she is concerned not only with the cause of firefighter/emergency responder fatalities and injuries but also with the proper use of protective clothing and respiratory protection equipment, establishment of rapid intervention crews, the use of PASS devices, the use of personnel accountability systems, and the establishment of rehabilitation services (**Figure 4.31**).

Case Study Reviews

Incident investigation and postincident analysis are used to develop detailed case studies that describe the incident and outline the recommended alterations in operating procedures or equipment. Case studies are used in training sessions, provided to NIOSH or other government agencies, and used to alert other emergency services providers of potential unsafe acts or equipment failures. The warnings published by NIOSH are in case-study formats.

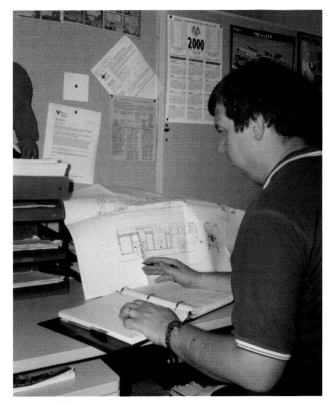

Figure 4.31 Once information on an incident is gathered from all sources, the health and safety officer analyzes it and develops a report that focuses on improving the safety aspect of future similar incidents.

Record Keeping

[NFPA 1500: 4.6.4, 4.12.4, 4.12.5, 4.12.6, 7.10.3, 7.10.4, 7.10.5]
[NFPA 1404: 6.1.2, 7.2.1, 7.3.1]
[NFPA 1852: 4.4.1, 4.4.2, 4.4.3, 4.4.4, 4.4.5, 4.4.6, 4.4.7, 4.4.8]

A variety of respiratory protection program records must be maintained by the fire and emergency services organization. These records are usually kept by various personnel or groups within the organization, including the SCBA maintenance section, health and safety officer, personnel office, training office, or organization's physician (**Figure 4.32**). The records that must be kept according to OSHA regulations and NFPA standards are as follows:

- Personnel medical records
- Hazardous materials exposure records
- Employee training records
- Facepiece fit-testing records
- Facepiece records
- Equipment inspection, maintenance, testing, and repair records

Personnel medical records. NFPA 1500 and Title 29 *CFR* 1910.134 require that all personnel assigned the use of respiratory protection be physically fit. Candidates for the fire and emergency services must pass both a medical examination and physical aptitude test to ensure their abilities to complete the tasks of firefighter or emergency services responder. Once hired, annual medical examinations for cardiovascular and pulmonary conditions are required (**Figure 4.33**). Medical records must be kept for all

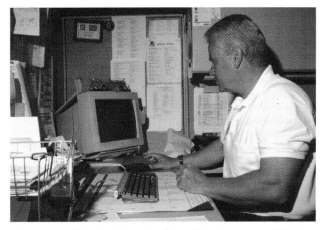

Figure 4.32 The health and safety officer is responsible for collecting and maintaining records related to the respiratory protection program.

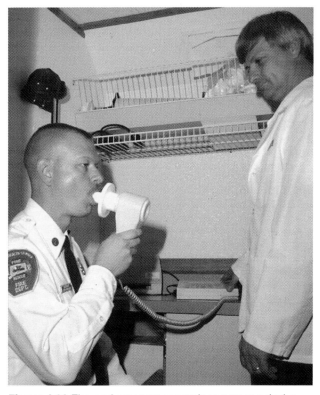

Figure 4.33 Fire and emergency services personnel who are expected to use respiratory protection equipment must be medically certified following a medical examination.

personnel and retained by the organization for 30 years past termination dates. This requirement ensures that long-term effects of hazardous or toxic chemicals can be traced to a source more effectively. All medical records are confidential. Only the employee or designated legal representative may have access to them.

Hazardous materials exposure records. Exposure records must be collected and retained on all personnel who are exposed to hazardous or toxic chemicals, bloodborne or airborne pathogens, contagious diseases, or carcinogens. This information is maintained with the medical records for 30 years following termination of an employee.

Employee training records. Respiratory protection training must be documented and records kept throughout the service career of all employees. This documentation ensures that training is provided and that employees have received it at least annually.

Facepiece fit-testing records. It is important to keep records of all facepiece fit tests. Information should include employees' names, types of tests used, facepiece brands and models, facepiece sizes of respiratory protection used, and results of tests. A fit test ensures that an individual is capable of getting a seal with a particular facepiece, brand, or model **(Figure 4.34)**. All facepiece fit-testing records should be retained for an extended period of time that is established by the organization's administra-

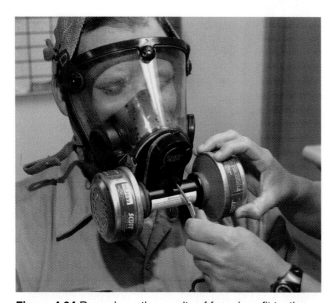

Figure 4.34 Records on the results of facepiece fit testing are maintained as part of an employee's file.

tion. This time frame may be based on either the service career of the employee or the time the employee is required to wear respiratory protection. Facepiece fit testing should be performed annually or whenever it is apparent that an individual has undergone the following changes:

● Weight gain or loss of 20 pounds (9 kg) or more

● Significant facial scarring in the area of the seal

● Significant dental changes

● Reconstructive or cosmetic surgery

Facepiece records. The department/organization officers are responsible for keeping accurate and complete records for each respiratory protection facepiece. These records should include inventory of serial numbers, dates of purchases, storage locations, dates of maintenance and repairs performed, parts replaced, dates of upgrades, and test performances. Facepiece records can be kept with the respiratory protection system records if the system is maintained as a single unit or in a separate file if the facepieces are issued to individuals.

Equipment inspection, maintenance, testing, and repair records. The department/organization is responsible for establishing a respiratory protection equipment maintenance program in accordance with NFPA 1404 and American National Standards Institute (ANSI) Z88.5 (Practices for Respiratory Protection for the Fire Service) in the United States and Canadian Standards Association (CSA) Z94.4-93 (Selection, Use, and Care of Respirators) in Canada. Records must be retained for the service life of the respiratory protection equipment. This program should be reflected in the SOPs of the department/organization and include the following record-keeping responsibilities:

● Maintain an inventory of respiratory protection equipment adequate to provide one unit to each department member on duty who may be exposed to respiratory hazards.

● Maintain individual records of each respiratory protection cylinder, regulator and harness assembly, and facepiece.

● Maintain annual testing, maintenance, and repair records on all respiratory protection components including the hydrostatic tests for cylinders **(Figure 4.35)**.

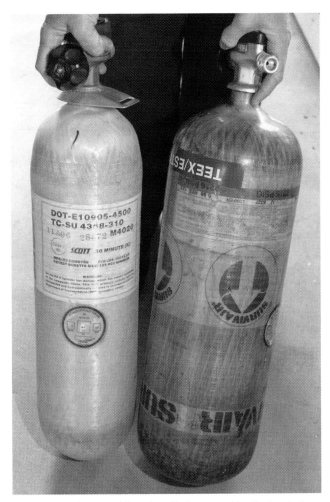

Figure 4.35 All breathing air cylinders must be hydrostatically tested and records must be maintained by the fire and emergency services organization. Both high-pressure (right) and low-pressure (left) cylinders must be marked with serial numbers and hydrostatic test data.

- Establish a replacement and upgrading program in compliance with NFPA 1981, *Standard on Open-Circuit Self-Contained Breathing Apparatus for the Fire Service.*

- Maintain records for each air compressor, each fill station, each cascade cylinder, each purification system, and related equipment used to produce or store breathing air. The record should contain the date of purchase, storage location, dates of inspection, dates of maintenance and repairs performed, and testing results of the device. NFPA requires that the equipment be tested at least quarterly. OSHA and Compressed Gas Association (CGA) standards as well as the local department of labor should be contacted to determine the requirements within the jurisdiction (**Figure 4.36**).

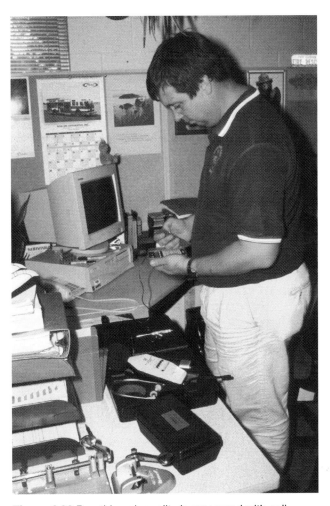

Figure 4.36 Breathing air quality is measured with calibrated instruments to ensure that the air meets the minimum standards.

Summary

The respiratory protection program is an essential part of the fire and emergency services safety and health program. The responsibility of developing and managing the respiratory protection program may be assigned to the health and safety officer or the safety and health program committee. Regardless, safety should be the primary consideration of the program and the risk management approach should be used in developing the program. The *NIOSH Respirator Decision Logic* process model is also helpful in selecting the proper respiratory protection based on the hazard. Together, these methods help ensure that maximum safety is provided for fire and emergency services personnel.

Respiratory Protection Equipment Selection and Procurement

This chapter provides information that will assist the reader in meeting the following job performance requirements from NFPA 1404, *Standard for Fire Service Respiratory Protection Training,* 2002 Edition; NFPA 1852, *Standard on Selection, Care, and Maintenance of Open-Circuit Self-Contained Breathing Apparatus,* 2002 Edition; and NFPA 1500, *Standard on Fire Department Occupational Safety and Health Program,* 2002 Edition.

NFPA 1404

6.1.2 Records of all respiratory protection training shall be maintained, including training of personnel involved in maintenance of such equipment, in accordance with Section 4.3 of NFPA 1852, *Standard on Selection, Care, and Maintenance of Open-Circuit Self-Contained Breathing Apparatus.*

6.2.1 Re-training shall be administered annually and when the following situations occur:

(1) Changes in the workplace or the type of respirator render the previous training obsolete

(2) Inadequacies in the member's knowledge or use of the respirator indicate that the member has not retained the requisite understanding or skill

(3) Any other situation arises in which re-training appears necessary to ensure safe respirator use

7.2.1 Inspection, maintenance, and repair records shall be maintained for SAR units used in training as required in Chapter 4 of this standard.

7.3.1 Inspection, maintenance, and repair records for FFAPR use in training shall be maintained as required in Chapter 6 of this standard.

NFPA 1500

7.9.1 The fire department shall adopt and maintain a respiratory protection program that addresses the selection, care, maintenance, and safe use of respiratory protection equipment, training in its use, and the assurance of air quality.

7.9.2 The fire department shall develop and maintain standard operating procedures that are compliant with this standard and that address the safe use of respiratory protection.

10.1.1 Candidates shall be medically evaluated and certified by the fire department physician.

NFPA 1852

4.1.1 As part of the respiratory protection program specified by Section 7.3 of NFPA 1500, *Standard on Fire Department Occupational Safety and Health Program*, the organization shall develop, implement, and apply the program component for the selection, care, and maintenance of open-circuit self-contained breathing apparatus (SCBA) used by the members of the organization in the performance of their assigned functions.

4.1.2 The program component shall have the following goals:

(1) To provide SCBA that is suitable and appropriate for the intended use.

(2) To maintain SCBA in a safe, useable condition to provide the intended protection to the user.

(3) To removing from use any SCBA that could cause or contribute to user injury, illness, or death because of its condition.

(4) To recondition, repair, or retire such SCBA.

4.1.3 The SCBA selection, care, and maintenance component of the organization's respiratory protection program shall be in accordance with Section 4.2.

4.4.8 The organization shall create, maintain, and disseminate the following as required:

(1) Written instructions for care, maintenance, and repair that correspond to those provided by the manufacturer

(2) Written instructions for checks while donning SCBA

(3) Written instructions for inspection, including procedures to be followed if defects are found

(4) Forms to document the findings during inspection

(5) Forms to record and to report defects, found during inspection, and to track the SCBA or cylinder as it is repaired

(6) Forms to document inspections, tests, and repairs by SCBA users and technicians that shall include the following:

  a. SCBA make, model, and serial number and other information to identify components.

  b. Documentation of the date, result of the inspection or test, and all actions taken as well as who acted.

(7) Written instructions for filling and for testing cylinders

(8) Written policy and procedure concerning training and authorization of SCBA technicians as well as documentation of that training and authorization

(9) Written procedures for the inspection of cylinders by technicians

(10) Written procedures for recording information about the inspection and repair of cylinders

(11) Stickers, tags, or other similarly effective means to alert users and technicians to defects, to document inspections, and to certify that tests, repairs, and other actions have been completed

(12) Written procedures for periodic tests and comprehensive inspections that comply with the SCBA manufacturer's instructions

(13) Documentation of the tests to verify SCBA performance

(14) Schedule for retention, disposition, and disposal of each report, record, and document

(15) Methods of identifying all SCBAs, cylinders, parts, and components so that these can be identified and tracked from initial receipt by the organization until removed from the possession and control of the organization

(16) Documentation when a defective or obsolete SCBA or component part is removed from service in accordance with the following:

    a. Until retirement and disposal of a defective or obsolete SCBA or component as specified in 4.6.3, a tag shall be conspicuously placed on the SCBA or component.

    b. The tag shall indicate the date and time the SCBA or component was removed from service, by whom, and for what reason.

    c. SCBA and components that are removed from service shall be stored separately from other SCBA and components and secured, as necessary.

    d. Access to tagged SCBA and components shall be limited, and only authorized persons shall remove tags after repair or service.

(17) Records for maintenance of each individual SCBA regulator, reducer, harness, cylinder including valve assembly, and facepiece including the following information:

    a. The manufacturer's serial number or other unique identifier

    b. Date of manufacture, receipt, service, inspection, test, maintenance, and repair

    c. Inspections, service, repairs, and tests

    d. Who performed the work

    e. Other comments

(18) Records of training provided to each user showing date(s) and subject(s) covered

(19) Such other reports, records, and documents including forms, tags, stickers, and other means necessary to effectuate the purposes of record keeping and the intent of this standard.

5.1.1 Prior to starting the procurement process of SCBA, a risk assessment shall be performed. The risk assessment shall include, but not be limited to, the expected hazards that can be encountered by users of SCBA based on the type of duties performed, frequency of use, the organization's experiences, and the organization's geographic location and climatic conditions.

5.1.2 The organization shall review the following standards as a minimum:

(1) NFPA 1981, *Standard on Open-Circuit Self-Contained Breathing Apparatus for the Fire Service*

(2) NFPA 1982, *Standard on Personal Alert Safety Systems (PASS)*

(3) NFPA 1500, *Standard on Fire Department Occupational Safety and Health Program*

5.1.2.1 Organizations in the United States shall also review 29 *CFR* 1910.134 and 29 *CFR* 1910.156.

5.1.2.2 Organizations outside the United States shall also review all applicable national, state/provincial, and local regulations.

5.1.3 The organization shall compile and evaluate information on comparative product strengths and weaknesses.

5.1.4 The organization shall ensure that the SCBA interfaces properly with other personal protective items already being used by the organization.

5.1.5 The organization shall also consider the following items during the selection process:

(1) Cross contamination between users and ease of cleaning/decontamination

(2) Legibility of remote pressure indicators in reduced visibility

(3) Size

(4) Weight

(5) Rated service time

(6) Breathing resistance

(7) Environment

(8) Ease of donning and doffing

(9) Comfort

(10) Fit range and available number of facepiece sizes

(11) The number and complexity of steps involved in operation and maintenance of the SCBA

(12) Design features that provide positive feedback to the user that required steps have been completed properly

(13) Design features that prevent steps from being performed improperly

(14) Operability by user wearing structural fire fighting gloves

(15) Facepiece vision area

(16) Cylinder fill station requirements

(17) Method for uniquely identifying the components of the SCBA

(18) Facepiece nose cup

(19) Vision correction needs of their personnel

(20) Characteristics of the end of service time indicators

(21) Communication capability such as speech diaphragms, voice amplifiers, radio interface, and so forth

(22) Supplied air compatibility

(23) Spare cylinders

(24) Rapid cylinder filling options

(25) Cylinder types

5.1.6 Where a field or laboratory evaluation is conducted, at least the following criteria shall be used for designing a systematic evaluation procedure.

(a) The organization shall develop an evaluation plan including, but not limited to, testing according to 7.4.2 prior to and after field evaluations.

(b) Participants for field evaluations shall be selected based on a cross section of personnel, willingness to participate, objectivity, and level of operational activity.

(c) Participants shall perform a field evaluation on each different product model being considered from each manufacturer for a particular SCBA. Participants shall be fitted for and instructed in the use of each product model being evaluated from each manufacturer.

(d) A product evaluation form shall be developed for each model.

(e) The organization shall solicit periodic reports from participants in the field evaluation.

(f) The organization shall conclude the evaluation process and analyze the results.

5.1.7 Purchase specifications shall require evidence that the SCBA to be purchased are certified as compliant with NFPA 1981, *Standard on Open-Circuit Self-Contained Breathing Apparatus for the Fire Service.*

5.1.7.1 Where SCBA-Integrated PASS are involved, the PASS portion of the SCBA-Integrated PASS shall be certified as compliant with NFPA 1982, *Standard on Personal Alert Safety Systems (PASS).*

5.1.7.2 For both NFPA 1981 and NFPA 1982, the edition of the respective standard(s) that is the current edition at the time of purchase, shall be the edition specified.

5.1.8 Where the organization develops purchase specifications, at least the following criteria shall be considered:

(1) All requirements developed by the organization in its evaluations conducted in accordance with paragraphs specified as 5.1.3, 5.1.4, 5.1.5, 5.1.6, and 5.1.7.

(2) Quantitative fit testing

(3) User training

(4) Maintenance training

(5) Manufacturer assistance to develop SOPs for maintenance

(6) SCBA testing on site prior to acceptance

(7) Maintenance schedule

(8) Complete parts list

(9) SCBA user and service manuals

(10) List of any specialized equipment or special tools needed for SCBA maintenance

(11) List of authorized service centers

(12) Warranty statement

(13) Procedures for returning items found defective upon initial receipt

5.2.1 Upon receipt, organizations shall inspect and test purchased SCBA, in accordance with 7.1.2, and 7.4.2 through 7.4.6 respectively. Organizations shall also verify that the equipment received is as specified.

5.2.2 Procedures shall be established for returning unsatisfactory products, if the organization's specifications are not met.

5.2.3 Organizations shall review information supplied with the products such as instructions, warranties, and technical data.

Chapter 5
Respiratory Protection Equipment Selection and Procurement

Whether a fire or emergency services organization is purchasing replacement units for an existing respiratory protection program, expanding an existing program, or establishing a new program, specific steps must be followed. First, a respiratory protection program must be developed and established, which requires the creation of a respiratory protection program committee. This committee should be composed of some of the members of the safety and health program committee. Then the respiratory protection program committee must establish an equipment selection process that results in the purchase of the best respiratory protection equipment to meet the needs of the organization **(Figure 5.1)**. The committee takes the following steps:

- Establish the equipment selection and procurement process.

- Research the respiratory hazards of the organization.

- Determine the regulatory requirements for respiratory protection.

- Research the available types of respiratory protection equipment.

- Develop respiratory protection equipment specifications.

- Perform physical evaluations of available respiratory protection equipment.

- Perform respiratory protection product reviews.

- Follow the jurisdiction's purchasing process.

- Implement the respiratory protection program.

- Perform ongoing evaluation of the respiratory protection equipment and program.

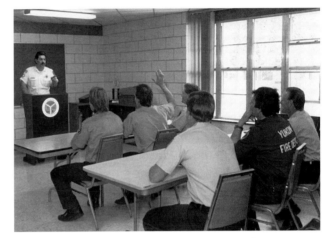

Figure 5.1 To ensure complete compliance and acceptance of the respiratory protection program, personnel who will use the equipment should be involved in the purchasing process by soliciting ideas, participating on the respiratory protection program committee, and helping to evaluate new equipment.

By following an established process, both the committee and the organization can justify the ultimate recommendations for purchases, which is especially important when purchases require a major capital outlay by a jurisdiction. This chapter provides a guide for the process of selection and procurement of respiratory protection equipment that can be applied to all types of protective equipment.

Respiratory Protection Responsibility

In the United States and Canada, the authority having jurisdiction (whether municipal, state/provincial, territorial, or some other level of authority) is required to provide respiratory protection for its employees. This responsibility is usually delegated to individual departments or organizations such as a fire and emergency services organization. The chief, chief executive officer (CEO), or department head may then assign the development and management of a respiratory protection program to a qualified member of the department/organization or a respiratory protection program committee.

Respiratory Protection Program

[NFPA 1500: 7.9.1, 7.9.2]

As explained in previous chapters, the primary requirement for a respiratory protection program is found in NFPA 1500, *Standard on Fire Department Occupational Safety and Health Program*, and OSHA Title 29 (Labor) *CFR* 1910.134 (Respiratory Protection) and 1910.156 (Fire Brigades). The respiratory protection program is part of the organization's safety and health program. Therefore, the health and safety officer (delegated by the fire chief, CEO, or department head) who chairs the safety and health program committee may have the authority for establishing and implementing the respiratory protection program. The health and safety officer may also have the responsibility for determining if and when respiratory protection equipment must be replaced or upgraded. Ultimately, the responsibility for the program rests with the department head, fire chief, or CEO. The department head, fire chief, or CEO must ensure that the program is established and implemented by providing the health and safety officer with the necessary authority and support to accomplish the task.

Respiratory Protection Program Committee

Representation on the respiratory protection program committee should be similar to that on the safety and health program committee. By including the personnel who will ultimately use and maintain the equipment, better results are achieved, which ensures that the program and the equipment will meet the actual needs of the organization (**Figure 5.2**). The membership of the respiratory protection program committee may include but is not limited to the following people:

- Health and safety officer
- Department/organization physician
- Department/organization administration official
- Training officer
- Emergency medical services officer
- Representatives of the member organization or association

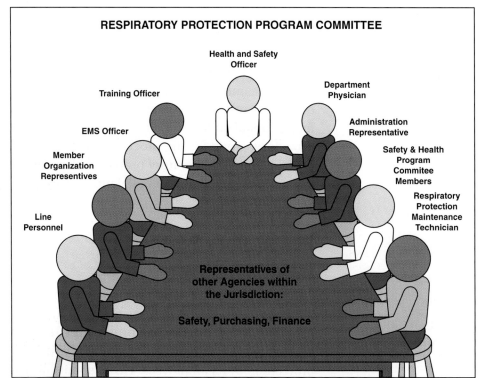

RESPIRATORY PROTECTION PROGRAM COMMITTEE

Health and Safety Officer

Training Officer

Department Physician

EMS Officer

Administration Representative

Member Organization Represenlives

Safety & Health Program Commitee Members

Respiratory Protection Maintenance Technician

Line Personnel

Representatives of other Agencies within the Jurisdiction:

Safety, Purchasing, Finance

Figure 5.2 The respiratory protection program committee should be composed of representatives of the organization including, among others, administrators, technical personnel, members representatives, and end users. The health and safety officer chairs the committee.

- Safety and health program committee members
- Line personnel (equipment users)
- Respiratory protection equipment maintenance technician
- Representatives of other agencies within the jurisdiction
- Purchasing department representative
- Safety department representative
- Finance department representative

Selection and Procurement Process

[NFPA 1852: 4.1.1, 4.1.2, 4.1.3]

The process for selecting and procuring respiratory protection equipment must be objective, logical, methodical, and repeatable. An *objective* process must be based on fact and not emotion or "gut-feelings." It must have a *logical*, stepping-stone pattern that allows each decision to be based firmly on the preceding decision. *Methodical* means that it adheres to an existing, well-established pattern that has been used successfully by other organizations. Finally, it must be *repeatable* by future committees who are given the task of replacing or upgrading respiratory protection equipment chosen through this process.

The selection and procurement process model given in this chapter is based on one developed and used by Scott Aviation. The model is reproduced in flow-chart form in Appendix G, Scott Aviation Flow Chart. Similar models may be available from other manufacturers. The process steps include the following:

- Determine the needs of the department/organization.
- Conduct research on respiratory protection equipment, manufacturers, and standards/regulations.
- Evaluate and field test proposed respiratory protection equipment.
- Review respiratory protection product data.
- Conduct the purchasing process.
- Implement the respiratory protection program.
- Evaluate the respiratory protection program results.

Determine Needs

[NFPA 1852: 5.1.1, 5.1.2, 5.1.2.1, 5.1.2.2]

The respiratory protection program committee must first be familiar with the applicable respiratory protection regulations that were outlined in Chapter 2, Regulations and Standards. Committee members must keep in mind that all standards and regulations require only a minimum level of protection. An increased level of protection may be established based on the research of the needs of the department/organization.

Next the committee must make an evaluation of the current level of respiratory protection and the current units in service. This information is necessary in determining whether upgrade or replacement is necessary. If the organization's current equipment is relatively new, then an upgrade to more recent standards may prove the most economical decision. In addition, manufacturers may offer extended warranties on upgraded equipment. Compatibility of existing units with new units must also be considered. An inventory of maintenance parts and accessories should also be included in an equipment survey (**Figure 5.3**).

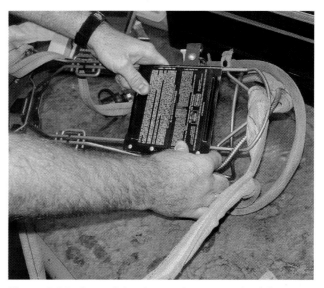

Figure 5.3 In determining the respiratory needs of the organization, existing equipment and replacement parts such as backpack frames should be inspected for condition and inventoried for quantity. *Courtesy of Kenneth Baum.*

The committee should now determine the respiratory protection hazards that the organization faces. The risk management model or the *NIOSH Respirator Decision Logic* model from the National

Institute for Occupational Safety and Health (NIOSH) may be applied. See Chapter 4, Safety and Risk Management, and Appendix C, NIOSH Decision Logic Flow Chart, for details. The NIOSH model helps to determine the appropriate respiratory protection against specific environmental conditions. Although it does not specifically address medical protection, it can be modified to include such hazards and the appropriate level of protection needed.

The next step of the process is to compare the existing respiratory protection equipment with the current state of respiratory protection technology. If an organization has not purchased equipment in many years or is just beginning to provide respiratory protection, this comparison provides an insight into what is currently available (**Figure 5.4**). Product literature, reviews in trade journals, and magazine articles on respiratory protection are valuable in this step.

With an understanding of the current design features of respiratory protection equipment, the committee can determine the compatibility with the organization's existing equipment. In some cases, the equipment provided by the same manufacturer is not compatible with older units. Changes in regulator, backpack, or facepiece designs may prevent the purchase of new components and compromise NIOSH or Mine Safety and Health Administration (MSHA) certification of the unit.

Compatibility concerns extend to the equipment interface with protective clothing, the apparatus mounting systems, and the storage areas for the respiratory protection equipment. As mentioned in Chapter 4, Safety and Risk Management, protective clothing interface is an important aspect in the selection of respiratory protection equipment. Information may be gathered from line personnel, safety investigations of injury incidents involving respiratory protection equipment, or manufacturers of protective clothing equipment. Particular concerns are the effects of compression on the thermal protection of the clothing, interface with the helmet and flashover hood, and restriction to user mobility caused by the respiratory protection unit (**Figure 5.5**).

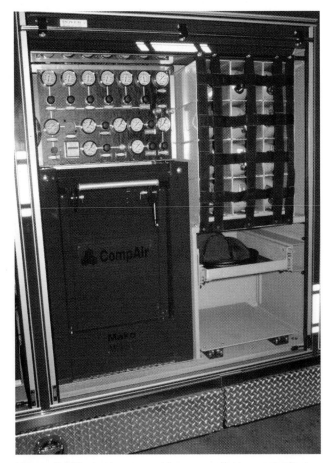

Figure 5.4 Trade shows provide an excellent opportunity to learn about and compare new products in the field of respiratory protection. As an example, apparatus-mounted breathing air systems found at trade shows permit committee members to gather information about equipment that might not be accessible in remote areas of the country.

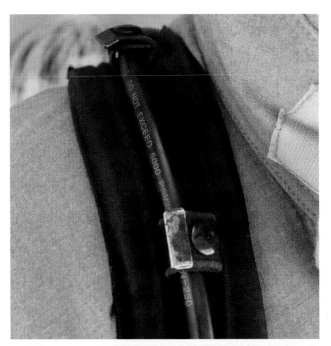

Figure 5.5 The committee should be aware of the effects that compressions caused by shoulder straps of SCBA units can have on reducing the thermal protection of protective coats. Clothing and SCBA manufacturers have been working together to reduce the effects of compression.

Other compatibility issues involve the interface between self-contained breathing apparatus (SCBA) and the apparatus storage systems. Apparatus jump seats and seat brackets must be able to securely hold the SCBA cylinder and still allow rapid donning of the unit (**Figure 5.6**). Storage space in compartments must also be considered. It must be decided if units will be secured in brackets or stored in cases. Supplied-air respirator (SAR) units require other considerations, especially if compressed-air cylinders or air compressors are permanently mounted on apparatus. Apparatus design then becomes a function of the decision process.

The committee must consider the organization's current equipment maintenance program and the parts inventory for the current respiratory protection system. Cost of maintenance (either in-house or contracted) must be considered, including the cost of retraining personnel on new equipment. The value of the current parts inventory and the annual parts budget should also be considered (**Figures 5.7 a and b**). This information is essential to justify replacement of existing units.

Once all the information has been gathered and evaluated, the committee must prepare a recommendation on the action to take. The choices

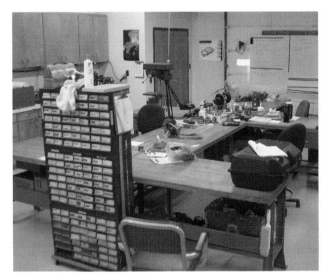

Figure 5.7a Another consideration that must be made during the selection process is the value of the current maintenance parts inventory. This inventory will include everything from small parts stored in bins (as shown here) to complete units used to replace damaged units. *Courtesy of Kenneth Baum.*

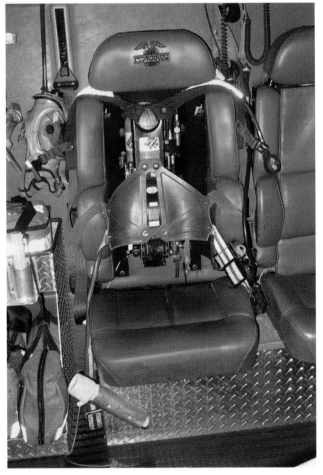

Figure 5.6 Respiratory protection program committee members must take into consideration how the respiratory protection systems are stored on apparatus. Incompatibility with existing brackets may create a logistics or maintenance problem or cause additional wear on the equipment if the problem is not addressed during the selection process. *Courtesy of Lloyd Lees.*

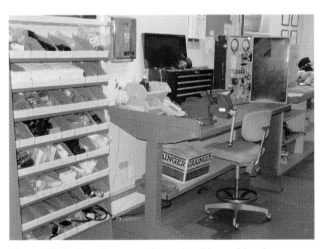

Figure 5.7b Also, the committee should consider the additional tools and certification training that will be required by each of the respiratory protection systems under consideration. Each type of respiratory protection system may require its own specialized tools, testing instrumentation like the unit shown at the far end of the work station, and ergonomically designed tools and work area. *Courtesy of Kenneth Baum.*

include the following: (1) purchase all new equipment, (2) upgrade the existing equipment, or (3) integrate new equipment with the existing equipment. Each option must be thoroughly described with benefits, deficits, costs, effects, and impacts. A cost/benefit analysis must also be provided for each option. Because the committee does not have the authority to make the final decision, this information has to be provided to the authority who has that responsibility. With this information, the chief, CEO, or department head can make the final decision and present it to the jurisdiction for funding and action.

Conduct Research

[NFPA 1852: 5.1.3, 5.1.4, 5.1.5]

Once the respiratory protection program committee has made its proposal to the chief/CEO/department head and the jurisdiction has approved the choice of options, the next step is to collect data on the available respiratory protection systems. The committee must provide sufficient time to gather and evaluate the information. An attainable timetable should be established with objectives firmly in place. The entire process may take from a few months to a few years. The research process includes surveying other jurisdictions, reviewing manufacturers' business histories, requesting references, reviewing standards and regulations, reviewing industry trends, comparing various products, determining equipment compatibility, reviewing purchasing ordinances and laws, and developing a request for proposal.

Survey Other Jurisdictions

Research can begin by surveying other jurisdictions about respiratory equipment used. Survey topics should include types of equipment used, problems encountered with the equipment, ability of the equipment to meet specifications, equipment service or maintenance difficulties, and after-sales support by manufacturers. The survey should be written and sent to various members of the organization, including the maintenance technician, training personnel, line personnel, the member organization or association, and the person in charge of the respiratory protection program. Allow each responder sufficient time to complete the survey. This approach provides a holistic view of the pro-

gram within other organizations/departments rather than the opinion of one individual. A sample survey form used for SCBA is included in Appendix H, SCBA Survey Form. This form can be used or adapted for purposes other than SCBA equipment.

Review Manufacturers' Business Histories

The committee should review the business histories of the various manufacturers and the vendors representing them. Annual reports, articles in trade journals, financial statements, and business reports published by companies like Dunn and Bradstreet can provide an image of the organization and provide some insight into the company's ability to supply the system or equipment. The share of the market that the manufacturers hold and why they have that share should be considered (**Figure 5.8**).

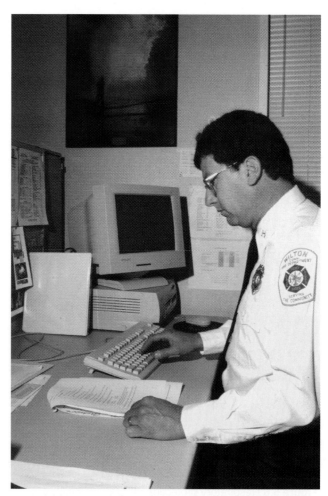

Figure 5.8 Research during the selection process includes the review of financial reports about the various vendors and manufacturers, annual reports, trade publications, and product reviews. Some of this material may be available on the Internet while other information may need to be requested directly from the companies.

Request References

References from other equipment purchasers are also an important source of information. The committee should request a list of the most recent purchasers of respiratory protection equipment similar to the type under consideration from the manufacturers. These references can be provided by other organizations within the area, including both public and private purchasers.

Review Standards and Regulations

Respiratory protection standards and regulations should also be reviewed. These standards/regulations include not only the equipment's operational requirements but also the design and testing requirements. This review allows the committee to develop specifications that meet or exceed the standards/regulations. A thorough understanding of the standards/regulations also allows the committee to better evaluate the products that are submitted for evaluation.

Review Industry Trends

Manufacturers are continuously making changes in the design of respiratory protection equipment to meet changes in the standards/regulations. In addition, changes are made to improve the equipment based on internal research projects. These changes must be submitted to NIOSH for approval before they can be incorporated into equipment certified for use by the fire and emergency services. Therefore, the committee must review the latest industry trends in equipment design. Trade journals, trade shows, and press releases by manufacturers' marketing divisions all provide opportunities to keep up with current developments. The committee may decide to delay purchase of a system if standard/regulation or industry changes are imminent. The committee must remember that all system components must be certified and that factor adds to the time before a system with a design change can reach the market **(Figure 5.9)**.

Compare Various Products

Competition is very strong among respiratory protection equipment manufacturers. Unlike the automobile industry, there are few respiratory protection equipment manufacturers and limited customers. Therefore, the committee must compare the various products based on similar characteristics, sales and technical support, parts availability, length of time before a unit becomes obsolete or has a major design change, available warranties and warranty support, local manufacturer representation, and a manufacturer's ability to fill orders within a specified time frame. This information can be entered into a matrix or database for ease of comparison. Competition in the marketplace can be used to an organization's advantage in negotiating the terms of contracts.

Determine Equipment Compatibility

Information gained during the needs assessment relating to compatibility can now be applied to the various respiratory protection systems on the market. Systems that would require a redesign of the apparatus jump seats or storage compartments may not be desirable for the department/organization. Some systems may work better with the

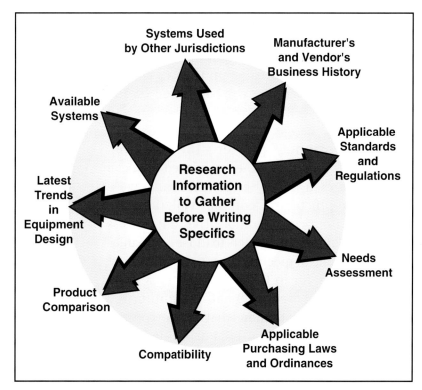

Figure 5.9 This illustration depicts many of the factors that the respiratory protection program committee must consider during the selection process.

organization's existing personal protective clothing than other systems. Compatibility also includes how the systems are used. The systems must meet the operational procedures of the department/organization without drastic changes in training and procedures. For example, if the organization is issuing individual facepieces that can be used with both SCBA and SAR units, compatibility concerns must be included in the evaluation.

Review Purchasing Ordinances and Laws

Once all of the essential data are collected, the committee should review the purchasing ordinances and laws of the jurisdiction. Some municipalities are bound by state/provincial purchasing requirements. Involving members of the finance or purchasing department in the process prevents any mistakes in specifications or bid development.

Develop Request for Proposal

If the jurisdiction permits, it is a good idea to develop a request for proposal (RFP) before sending bid notices. An RFP defines the needs of the department/organization and allows manufacturers or their authorized distributors to decide if they can meet bid specifications. An RFP must have a specific schedule outlined, including bid dates, delivery dates, provisions for supplying units for scheduled evaluations, and training dates for technicians and training officers. An RFP also allows the jurisdiction to have control over the companies that can bid based on the response to the RFP and participation in pre-bid meetings. Companies who cannot meet delivery deadlines, cannot provide the required performance bonds, lack the established financial support to complete the contract, or have a documented history of contract violations are eliminated from consideration. The RFP process reduces the number of bidders to those companies who are capable of meeting the bid specifications. Before writing an RFP, the committee should consult both legal counsel and the authority's purchasing laws to determine what kinds of controls can legally be placed on bids or bidders. The selection of bidders may not be subjective or arbitrary. A sample RFP is found in Appendix I, Sample Request for Proposal.

NOTE: Fire and emergency services organizations cannot be subjective or arbitrary in the selection of bidders for respiratory protection equipment. All governmental organizations are regulated by open and fair purchasing laws. Respiratory protection program committees must respect these laws and operate within them.

Although the bid process is designed for major equipment systems such as the purchase of SCBAs, it can be applied to any component of the respiratory protection program. High efficiency particulate air (HEPA) filter masks, air-purifying respirators (APR), and dust masks can all be purchased through this process. Once a specific product is determined to be the most appropriate for the department/organization, it can be established as the "standard" for the department/organization. Thus the department/organization does not have to rewrite specifications the next time equipment needs to be purchased. Another approach is to establish a renewable contract in the bid specifications. The contract may be negotiated for 1 year with three subsequent annual renewals based on a set increase for inflation if both parties agree. However, due to rapid changes in the standards/regulations for respiratory protection, the purchasing organization must be prepared to rewrite the specifications. Contract language should also reflect this possibility.

Evaluate Equipment
[NFPA 1852: 5.1.6, 5.2.3]

The RFP should contain language requiring a physical evaluation of all respiratory equipment units and accessories that each manufacturer is planning to submit for bid. This physical evaluation is an opportunity for the department/organization to test the proposed equipment in controlled training exercises and in actual daily operations.

The physical evaluation, like the pre-bid conference, should be a requirement for participation in the official bid process. Companies that do not participate should not be certified to continue the bidding process. Each manufacturer should be required to provide a specified number of units, usually enough to outfit at least one company. Before the actual evaluations, the manufacturer must provide training for personnel participating in the testing of the equipment. Individual facepieces must be supplied for the testing personnel and properly fit tested. The facepieces must be provided in a variety of sizes in order to fit all possible facial configurations (**Figure 5.10**). All accessories that are available for the system should be provided, including integrated personal alert safety system (PASS) devices, air-supply line covers, quick-fill valves, and facepiece fit-testing accessories. A manufacturer's sales or technical representative should be present during the equipment evaluations to answer questions or provide additional training.

The physical evaluation should include both training evolutions and actual field tests. Therefore, the RFP must specify the total amount of time that the units are needed for evaluation, the specific date and time for the training evolutions, and language releasing the department/organization from responsibility for any damage or wear to the units.

Depending on the number of units evaluated, the committee may wish to specify one or more days for the training evolutions (**Figure 5.11**). These tests must be performed under controlled conditions. Therefore, the same personnel must be used to test all of the evaluation units under the identical conditions. For example, emergency response personnel may be used for the evaluation. They are given a set of activities to perform that simulate actual operation conditions. These activities depend on the tasks that personnel perform and the hazard that the equipment is intended to protect against. The activities may include a smoke building search and rescue, live burn exercise, salvage and overhaul operation, confined-space rescue, or stair climb. Evaluations of medical respiratory protection equipment may involve working with a patient in a confined space, wearing the respiratory protection facepiece for a prolonged period, or wearing the facepiece during strenuous respiratory activity.

Regardless of the types of training evolutions, the committee must have an objective grading system for the units. Criteria should be established and points assigned based on the unit's ability to meet the standard/regulation. The grades may be numerical from best to worst or terms such as *excellent, good, fair,* or *poor.* A comments section should be included on the grade form for any

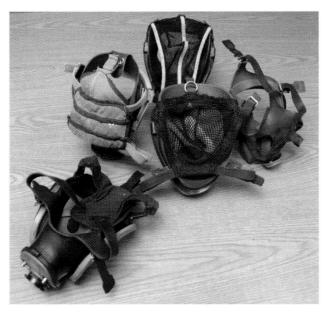

Figure 5.10 The committee has to evaluate the wide variety of options offered by the manufacturers of respiratory protection equipment. This photo shows just a few of the facepiece head strap and net assemblies that are available.

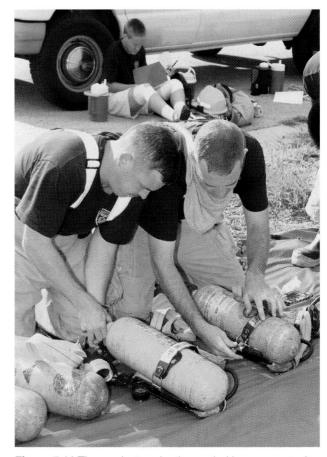

Figure 5.11 The product evaluation period is an opportunity for committee members to physically operate the equipment they are reviewing. By comparing the operation of various parts of each system, the committee will be able to recommend the best system for the organization's needs. *Courtesy of Bob Parker.*

additional information or opinions by the users. A sample form is included in Appendix J, Equipment Evaluation Form. Evaluation criteria may include but are not limited to the following factors:

- Maneuverability
- Flexibility
- Impact on vision
- Ease of donning
- Ease of doffing
- Impact on workload
- Comfort

Once the controlled training evaluations are complete, the evaluation units should be assigned to active emergency response companies (**Figure 5.12**). Depending on the activity level of the companies, this portion of the evaluation may take up to a month or more. Equipment evaluation forms should be supplied for personnel to complete after each use. Field evaluations under actual use conditions provide additional data for the committee and also allow personnel who will be using the final product an opportunity to have a part in the selection process. Therefore, personnel other than those who participated in the controlled training evaluations should be selected to conduct field tests.

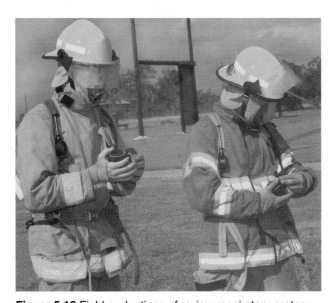

Figure 5.12 Field evaluations of review respiratory protection systems provide an opportunity for company or line personnel to use the equipment in actual emergency situations. However, personnel must be thoroughly trained in the use of the equipment before placing it in service. *Courtesy of Bob Parker.*

The information gained from the physical evaluations must be compiled and analyzed by the committee. All grading forms and comments should be retained in the committee files in case the final purchase decision is questioned. The importance of maintaining thorough and complete records cannot be overstressed.

Review Product Data

Once the field evaluations are complete, the committee can consider other facts about the various equipment systems (**Figure 5.13**). Some areas of concern and factors to consider are as follows:

- *Features* — List the various features and accessories available with the particular units such as quick-fill and buddy-breathing connections, integrated PASS devices, amplified speaking diaphragms, etc.

- *Durability* — Answer the following questions: How sturdy is the unit? Are plastic parts easily broken? Will the unit stand up to rough treatment?

- *Lifecycle cost* — Include the initial purchase price (which may have to be estimated based on the list price) and the cost of annual maintenance, parts, and support amortized over the life expectancy of the unit to determine lifecycle cost.

- *Maintenance requirements* — Determine maintenance requirements by considering the manufacturer's suggested maintenance schedule, the level of technician certification and training, and whether maintenance can be done in-house or by a contract vendor approved by the manufacturer.

- *Infrastructure* — Answer the following questions: What is the existing infrastructure that supports the current brand of respiratory protection equipment? What changes or investments are required to reequip the respiratory protection equipment maintenance facility, modify existing cascade systems, and retrofit apparatus mounting hardware?

When all the data is collected and reviewed, the committee should select the systems that best meet the established needs of the organization. Units that do not meet the criteria should be eliminated from consideration. The committee must be fully aware of purchasing ordinances or laws in the event that specifications are too restrictive and legally prohibited. If specific equipment is determined to meet the organization's needs, thereby precluding an open-bid process, a variance or exemption from the approved purchasing process may be required from the purchasing and legal departments. See Create Bid Specifications section for more information.

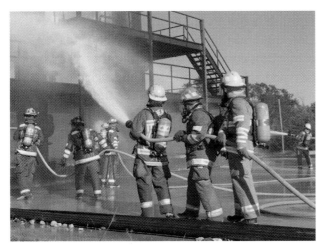

Figure 5.13 The committee must consider the durability, lifecycle cost, and features of the review equipment. For instance, equipment used continuously for training such as the units shown being used for petroleum fire fighting training need to be evaluated differently than units that are only used periodically.

Conduct Purchasing Process

The purchasing procedure for respiratory protection equipment depends on the process adopted and regulated by the authority having jurisdiction. Most respiratory protection equipment such as SCBA and SAR systems are considered capital purchases and must have funds specifically allocated for those purposes. Other items such as HEPA masks, equipment parts, APR cartridges, and equipment accessories may be purchased from operating funds. Some purchases may require a formal bid process while others may be purchased on a purchase order form that does not require an official bid. The committee must be aware of the process and conform to it. Generally, the purchasing process consists of the following steps: Determine the funds available and the source of the funds, create bid specifications based on the evaluation process, evaluate the certified bid proposals, score the bid proposals, and award the contract for purchase.

Determine Funding Sources

The first step in the purchase process is to determine the funding source. Some of the more common sources are operating funds, capital funds, bonds, grants, and lease or lease/purchase arrangements (**Figure 5.14**).

Operating funds. Operating funds are designated in an annual budget for purchasing perishable items. Perishable items are those things that are used up quickly such as disposable filter masks, cartridges, and repair parts (**Figure 5.15**). A projection of the cost and quantity of perishable items must be made and submitted to the finance section of the department/organization prior to the

Funding Sources	
Operating Funds	Bonds
Capital Funds	Grants
Lease or Lease/Purchase	

Figure 5.14 The respiratory protection program committee should consider all funding options available to the jurisdiction during the selection process.

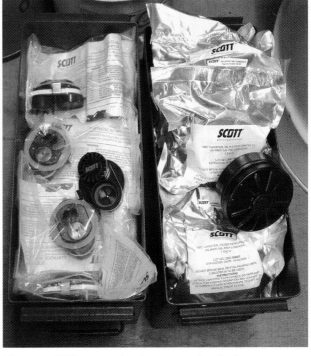

Figure 5.15 The cost of replacements for single-use cartridges, canisters, and filters such as these stored in a ready-to-use case must be calculated during the selection process. The impact of these costs on the annual operating budget must be considered. *Courtesy of Kenneth Baum.*

approval of the annual budget. The value of a purchased item is usually restricted to a specific value such as "less than $1,000."

Capital funds. Capital purchase funds are designated in an annual budget for purchasing capital items. Capital purchases consist of those items over a fixed value such as "more than $1,000" with a life expectancy of more than 1 year. Capital purchases include items such as SCBAs, SAR systems, air compressors, and apparatus (**Figure 5.16**). These items are requested specifically during budget preparation and purchased through the bid process if approved

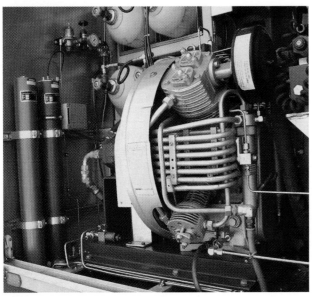

Figure 15.16 Breathing air compressors like this apparatus-mounted unit are usually considered capital purchase items and may require a different purchasing process than perishable items that are purchased through the operating budget. *Courtesy of Lloyd Lees.*

Bonds. While both capital purchase and operating funds usually come from the jurisdiction's primary funding source such as sales or property taxes, bonds provide specific funds for specific projects or purchases. Bonds that are issued by a jurisdiction and purchased by investors must be approved by a vote of the population. Bonds are set for a fixed amount, a specified time period, and specific items. Bond issues are used for large-cost projects such as the replacement of the entire respiratory protection system in use by a department/organization. Because they depend on the approval of voters, bond proposals must be supported by good documentation and justified to the population.

Grants. Grants are a source of funds provided by governmental agencies and nongovernmental organizations. Grants are intended to provide equipment that an organization may not have the funds to purchase. For instance in the United States, an organization that must respond to transportation incidents that involve hazardous materials on an interstate highway can apply for a grant from the U.S. Department of Transportation for funds to purchase hazardous materials response protective clothing and the appropriate level of respiratory protection equipment. Grant funds do not have to be paid back, but the jurisdiction receiving the grant must be accountable for how the funds are spent.

Lease or lease/purchase. Although not a funding source as such, a lease or lease/purchase is another method of obtaining or purchasing capital items. Again, the purchasing ordinances and laws of the jurisdiction govern this method. In some cases it may be illegal to encumber funds in the subsequent budget cycle, thereby preventing a lease. The committee must research this form of acquisition or purchase before including it in bid specifications. A lease can be used when equipment is needed only for a short duration or for extended evaluations. A lease/purchase arrangement allows the cost to be spread over 3 to 5 years. A cost/benefit analysis must be made to compare the direct purchase of equipment with the lease/purchase process cost.

Create Bid Specifications
[NFPA 1852: 5.1.7, 5.1.7.1, 5.1.7.2, 5.1.8]

Once the funding source is established and committed, the committee must develop the actual bid specifications (**Figure 5.17**). The bid specifications include the specific respiratory protection equipment requirements of the department/organization plus the legal requirements of the finance or purchasing officer of the jurisdiction. The legal requirements, sometimes referred to as *boiler plate*, are prepared by the purchasing department and define the legal obligations that are necessary to meet the specifications and are required in all bid specifications. These requirements may include vendor attendance at a pre-bid meeting, warranties, liability or performance bonds, specified delivery times, payment schedules, and financial statements. The respiratory protection program

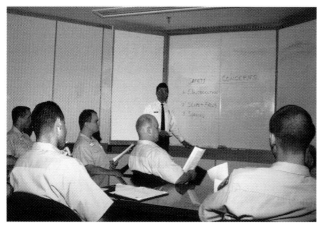

Figure 5.17 When all the information on various products, legal requirements, and purchasing considerations is gathered, the committee must develop specifications for the respiratory protection system to be purchased. The committee may wish to use a consensus approach by listing on a chalkboard the important features of each model and then voting on them.

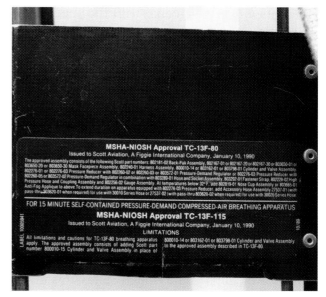

Figure 5.18 One important element of the specifications for fire fighting respiratory protection equipment is the requirement that it be NIOSH/MSHA approved for that use. The equipment, such as this SCBA harness, must carry the appropriate label.

committee does not develop these particular sections of the specifications but should be aware of them and their impact on potential bidders.

The development of the product-specific specifications is the responsibility of the respiratory protection program committee. The language must be clear and concise. Each detail of the design requirement must be included and nothing should be assumed. Some of the topics that should be included in bid specifications are as follows:

- NIOSH/MSHA (current standard) or American National Standards Institute (ANSI) certification for the intended use (**Figure 5.18**)
- NFPA compliance
- Number to be purchased
- Design requirements
- Delivery date
- Warranty
- Accessories
- Training for maintenance technicians
- Training for operational personnel
- Spare cylinders
- Facepiece fit-testing kit
- Startup parts inventory
- Acceptance testing
- Technical support
- Replacement or loaner units

If a specific feature that meets valid operational requirements is only available from a single manufacturer, an option for bidding an equal alternative or a method to take exception to the specifications must be included. Including too many specifications that only one manufacturer can meet results in a restrictive bid that may be prohibited by the purchasing ordinances or laws of the jurisdiction. If a specific brand is the only type that meets the needs of the department/organization, then the finance or purchasing officer of the jurisdiction may be able to grant a variance or exemption for a sole-source bid and declare that specific brand as the jurisdiction's standard.

Most manufacturers provide sample specifications forms as a guide. Specifications usually have to be approved by the jurisdiction's finance or purchasing officer. Once approved, the purchasing department issues the bid requests to the qualified bidders and sets a date for the opening of the bids. The bids may only be returned to and handled by the purchasing department. Once received, the qualified bids are turned over to the respiratory protection program committee for evaluation.

Evaluate and Score Proposals

The evaluation process of the qualified bids is based on the original bid specifications. A matrix or spreadsheet can be created with the specific requirements listed down the side and individual bidders listed across the top (**Figure 5.19**). Values can be assigned to each requirement and filled into the corresponding box, depending on whether or not the bidder exceeded, met, or failed to meet the specification.

Once the grid is filled, the scores are added. If certain specifications outweigh others, the scoring can be weighted in favor of the more important specification. For example, a buddy-breathing accessory or integrated PASS device would receive more points than a carrying case or neck strap. Scoring must be equitable and well documented. In most jurisdictions in the United States, this material may be subject to the Freedom of Information Act and, therefore, subject to outside review.

Evaluation Matrix						
Critieria	**A**	**B**	**C**	**D**	**E**	**F**
NIOSH/MSHA Certified						
Warranty						
Training Provided						
Accessories						
Facepiece Fit Test Kit						
Technical Support						
Spare Cylinder						
Maintenance Contract						
Loaner Units						
Delivery Date						
Meets Specifications						

Figure 5.19 A matrix such as this one may be of assistance in the bid evaluation process.

Award Contract

After the committee has reviewed the bids and made their recommendation to the chief, CEO, or department head, the bid must be awarded by the jurisdiction. Usually the legal department writes a contract and then awards it to the winning supplier. The contract binds both the supplier to meet the specifications and the jurisdiction to pay for the goods or services. Administration of the contract is the responsibility of the purchasing department on behalf of the emergency services organization that receives the goods or services. The emergency ser-

vices organization, through the respiratory protection program committee, is responsible for implementing the respiratory protection program for which the equipment was purchased.

Implement Respiratory Protection Program

The implementation of the respiratory protection program may be assigned to the entire respiratory protection program committee or to a single individual such as the health and safety officer, training officer, or logistics officer. Implementation consists of conducting personnel medical evaluations, facepiece fit testing, and training of operational and maintenance personnel. It also involves establishing a record-keeping process, inventorying and acceptance testing new equipment, identifying required support needs, purchasing additional accessories, and making a transition to the new or upgraded equipment.

Conduct Medical Evaluations

[NFPA 1500: 10.1.1]

All personnel who are expected to use respiratory protection equipment must have a full medical examination and be certified to perform firefighter/emergency responder duties. Medical examinations and evaluations can take place prior to the receipt of the respiratory protection equipment. Medical records are confidential and result in only a "pass/fail" determination report (**Figure 5.20**). Medical requirements are covered in detail in Chapter 6, Medical Requirements and Facepiece Fit Testing.

Conduct Facepiece Fit Testing

To ensure a complete face seal, every individual who wears respiratory protection equipment must undergo facepiece fit testing. Like the medical examination, this testing is mandatory (**Figure 5.21**). Facepiece fit testing is also covered in Chapter 6, Medical Requirements and Facepiece Fit Testing.

Conduct Training

[NFPA 1404: 6.2.1]

Training in the use, care, cleaning, and storage of the respiratory protection equipment can begin with the training personnel and the evaluation units

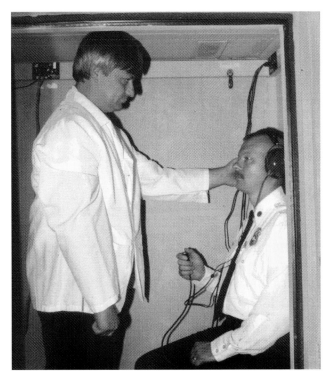

Figure 5.20 All personnel who are required to use respiratory protection equipment must undergo both medical evaluations and examinations. Medical examinations require hearing tests such as the one shown.

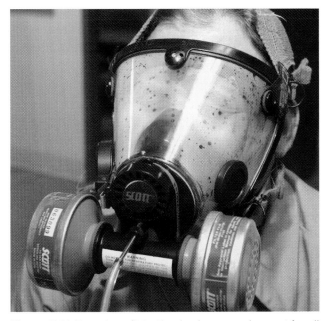

Figure 5.21 Facepiece fit testing is also a requirement for all personnel who use respiratory protection equipment. Fit testing must be performed on every type of facepiece worn by individuals.

if they are still available. The manufacturer's representatives conduct this initial training. The training staff then develops training programs and schedules for the remaining emergency response

employees of the department/organization (**Figure 5.22**). Chapter 7, Training, discusses this phase of the process.

Maintenance personnel must also be trained and certified by the manufacturer to work on the specific brand and model purchased by the organization. Whether equipment maintenance, testing, and repair are performed within the emergency response organization or through a separate department of the jurisdiction, maintenance personnel must be trained and certified. If the work is contracted to an outside vendor, that vendor must provide documentation that its technicians are certified (**Figure 5.23**). Manufacturers usually provide certification courses with the purchase of

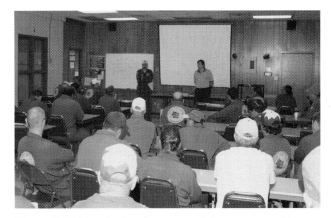

Figure 5.22 Manufacturer's representatives can provide initial training on new equipment as well as maintenance training for the organization's respiratory protection equipment maintenance technicians.

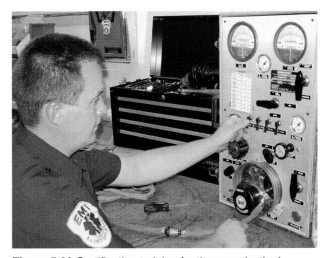

Figure 5.23 Certification training for the organization's maintenance personnel includes trouble-shooting problems, repair techniques, and the use of testing equipment such as the one shown. The manufacturer may require periodic recertification training.

equipment or at an additional charge. Manufacturers also require periodic recertification of maintenance personnel. This potential cost must be considered when determining the best source for respiratory protection equipment maintenance and testing.

Establish Record Keeping and Tracking Process
[NFPA 1404: 6.1.2, 7.2.1, 7.3.1]
[NFPA 1852: 4.4.8]

A complete record for each respiratory protection unit must be kept by the organization. The units may be tracked by a fixed asset number provided by the department/organization or by the serial number on the regulator (**Figure 5.24**). Individual reusable facepieces and masks may be tracked by either a fixed asset number or an employee number when the equipment is assigned to a person. Disposable masks and cartridges do not require this type of record keeping. Records are usually retained by the respiratory protection equipment maintenance section, training officer, or health and safety officer. Records must be available for periodic reviews by any authority having jurisdiction such as OSHA. Records on SCBAs and SAR units must include the following information:

- Purchase date
- Acceptance testing results
- Unit assignment
- Facepiece assignment
- Annual testing results
- Maintenance performed
- Disposal date

Unpack and Conduct Acceptance Testing
[NFPA 1852: 5.2.1, 5.2.2]

When the respiratory protection equipment is delivered, it must be inventoried and tested. It is advisable to assign the unpacking and inventorying to two- or three-person teams in a secure and clean area. As part of the team unpacks the equipment, one member checks the packing slip for accuracy (**Figure 5.25**). The packing slip then is checked against the original order to ensure that the order is complete. The manufacturer's representative must be notified immediately if items appear to be missing or damaged. If possible, the manufacturer's representative should be present

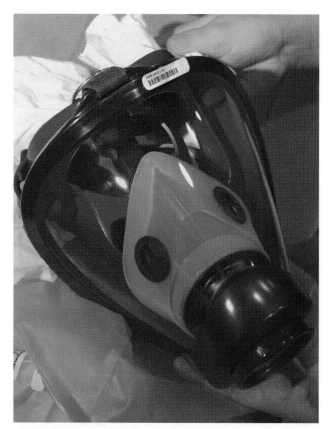

Figure 5.24 All elements of the respiratory protection system should be inventoried for maintenance and tracking purposes. This facepiece is bar coded with a tracking number.

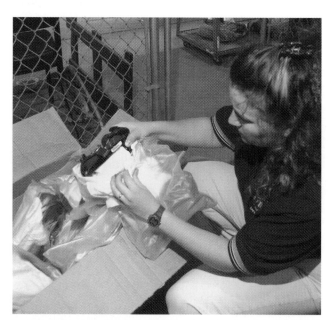

Figure 5.25 New respiratory protection equipment should be carefully unpacked, checked for defects and accuracy of the shipment, and then placed into the organization's inventory database.

during the unpacking of the equipment. When all the equipment is checked in, temporary inventory numbers can be assigned. These numbers become permanent once the units pass the acceptance testing.

Acceptance testing follows a variety of methods depending on the type of equipment purchased. These equipment types and procedures are as follows:

- *Respiratory protection systems* — Systems such as SCBA, combination SCBA/SAR units, or SAR units should be inspected visually, assembled, charged with air, given a dynamic breathing or Posi-Chek® bench test, and worn in a simulated exercise. Each unit should be given the same test to ensure that they all work properly. NFPA 1852, *Standard on Selection, Care, and Maintenance of Open-Circuit Self-Contained Breathing Apparatus*, establishes the testing criteria for these units.

- *Air-purifying respirators* — These units should be given a visual inspection. A representative selection of the units should be worn in a simulated exercise. Because the exposure to air may reduce the life of the cartridges, they should not be opened before use.

- *Disposable filter masks* — Masks should be inspected visually. Because the exposure to air may reduce the life of the filter, individually wrapped masks should not be opened until time of use.

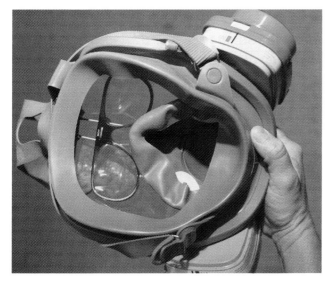

Figure 5.26 Perishable parts such as air-purifying filters and accessories like the eyeglass kit shown here installed in a facepiece require only a visual inspection before placing into storage or use.

- *Parts and accessories* — These items need only a visual inspection to ensure compliance with the specifications (**Figure 5.26**).

Once all the equipment has satisfactorily passed the acceptance test or visual inspection, the purchase order may be approved and forwarded to the financial or purchasing department for payment. The manufacturer and the purchasing department should be notified immediately if any of the equipment does not pass the acceptance test. It is the responsibility of the manufacturer to correct the deficiencies. The purchasing department determines whether it is appropriate to withhold payment until the situation is resolved (**Figure 5.27**).

Identify Required Support Needs

Depending on the type of respiratory protection equipment purchased, a variety of support equipment or materials may be required. These items should have been identified during the research phase of the process. If an item is a major purchase such as the breathing-air compressor, it needs to be included with the purchase of the respiratory protection system. Other items like cleaning supplies may already be available through the operating budget. Among support products that may be required are the following:

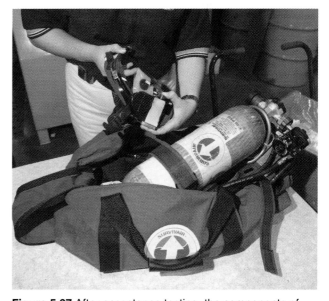

Figure 5.27 After acceptance testing, the components of the new respiratory protection system should be assembled into complete units, including all the accessories that will be provided with each unit, in this case a soft-sided carrying bag.

- Breathing-air compressor
- Breathing-air fill station
- Mobile breathing-air system (**Figure 5.28**)
- Specialized maintenance tools
- Clean room for respiratory protection equipment maintenance
- Computer inventory database program
- Airflow breathing machine
- Secure equipment inventory storage area
- Disinfecting sinks (**Figure 5.29**)
- Cleaning products/supplies

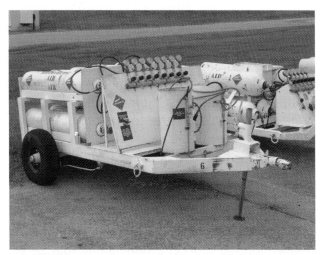

Figure 5.28 The need for support equipment such as this mobile trailer-mounted breathing air cascade system should be taken into consideration during the research phase of the purchasing process.

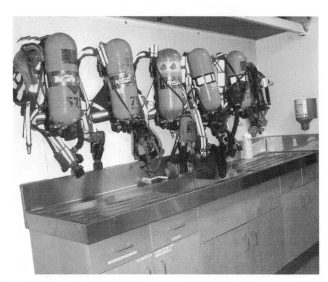

Figure 5.29 Changes and additions to the organization's facilities may include respiratory protection maintenance "clean rooms," cylinder storage areas, and disinfecting and drying areas like the one shown. *Courtesy of Lloyd Lees.*

Purchase Accessories

The respiratory protection system accessories should have been identified and purchased with the systems. However, acceptance testing and initial deployment of the equipment may identify further requirements. Accessories are not usually expensive and can be purchased from the operating budget. Apparatus mounting hardware, storage containers, eyeglass holders, and air-supply line covers can be purchased as needed (**Figure 5.30**). More expensive items such as spare cylinders may have to be added to the next budget request cycle.

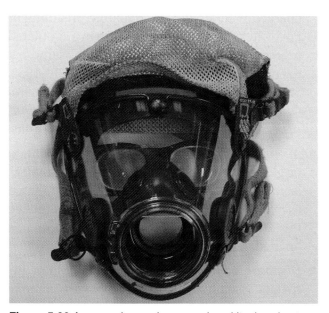

Figure 5.30 Accessories such as eyeglass kits, head nets, or facepiece bags may be purchased from the annual operating budget as the need arises.

Make Transition to New or Upgraded Equipment

Deployment of the respiratory protection equipment depends on the type of equipment and whether it is new or replacing an existing system. Training is the first step in the deployment process. Training may begin with the evaluation units or as units are prepared for service. The manufacturer's representative or a department/organization training officer is responsible for this function. The health and safety officer or members of the respiratory protection program committee may need to answer questions and assist in the process. In departments/organizations where personnel are assigned to rotating shifts, all shifts should be trained prior to placing the equipment in service. See Chapter 10, Emergency Scene Use, for information on developing operational protocols.

If the new equipment is replacing a different equipment type, model, or brand, the transition process requires a systematic approach. This approach may involve deploying the new equipment by battalion or district to prevent the possibility of confusion among personnel. If high-pressure SCBA systems are intermixed with standard pressure units, it is essential that personnel understand the difference and units are marked appropriately (**Figure 5.31**). In any case, the transition requires supervision and control from the respiratory protection program committee, training officer, or health and safety officer.

Evaluate Respiratory Protection Program

The duties of the respiratory protection program committee do not end with the deployment of new equipment. Because the respiratory protection program is a continuous process, the committee must be available to monitor the program. Comments from field personnel, incidents involving the equipment, comments from maintenance personnel, frequency of repairs, maintenance costs, manufacturer support, and changes in operational procedures must be recorded, analyzed, and addressed. Should the respiratory protection system prove inadequate or if operational procedures need to be altered, the committee must be available to make recommendations to the chief, CEO, or department head. The program should be reviewed annually by starting at step one of the selection justification and procurement process.

Summary

The development of a respiratory protection program can be a long and involved process. The project can be efficient and effective with administrative commitment, membership participation, leadership, and a process model. A respiratory protection program is mandatory, and it protects both the membership and the organization. Thorough record keeping is an essential part of both the program and the process. Finally, the respiratory protection program is an ongoing process and not a one-time event.

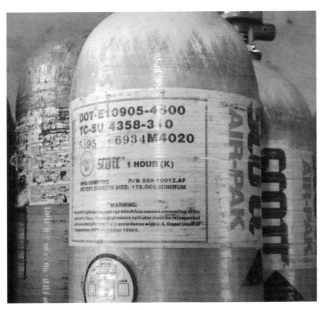

Figure 5.31 If the organization is transitioning into a system that is not compatible with the current system, personnel must be trained to recognize differences between the systems to prevent mixing the unit components. High-pressure cylinders shown here must be distinctly marked to prevent use with low-pressure systems.

Medical Requirements and Facepiece Fit Testing

This chapter provides information that will assist the reader in meeting the following job performance requirements from NFPA 1404, *Standard for Fire Service Respiratory Protection Training*, 2002 Edition, and NFPA 1500, *Standard on Fire Department Occupational Safety and Health Program*, 2002 Edition.

NFPA 1500

4.6.1   The fire department shall establish a data collection system and maintain permanent records of all accidents, injuries, illnesses, exposures to infectious agents and communicable diseases, or deaths that are job related.

4.6.2   The data collection system shall also maintain individual records of any occupational exposure to known or suspected toxic products or infectious or communicable diseases.

4.6.3   The fire department shall assure that a confidential health record for each member and a health database is maintained.

4.13.2   The health and safety officer shall assist and make recommendations regarding the evaluation of new equipment and its acceptance or approval by the fire department in accordance with the applicable provisions of Chapter 6.

4.13.3   The health and safety officer shall assist and make recommendations regarding the service testing of apparatus and equipment to determine its suitability for continued service and in accordance with Chapter 6.

4.13.4   The health and safety officer shall develop, implement, and maintain a protective clothing and protective equipment program that will meet the requirements of Chapter 6, and provide for the periodic inspection and evaluation of all protective clothing and equipment to determine its suitability for continued service.

4.16.1   The health and safety officer shall be a member of the fire department occupational safety and health committee.

4.16.5   The health and safety officer shall maintain a liaison with staff officers regarding recommended changes in equipment, procedures, and recommended methods to eliminate unsafe practices and reduce existing hazardous conditions.

4.16.6   The health and safety officer shall maintain a liaison with equipment manufacturers, standards-making organizations, regulatory agencies, and safety specialists outside the fire department regarding changes to equipment and procedures and methods to eliminate unsafe practices and reduce existing hazardous conditions.

4.16.7   The health and safety officer shall maintain a liaison with the fire department physician to ensure that needed medical advice and treatment are available to the members of the fire department.

7.12.1   The facepiece seal capability of each member qualified to use respiratory protection equipment shall be verified by qualitative or quantitative fit testing on an annual basis and whenever new types of respiratory protection equipment or facepieces are issued.

7.12.2   The fit of the respiratory protection equipment of each new member shall be tested before the members are permitted to use respiratory protection equipment in a hazardous atmosphere. Only members with a properly fitting facepiece shall be permitted by the fire department to function in a hazardous atmosphere with respiratory protection equipment.

7.12.3   Fit testing of tight-fitting atmosphere-supplying respirators and tight-fitting powered air-purifying respirators shall be accomplished by performing quantitative or qualitative fit testing in the negative-pressure mode, regardless of the mode of operation (negative or positive pressure) that is used for respiratory protection.

7.12.4   Qualitative or quantitative test protocols shall be conducted as required by the authority having jurisdiction.

7.12.5   Records of facepiece fitting tests shall include at least the following information:

(1)   Name of the member tested

(2)   Type of fitting test performed

(3)   Specific make and model of facepieces tested

(4)   Pass/Fail results of the tests

7.12.6   For departments that perform quantitative fitting tests, the protection factor produced shall be at least 500 for negative-pressure facepieces for the person to pass the fitting test with that full facepiece.

10.1.1   Candidates shall be medically evaluated and certified by the fire department physician.

10.1.2   Medical evaluations shall take into account the risks and the functions associated with the individual's duties and responsibilities.

10.1.3   Candidates and members who will engage in fire suppression shall meet the medical requirements specified in NFPA 1582, *Standard on Medical Requirements for Fire Fighters and Information for Fire Department Physicians*, prior to being medically certified for duty by the fire department physician.

10.4.1   The fire department shall ensure that a confidential, permanent health file is established and maintained on each individual member.

10.4.2   The individual health file shall record the results of regular medical evaluations and physical performance tests, any occupational illnesses or injuries, and any events that expose the individual to known or suspected hazardous materials, toxic products, or contagious diseases.

10.4.3   Health information shall be maintained as a confidential record for each individual member as well as a composite database for the analysis of factors pertaining to the overall health and fitness of the member group.

10.6.1   The fire department shall have an officially designated physician who shall be responsible for guiding, directing, and advising the members with regard to their health, fitness, and suitability for various duties.

10.6.3   The fire department physician shall be a licensed medical doctor or osteopathic physician qualified to provide professional expertise in the areas of occupational safety and health as they relate to emergency services.

NFPA 1404

6.1.4 Fit-testing procedures as provided in NFPA 1500, *Standard on Fire Department Occupational Safety and Health Program*, shall be required for all recruits who are expected to use a tight-fitting facepiece respirator, including SCBA, SAR units, and FFAPRs that use a full facepiece, prior to training in contaminated atmospheres.

6.1.5 Prior to initial training, members shall be examined and certified by a physician as being medically and physically fit in accordance with the following:

(1) NFPA 1500, *Standard on Fire Department Occupational Safety and Health Program*

(2) NFPA 1582, *Standard on Medical Requirements for Fire Fighters and Information for Fire Department Physicians*

(3) Physical fitness requirements developed and validated by the authority having jurisdiction for entry level personnel

Chapter 6
Medical Requirements and Facepiece Fit Testing

The effectiveness of a respiratory protection program is determined by the following factors:

- Administrative commitment
- User commitment
- Accurate risk assessment
- Selection and purchase of the appropriate respiratory protection equipment
- Thorough inspection and maintenance programs
- Effective training program
- Personnel medical testing and record keeping
- Facepiece fit testing

A critical component of the respiratory protection program is the medical testing and certification for all individuals who use respiratory protection equipment. To ensure the maximum level of respiratory protection, facepiece fit testing must be provided for each member and for each type of respiratory protection facepiece or mask that members will wear. This chapter outlines the requirements for medical testing and facepiece fit testing.

Medical Requirements

As mentioned in Chapter 2, Regulations and Standards, the medical requirements for a respiratory protection program are found in the following documents:

- NFPA 1404, *Standard for Fire Service Respiratory Protection Training*
- NFPA 1500, *Standard on Fire Department Occupational Safety and Health Program*
- NFPA 1582, *Standard on Medical Requirements for Fire Fighters*

- ANSI Z88.2-1992, Practices for Respiratory Protection
- ANSI Z88.6-1984, For Respiratory Protection — Respirator Use — Physical Qualifications for Personnel
- ANSI Z88.10-2001, Fit Testing Methods
- CSA Z94.4-1993, Selection, Use, and Care of Respirators
- OSHA Title 29 (Labor) *CFR* 1910.134, Respiratory Protection Requirements

Areas of concern are medical evaluations/examinations, the role of the physician or licensed health-care professional, record keeping, medical confidentiality, the role of the health and safety officer in the process, and the requirement for a letter of certification for personnel assigned to use respiratory protection equipment.

Physician/Licensed Health-Care Professional Role
[NFPA 1500: 10.6.1, 10.6.3]

Both NFPA 1500 and NFPA 1582 require the fire department and/or emergency services organization to designate a physician to provide medical direction in the areas of occupational safety and health as it pertains to emergency services. NFPA 1582 requires the physician to "be a licensed doctor of medicine or osteopathy who shall be responsible for guiding, directing, and advising the members with regard to their health, fitness, and suitability for duty as required by NFPA 1500, *Standard on Fire Department Occupational Safety and Health Program*." At the same time, OSHA Title 29 *CFR* 1910.134 designates a physician or licensed health-care professional as being responsible for medical evaluations for personnel assigned the use of respiratory protection equipment. The authority having jurisdiction determines which definition applies.

Physicians or licensed health-care professionals must understand the pertinent physiological and psychological aspects of the emergency response personnel they serve. The physician/licensed health-care professional must be provided with job descriptions for all organizational positions. The physician/licensed health-care professional shall evaluate and medically certify all personnel within the organization whose job descriptions require the use of respirators. The organization's physician/licensed health-care professional shall review medical evaluations that are conducted by a physician (personal or otherwise) other than the organization's physician/licensed health-care professional. Contract services are available for those organizations that do not or cannot provide medical evaluations that comply with NFPA 1582 or OSHA Title 29 *CFR* 1910.134.

Medical Evaluations/Examinations
[NFPA 1500: 10.1.1, 10.1.2, 10.1.3, 10.4.2]
[NFPA 1404: 6.1.5]

NFPA 1404 establishes the requirement for an initial medical examination and certification for all fire service candidates in accordance with the requirements of NFPA 1001, *Standard for Fire Fighter Professional Qualifications*. In turn, NFPA 1001 refers to the medical testing and certification requirements of NFPA 1582. NFPA 1404 also references NFPA 1500 in requiring that all fire and emergency services personnel who are required to use respiratory protection equipment be certified as medically fit. The basic criteria for medical fitness are outlined in NFPA 1582.

Once a candidate has been certified by a physician/licensed health-care professional and has been hired by the organization, annual medical evaluations are required (**Figure 6.1**). These periodic evaluations include the following items:

• Interval medical history

• Interval occupational history including any hazardous materials/disease exposure reports

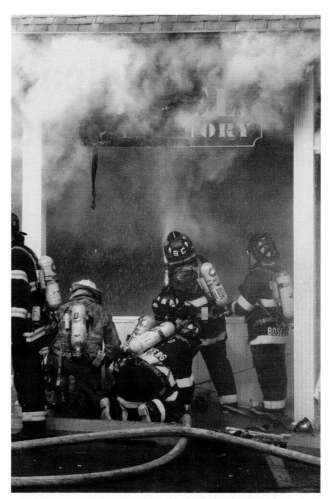

Figure 6.1 The strenuous nature of emergency response mandates that personnel be healthy and physically fit. Periodic medical examinations and evaluations are means to monitor the health of fire and emergency services personnel. *Courtesy of Chris Tompkins.*

• Recording of current height and weight

• Recording of current blood pressure

In addition, medical evaluations are required when an employee has been off duty with an illness or injury and is ready to return to duty. The fire department/emergency services organization physician may also require a medical examination before the employee returns to duty.

Emergency services organizations that are regulated by the Occupational Safety and Health Association (OSHA) will find a medical evaluation form in Title 29 *CFR* 1910.134, Appendix C (OSHA Respiratory Medical Evaluation Questionnaire). The organization's physician may administer this form or a medical examination that determines the answers to the questions on the form. The results of OSHA-mandated medical evaluations are transmitted to the emergency services organization in the form of a "pass/fail" report. If the candidate/member is unable to pass the medical evaluation/examination, then that person is simply not certified to perform the tasks of the organization. No reason can be given due to the patient-physician confidentiality agreement.

In addition to the annual medical evaluations, medical examinations are required periodically, depending on the employee's age (**Figure 6.2**). The age requirements are as follows:

- Under 29 years of age, a medical examination is required every three years.
- Between 30 and 39 years of age, a medical examination is required every two years.
- Over 40 years of age, a medical examination is required every year.

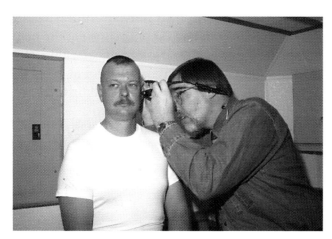

Figure 6.2 The frequency of periodic medical evaluations is based on the age of the individual responder.

Medical examinations are more thorough than medical evaluations. Of particular importance to the respiratory protection program is the pulmonary function testing of the respiratory system. Examinations consist of the following items:

- Vital signs recordings: pulse, respiration, blood pressure, and temperature if needed
- Dermatological system examination
- Ears, eyes, nose, throat, and mouth examinations
- Cardiovascular system examination
- Gastrointestinal system examination
- Respiratory system examination
- Genitourinary system examination

- Endocrine and metabolic system examination
- Musculoskeletal system examination
- Neurological system examination
- Audiometry testing
- Visual acuity and peripheral vision testing (**Figure 6.3**)
- Pulmonary function testing
- Laboratory testing if needed
- Diagnostic testing if needed
- Electrocardiography testing if needed

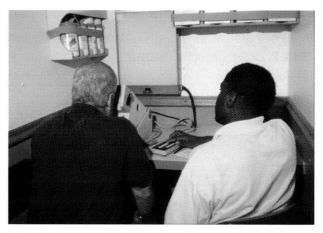

Figure 6.3 Medical examinations are more thorough than medical evaluations and include visual acuity and peripheral vision tests.

Medical Record Keeping
[NFPA 1500: 4.6.1, 4.6.2, 4.6.3]

A complete medical history of each member of the fire and emergency services organization must be maintained by the organization according to NFPA 1500 and 1582. The information maintained in this medical history includes the following reports/results:

- Results of periodic medical evaluations
- Results of physical performance tests
- Reports on occupational illnesses or injuries
- Reports of any exposures to hazardous materials, toxic products, or contagious diseases

The fire and emergency services organization or the jurisdiction's physician maintains these records. The organization's health and safety officer maintains similar records, including information on occupational deaths, injuries, illnesses, and exposures to hazardous materials or diseases. See the Health and Safety Officer Role section later in this chapter.

Medical Confidentiality

[NFPA 1500: 10.4.1, 10.4.3]

All member medical records and analysis of those records are confidential. They may only be released to the individual member or to a designated individual or organization authorized in writing by the individual member (**Figure 6.4**). Medical confidentiality is guaranteed by OSHA Title 29 *CFR* 1910.134 and 1910.1020 (Access to Employee Exposure and Medical Records). A sample authorization for release of medical information letter is provided in 1910.1020, Appendix A (Sample Authorization Letter for the Release of Employee Medical Record Information to a Designated Representative).

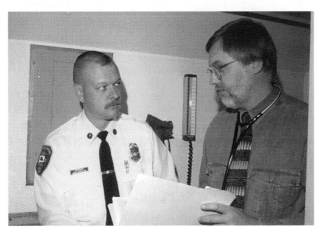

Figure 6.4 The results of medical examinations and evaluations and the contents of an individual's medical records are confidential. The records may only be released by the physician to the individual or a person/organization that is designated in writing by the individual.

Health and Safety Officer Role

[NFPA 1500: 4.13.2, 4.13.3, 4.13.4, 4.16.1, 4.16.5, 4.16.6, 4.16.7]

The organization's health and safety officer can play an instrumental role in the respiratory protection program. When the organization adheres to the NFPA standards, the health and safety officer is assigned the following duties that relate to respiratory protection:

- Act as liaison between the administration and the safety and health program committee and the respiratory protection program committee.

- Act as liaison between the organization and manufacturers, standards-writing organizations, and regulatory agencies.

- Function as the organization's infection control officer or act as liaison with that position.

- Make recommendations regarding the specifications, evaluation, and service testing of equipment, including respiratory protection equipment.

- Develop, implement, and maintain the organization's personal protective equipment program (**Figure 6.5**).

- Act as liaison with the organization's medical officer or physician.

- Collect and maintain data related to issues of safety and health, including the respiratory protection program.

Organizations that do not fall under legally adopted NFPA standards should consider the benefits of having a health and safety officer within their organization. Officials can consult the requirements of their regulatory agency or the authority having jurisdiction for more information.

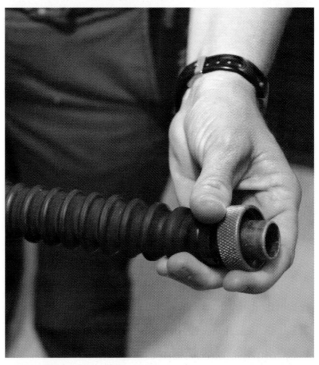

Figure 6.5 As part of the organization's safety and health program, the health and safety officer is responsible for inspecting the organization's personal protective clothing and equipment such as low-pressure hoses and fittings used on belt-mounted regulators.

Letter of Certification

In the United States, OSHA mandates that the organization's medical authority must determine the employee's ability to use a respirator and then provide the organization with a letter of certification to that effect. The written recommendation, which becomes part of the employee's personnel file, must provide the following information:

- Limitations on respirator use related to the medical condition of the employee

- Limitations relating to the workplace conditions in which the respirator will be used

- Whether or not the employee is medically able to use the respirator

- Need (if any) for follow-up medical evaluations

- Statement that the employee has been provided with a copy of the written recommendations

If the respiratory protection equipment worn is a negative-pressure type and the medical authority finds a medical condition that may place the employee's health at increased risk by using the respirator, the organization must provide the employee with a powered air-purifying respirator (PAPR). Employees who fail to pass the medical evaluation are prohibited from using respiratory protection and need to be reassigned to duties that do not contain respiratory hazards.

Facepiece Fit Testing

Because respiratory protection equipment depends on a full and complete seal between the facepiece and the wearer, facepiece fit testing is essential to the respiratory protection program **(Figure 6.6)**. The primary purpose of fit testing is to determine that the make, model, and size of respirator facepiece provides a full and complete seal. The test procedures, test protocols, and record keeping of the facepiece fit-test program are discussed in the sections that follow. In addition, information about equipment calibration, new testing technology, testing types of respiratory protection equipment, and third-party or outside testing contractors is also provided.

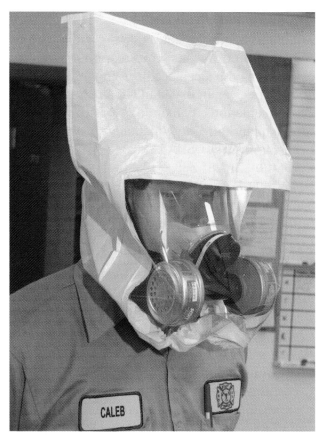

Figure 6.6 Fit testing of individuals who are required to wear respiratory protection equipment ensures that the facepiece will provide complete protection. Both quantitative (shown here) and qualitative protocols for testing may be used in the fit-test process.

Test Procedures

[NFPA 1500: 7.12.1, 7.12.2, 7.12.3, 7.12.4, 7.12.5, 7.12.6]

[NFPA 1404: 6.1.4]

OSHA and NFPA require facepiece fit testing when an employee is hired or transferred into a position that requires performing tasks that expose the employee to hazardous atmospheres. Once the medical evaluation and the letter of certification have established that the employee is physically fit to perform the tasks, an entry-level facepiece fit test is performed using the type or types of respiratory protection equipment that the employee will wear.

Annual retests are required to ensure that no changes have occurred that may compromise the fit of the facepiece. Potential changes include gain or loss of weight, major dental work, facial injuries, a change in facepieces, or a change in respiratory hazards. Along with the fit test, a medical evaluation is also required annually.

Standard Test Protocols

Although NFPA 1500 states that the authority having jurisdiction has the responsibility for establishing the facepiece fit-testing protocol, the guidelines given in that standard are based on the OSHA regulations. Two options for fit-testing protocols (quantitative and qualitative methods) have been approved by OSHA Title 29 *CFR* 1910.134, CSA Z94.4-1993, ANSI Z88.2-1992, Z88.10-2001, and NFPA 1500. Both options check the amount of leakage through the respirator facepiece seal. Of the two options, quantitative fit testing is the most accurate because it measures the concentration of test agent within the mask. The qualitative fit-test method depends on the wearer's senses to detect any leakage. Regardless of the protocol chosen, have the test subject don the facepiece before the fit testing and collect data based on the following observations:

- Assess the comfort of the facepiece by positioning the facepiece on the nose (half mask), ensuring room for eye protection (half mask), ensuring room for communication, and positioning the facepiece on the face and cheeks (**Figure 6.7**).

- Determine the adequacy of the facepiece fit. Address the following items:
  — Chin properly placed in facepiece
  — Adequate strap tension, not overly tight
  — Proper fit across bridge of nose
  — Proper-size facepiece to cover distance from nose to chin
  — Potential slippage of facepiece
  — Self-observation in a mirror to evaluate fit and position

- Have the test subject perform a negative-pressure or positive-pressure user seal check (**Figure 6.8**). See sidebar for instructions.

- Ensure that facial hair does not interfere with the facepiece seal.

- Provide the test subject with an alternate size facepiece if a facepiece fit is unacceptable.

- Give the test subject a description of the fit-test exercises and the subject's responsibilities during the test before beginning the exercises.

- Have the test subject wear the facepiece for at least 5 minutes before beginning the test exercises to allow ambient particles trapped in the facepiece to purge before starting the test (**Figure 6.9**).

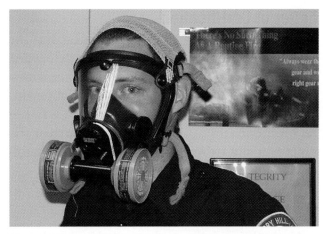

Figure 6.7 The first step in any fit-test protocol is to test for facepiece comfort when the straps are properly adjusted. *Courtesy of Kenneth Baum.*

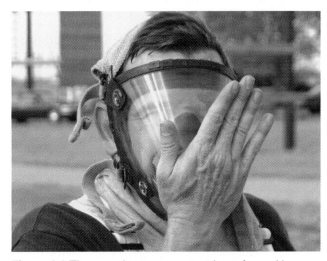

Figure 6.8 The negative-pressure test is performed by placing the hand over the inhalation opening of the facepiece (or end of the low-pressure hose) and inhaling. If the seal is good, the facepiece will collapse against the face. *Courtesy of Bob Parker.*

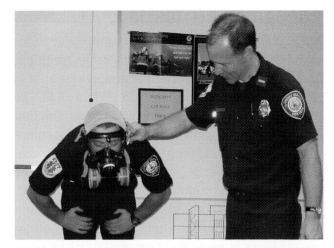

Figure 6.9 Before the fit test, the test subject should wear the facepiece for 5 minutes. During this time, the evaluator should observe the subject for any signs of stress such as shortness of breath or hyperventilation. *Courtesy of Kenneth Baum.*

Facepiece Positive- and/or Negative-Pressure Checks

- **Positive-pressure check** — Close off the exhalation valve and exhale gently into the facepiece. The face fit is considered satisfactory if a slight positive pressure can be built up inside the facepiece without any evidence of outward leakage of air at the seal.

- **Negative-pressure check** — Close off the inlet opening of the facepiece or canister/cartridge by covering with the palm of the hand or by replacing the filter seal(s), inhale gently so that the facepiece collapses slightly, and hold the breath for 10 seconds. The design of the inlet opening of some cartridges cannot be effectively covered with the palm of the hand. The test can be performed by covering the inlet opening of the cartridge with a thin latex or nitrile glove. If the facepiece remains in its slightly collapsed condition and no inward leakage of air is detected, the tightness of the seal is considered satisfactory.

The test subject must wear any personal protective equipment normally worn with the facepiece. Include the required level of personal protective clothing (head protection, eye protection, protective hood, and protective coat and pants) when the test involves a self-contained breathing apparatus (SCBA) facepiece (**Figure 6.10**).

NOTE: To ensure a proper fit of the facepiece during fit testing, training, and emergency use, the wearer should perform a user seal check every time the facepiece is donned.

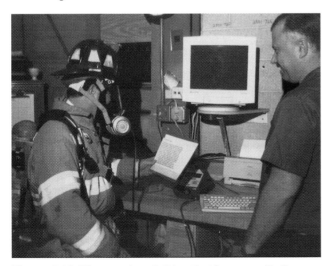

Figure 6.10 All protective clothing that is worn with the respiratory protection equipment must be worn during the fit test.

Use the following standard test exercise sequence with all qualitative and quantitative test protocols *except* the quantitative controlled negative-pressure (CNP) test protocol. The exercise program used with the CNP protocol is listed later in the chapter (see Quantitative Fit-Test Method section). The text subject performs each exercise for 1 minute with the exception of the grimace, which is performed for 15 seconds. The test exercise sequence is as follows:

- **Breathe Normally** — Perform while standing in a normal position without talking.

- **Breathe Deeply** — Perform while standing in a normal position without talking. Take slow, deep breaths.

- **Turn Head from Side to Side** — Perform while standing in a normal position without talking. Rotate the head to its fullest extent from side to side. Inhale at the extreme points of rotation (**Figure 6.11**).

- **Move Head Up and Down** — Perform while standing in a normal position without talking. Move the head slowly up and down on the center axis of the body. Inhale when looking up (**Figure 6.12**).

- **Talk** — Perform while standing in a normal position. Talk out loud slowly. Read from a prepared text (see sidebar on p. 136 for example), count backward from 100, or quote a memorized passage or verse (**Figure 6.13**).

  NOTE: The test administrator must hear the test subject clearly.

- **Grimace** — Perform while standing in a normal position. Frown or smile to create a facial grimace.

  NOTE: The grimace is only used in the quantitative test protocol and not the qualitative test protocol. The grimace exercise tests the respirator's ability to reseal to the wearer's face, and the results are used to calculate the fit factor (see Quantitative Fit-Test Method section).

- **Bend Over** — Perform while standing in a normal position without talking. Bend at the waist as though attempting to touch the toes (**Figure 6.14**).

NOTE: If the shroud-type test unit that does not permit this movement is used, jogging in place is permitted.

- *Breathe Normally* — Perform while standing in a normal position without talking.

At the end of the test protocol, the test subject is questioned about the comfort of the facepiece. If the comfort level is unacceptable, the test is repeated with a different size or type of facepiece. Any adjustment to the facepiece during the test protocol voids the test and causes it to be repeated.

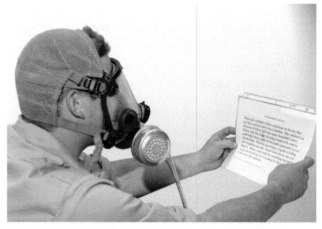

Figure 6.13 The talking portion of the fit test requires the subject to read a passage (such as the Rainbow Passage) loud enough for the test administrator to understand the material.

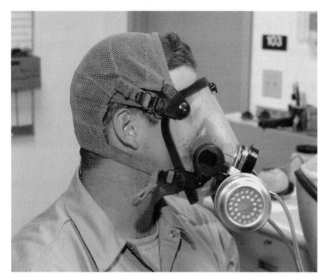

Figure 6.11 The fit test requires that the subject rotate the head from side to side, inhaling at the extreme points of rotation.

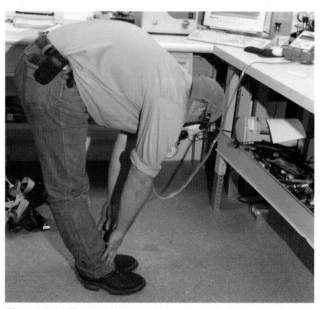

Figure 6.14 The subject must bend over and attempt to touch the toes during the fit-test protocol.

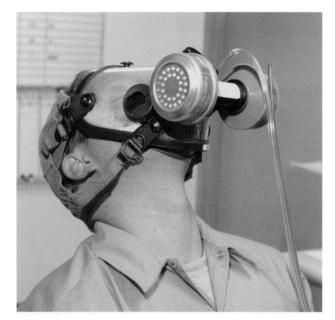

Figure 6.12 The head is raised and lowered on the center of the body's axis, with inhalation taking place when the subject is looking up.

Rainbow Passage

The following paragraph is the OSHA-recommended prepared text for the talk portion of the test exercise:

When the sunlight strikes raindrops in the air, they act like a prism and form a rainbow. The rainbow is a division of white light into many beautiful colors. These take the shape of a long round arch, with its path high above and its two ends apparently beyond the horizon. There is, according to legend, a boiling pot of gold at one end. People look, but no one ever finds it. When a man looks for something beyond reach, his friends say he is looking for the pot of gold at the end of the rainbow.

Quantitative Fit-Test Method

The measurement of the effectiveness of a respirator seal in the ambient atmosphere is determined most accurately by a quantitative fit test. Because all qualitative fit testing is subjective, a quantitative fit test (QNFT) is the preferred method of testing facepiece seal. Two types of quantitative tests are found in the OSHA guidelines: condensation nuclei counting (CNC) and controlled negative pressure. The controlled negative pressure protocol is discussed later in this section. In the CNC quantitative tests, the amount of particulates within the facepiece is compared to the amount in the ambient air outside the facepiece. This protocol may be performed within a test chamber or without a test chamber. The facepiece is equipped with a sampling probe that is connected with flexible tubing to a portable or nonportable test instrument such as the PortaCount® respiratory fit tester or similar device. The test facepiece must be constructed so that no leakage occurs around the port where the probe is attached. The probe must be midway between the nose and mouth and at least ¼ inch (6.4 mm) into the facepiece cavity. While wearing the probe-equipped facepiece in a controlled test atmosphere (a test chamber or shroud containing a required concentration of test agent), the wearer performs the test exercises mentioned earlier. The test instrument records test-agent facepiece penetration values in parts per million (ppm). These values are then converted to a protection factor or *fit factor:* the ratio of the test-agent concentration outside the facepiece to the test-agent concentration inside the facepiece (see sidebar). The ratio indicates how well the facepiece is sealed.

Fit Factor

The fit factor is the concentration within the facepiece divided by the concentration outside the facepiece. For full facepiece units the minimum factor allowed is 500. For half facepiece units the minimum factor allowed is 100. If the ratio is equal to or greater than these respective quantities, the quantitative fit test (QNFT) has been passed with that respirator.

Both quantitative test protocols are approved by OSHA in Title 29 *CFR* 1910.134, Appendix A, Fit Testing Procedures (Mandatory). OSHA requirements for the quantitative fit-test protocols include trained personnel, a test chamber for nonhazardous test aerosols, instrumentation equipment, and test agents. Testing personnel must be able to calibrate the equipment, perform the test protocol, recognize invalid tests, calculate fit factors, and maintain the equipment in clean working order. The test chamber must be large enough for the test subject to freely perform all required exercises without disturbing the instrumentation arrangement or the test-agent concentration. The test setup must allow the test administrator to view the test subject inside the chamber. Instrumentation equipment may be the PortaCount® condensation nuclei counter, a controlled negative-pressure instrument, or some other approved fit-test instrument. It must be operated, calibrated, and maintained according to the manufacturer's instructions (**Figure 6.15**). It must produce a printed record that shows the increase and decrease of the test concentration with each inspiration and expiration at fit factors of at least 2,000. Testing agents may be corn oil, polyethylene glycol 400, di-2-ethyl hexyl sebacate, or sodium chloride. Facepieces that are used in the fit-test protocol must be the same model that will be worn during emergency operations. Any accessories, such as eyeglass kits, must be installed in the facepieces used for fit testing (**Figure 6.16**).

Because quantitative fit testing is highly technical and requires specific testing agents, test atmospheres, test-booth designs, test instrumentation, and exacting mathematical computations, it is recommended that fire and emergency services

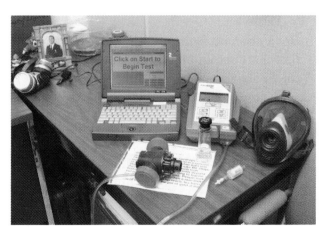

Figure 6.15 All approved fit-test instruments (such as the PortaCount® condensation nuclei counter shown) must be operated, calibrated, and maintained in accordance with the manufacturer's instructions.

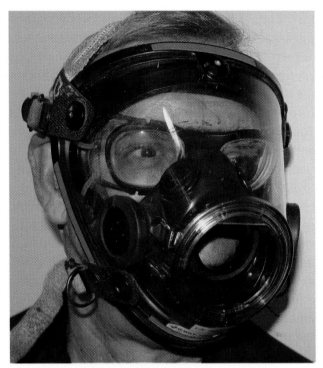

Figure 6.16 If the test subject will use accessories such as eyeglass kits with the facepiece, those accessories must be in place during the fit test. *Courtesy of Kenneth Baum.*

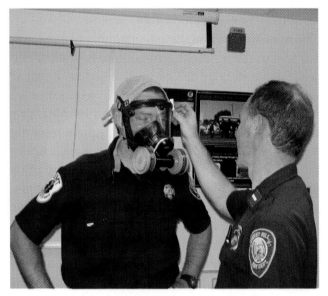

Figure 6.17 The test administrator may use an abbreviated qualitative fit test to identify poorly fitting facepieces before the beginning of a quantitative fit test. *Courtesy of Kenneth Baum.*

have the testing done by personnel trained by the test machine manufacturer. These personnel may be members of the fire and emergency services organization or employees of a firm under contract to perform the fit testing. The accuracy of the quantitative fit-testing protocol is offset by the high cost of the equipment, training, materials, and test personnel or an outside contractor.

Information specific to each of the three accepted quantitative fit-test protocols approved by OSHA (CNC with test chamber, CNC without test chamber, or controlled negative pressure) is as follows:

1. **Use a nonhazardous test aerosol generated in a test chamber and instrumentation to quantify the fit of a facepiece.**

   • When the initial facepiece seal check is made, the sampling hose must be crimped closed during the positive- or negative-pressure test.

   • Either an abbreviated qualitative test or a CNC quantitative test instrument in the count mode may be used to identify poorly fitting facepieces prior to beginning the quantitative test (**Figure 6.17**).

   • When the test subject enters the test chamber, the concentration of the test agent is

measured. The peak concentration must not exceed 5 percent for a half mask or 1 percent for a full facepiece. If this peak level exceeds these percentages during the test, the test must be terminated immediately.

   • A stable concentration of the test agent must be obtained in the test chamber before beginning the test.

   • The fit factor is determined by the ratio of the average chamber concentration to the concentration measured in the facepiece for each exercise *except* the face grimace.

   • The concentration of test agent inside the facepiece is determined by one of three methods: (1) an average peak penetration based on a computer calculation, (2) the maximum peak penetration based on a strip chart of the highest peaks for each exercise, or (3) integration by calculation of the area under each individual peak for each exercise.

   • The calculation of the overall fit factor involves converting the exercise fit factors to penetration values, determining the average, and then converting that result back to a fit factor.

   • The test subject does not pass unless a fit factor of 100 or better is achieved for a half or quarter mask or a minimum fit factor of 500 is achieved for a full facepiece.

2. **Use ambient atmosphere as the test agent and appropriate instrumentation such as the PortaCount® condensation nuclei counter to quantify the fit of a facepiece (Figure 6.18).**

- The CNC test does not require the use of a test chamber or shroud or test agents. It depends on the particulates in the ambient atmosphere.

- The probe attaches to the test facepiece as indicated earlier.

- The test exercise protocol is the same as that outlined earlier.

- The CNC instrument automatically calculates the overall fit for each of the exercises. The result is indicated by a "pass/fail" message.

- Test agents may be used with the CNC instrument in a test chamber, but the unit has to be thoroughly cleaned following the test.

3. **Use the controlled negative-pressure protocol and exercises and appropriate instrumentation to measure the volumetric leak rate of a facepiece to quantify its fit.**

- The test is based on the theory of exhausting air from a temporarily sealed facepiece to generate and then maintain a constant negative pressure inside the facepiece. This method measures leak rates through the facepiece.

- The CNP instrumentation is available from Dynatech Nevada and is calibrated to a nonadjustable test pressure of -1.5 millimeters of

water (-0.058 inches of water) and modeled inspiratory flow rate of 53.8 liters per minute for performing fit tests. The system default values may also be used to provide greater accuracy for workload and gender differences.

- The test instrument is equipped with an audio warning device that sounds when test subjects fail to hold their breaths during the test.

- The individual who conducts the CNP fit testing must be thoroughly trained in the use of the equipment.

- The test subjects must be trained to hold their breaths for at least 20 seconds.

- To perform the test, test subjects close their mouths and hold their breaths while an air pump removes the air from the facepiece creating a predetermined constant pressure. The fit factor is expressed as the leak rate measured in millimeters per minute (mm/min).

- The fit factor of 100 or better is required for the half and quarter masks and 500 for full facepieces.

- Respirators that are equipped with filters or cartridges must have these parts replaced with the CNP test manifold (**Figure 6.19**).

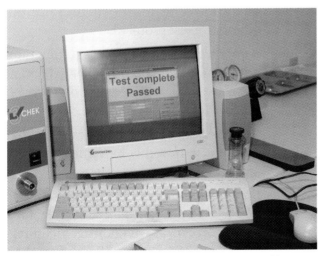

Figure 6.18 The condensation nuclei counting (CNC) test instrumentation depends on a computer with fit-test software installed to calculate the fit of the facepiece.

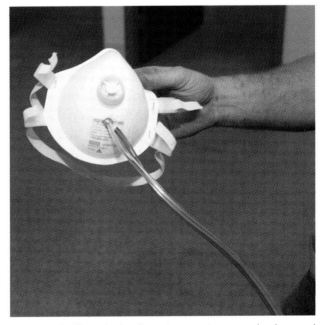

Figure 6.19 Quantitative fit-test apparatus may also be used when testing the fit of high-efficiency particulate air (HEPA) filters and air-purifying respirators (APR) by attaching the test apparatus to the facepiece.

- The general test protocol for all quantitative fit testing must be followed *except* the test exercises for the CNP protocol differ from the ones previously mentioned. Note that the last part of each exercise involves holding the breath, which is not part of the non-CNP testing. CNP exercises are as follows:

  — *Breathe Normally*: Perform while standing in a normal position without talking. Breathe normally for 1 minute. Following the normal breathing, hold the head straight ahead and then hold the breath for 10 seconds while the measurement is taken.

  — *Breathe Deeply:* Perform while standing in a normal position without talking. Take slow, deep breaths for 1 minute. Following the deep breathing, hold the head straight ahead and then hold the breath for 10 seconds while the measurement is taken.

  — *Turn Head from Side to Side:* Perform while standing in a normal position without talking. Rotate the head to its fullest extent from side to side for 1 minute. Inhale at the extreme points of rotation. Following the head rotation exercise, hold the head straight ahead and then hold the breath for 10 seconds while the measurement is taken. Next, turn the head to the extreme right and hold the breath for 10 seconds (**Figure 6.20**).

  — *Move Head Up and Down:* Perform while standing in a normal position without talking. Move the head slowly up and down on the center axis of the body. Inhale when looking up for 1 minute. Following the moving exercise, hold the head straight ahead and then hold the breath for 10 seconds while the measurement is taken. Then hold the head in the full down position and hold the breath for 10 seconds.

  — *Talk:* Perform while standing in a normal position. Talk out loud slowly. Read from a prepared text, count backward from 100, or quote a memorized passage or verse for 1 minute. Following the talking exercise,

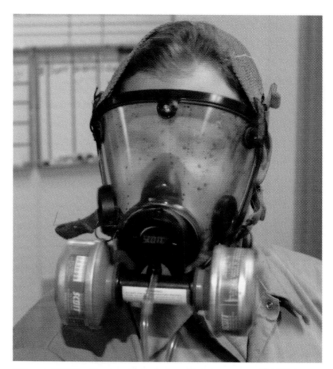

Figure 6.20 In the controlled negative-pressure (CNP) test, the subject rotates the head from side to side for 1 minute. Measurements are taken while the subject holds the breath for 10 seconds.

hold the head straight ahead and then hold the breath for 10 seconds while the measurement is taken.

NOTE: The test administrator must hear the test subject clearly.

  — *Grimace:* Perform while standing in a normal position. Frown or smile to create a facial grimace for 15 seconds (**Figure 6.21**).

NOTE: The grimace is only used in the quantitative test protocol and not the qualitative test protocol.

  — *Bend Over:* Perform while standing in a normal position without talking. Bend at the waist as though attempting to touch the toes for 1 minute.

NOTE: If the shroud-type test unit that does not permit this movement is used, jogging in place is permitted.

  — *Breathe Normally:* Perform while standing in a normal position without talking for 1 minute. Following the normal breathing, hold the head straight ahead, and then hold the breath for 10 seconds while the measurement is taken.

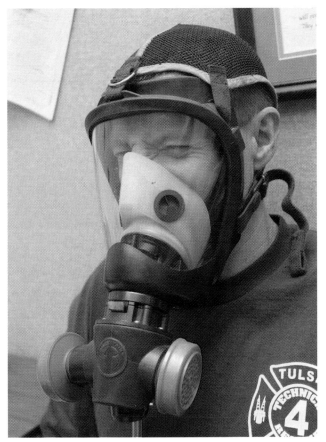

Figure 6.21 In the CNP fit-test protocol, the test subject creates a facial expression with an exaggerated frown or smile that is intended to test the effectiveness of the facepiece seal.

Qualitative Fit-Test Method

Another test procedure usually performed during the fitting process to determine the effectiveness of the seal between the facepiece and the wearer's face is the qualitative fit test (QLFT). It involves a test subject's response (either voluntary or involuntary) to a chemical outside the respirator facepiece. These tests are fast to conduct, easy to perform, and use inexpensive equipment. However, because they are based on the respirator wearer's subjective response to the test substance, accuracy may vary. Although all full facepiece SCBA, supplied-air respirator (SAR), and air-purifying respirator (APR) units may be tested with this method, qualitative fit testing may only be used to fit negative-pressure air-purifying respirators that must achieve a fit factor of 100 or less. Three of the most popular qualitative facepiece fit test methods are the irritant smoke test, the odorous vapor test, and the taste test.

Irritant smoke test. This qualitative fit test is a subjective test that uses the test subject's response

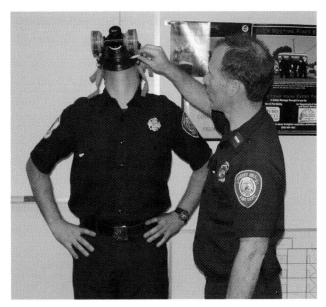

Figure 6.22 Stannic chloride smoke tubes are used to test facepiece seals in the irritant smoke test. The tube is held close to the facepiece while the subject performs the fit-test protocol. *Courtesy of Kenneth Baum.*

to irritating chemicals that are released into the atmosphere. The test is conducted in a well-ventilated room, and the smoke for the test usually comes from a stannic chloride smoke tube (**Figure 6.22**). Because the test agent or smoke is irritating to the eyes, lungs, and nasal passages, care must be taken to minimize the test subject's exposure to the material. Recent research has indicated that stannic chloride contains chemical agents that may cause cancer in a portion of the population. This potential may cause some organizations to reconsider the use of the irritant smoke test. The irritant smoke test protocol is as follows:

● Perform an odor sensitivity-screening test on the test subject first.

— Expose the test subject to a small, diluted concentration of the test material to ensure the ability to detect the irritant.

— Open the stannic chloride smoke tube and attach it to a low-flow air pump that delivers 200 milliliters per minute or an aspirator squeeze bulb.

— Advise the test subject that the smoke can irritate the eyes, lungs, and nasal passage and to keep the eyes shut during the test.

— Spray a small amount of the smoke toward the test subject and ask if the test subject can smell it.

- Have the test subject don the respirator facepiece and perform the user seal check mentioned earlier.

- Direct a stream of the smoke toward the facepiece seal beginning at 12 inches (305 mm) and moving to within 6 inches (152 mm) while making two passes (**Figure 6.23**).

- Have the test subject perform the exercise regimen while the smoke is directed at the facepiece.

- Note test results.
  — If the test subject reports detecting the odor of the smoke, then the test is a failure.

  — If the test subject passes the test without evidence of leakage, then give a second odor sensitivity-screening test to ensure reaction to the smoke. Failure to react voids the test.

Odorous vapor test. The odor test is another simple check for proper facepiece seal. It depends on the test subject's ability to detect the odor of isoamyl acetate, also known as *isopentyl acetate* or *banana oil*. Most people can detect a concentration of less than 1 ppm of banana oil (**Figure 6.24**). However, the isoamyl acetate protocol has its drawbacks. The test agent must be prepared in the exact solution established in the OSHA guidelines and must be used the day it is mixed. An organic vapor filter must be connected to the facepiece to filter out the odor of the isoamyl acetate. If the test subject smells the test agent, the test ends and the subject returns to the selection room to start the process with a new facepiece. The testing room must be well ventilated, and test subjects must be kept in the separate, uncontaminated selection room. Facepieces must be cleaned and decontaminated between tests to prevent the transmission of germs (**Figure 6.25**). The test protocol is as follows:

- Administer a pretest odor sensitivity screening to the test subject. Ensure that the subject correctly identifies the test solution contained in a jar as described in the OSHA guidelines.

- Use an enclosed test chamber constructed from a 55-gallon (208 L) plastic drum liner suspended over a 2-foot (0.6 m) diameter frame. Ensure that the chamber, or shroud, is 6 inches (152 mm) above the test subject's head.

- Fit test facepieces with an organic vapor cartridge or filter.

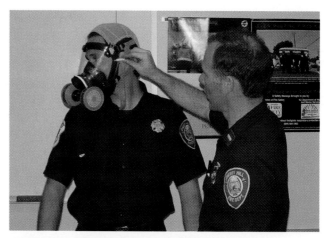

Figure 6.23 The test administrator moves the stannic chloride tube from 12 inches (305 mm) to within 6 inches (152 mm) of the facepiece. *Courtesy of Kenneth Baum.*

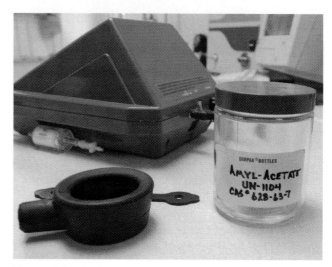

Figure 6.24 The odorous vapor qualitative fit test is performed with isoamyl acetate, also known as banana oil, to determine the effectiveness of the facepiece seal.

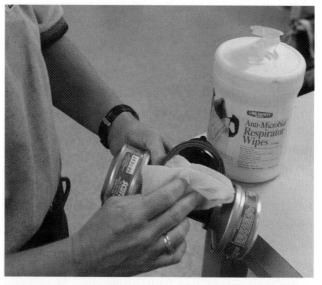

Figure 6.25 Antiseptic alcohol swabs may be used to clean the test facepiece between uses.

- Ensure that a copy of the test exercises is taped inside the test chamber.

- Have the test subject don the facepiece in the selection room, enter the fit-testing room, and go into the test chamber.

- Give the test subject in the test chamber a 6- by 5-inch (152 mm by 127 mm) paper towel that is folded in half and wetted with 0.75 milliliter of pure isoamyl acetate.

- Allow 2 minutes for the test agent to completely stabilize within the chamber before beginning the test exercises.

- Explain the fit-test protocol during this time. Explain the importance of the test subject's cooperation and the purpose of the test exercises. Demonstrate the exercises if necessary.

- Note test results.

    — If the test subject detects the odor of the test agent at anytime during the fit test, the test subject must immediately leave the test chamber and test room and move to the selection room. Consider the test a failure and provide a new facepiece. Begin a new test at least 5 minutes later.

    — If the test is a success, the test subject must demonstrate the success of the test by removing the facepiece while in the test chamber and taking a deep breath.

- Remove the used paper towel from the chamber and place it in a sealed plastic bag for disposal.

One of the obvious benefits of the isoamyl acetate fit test is that it is portable. It may be conducted at a central location or taken to remote sites that have sufficient ventilation in the fit-test room. It also requires less expensive equipment than the quantitative fit-test protocol and has been shown to perform as designed.

Taste test. The taste test is another simple qualitative test that relies on the test subject detecting the taste of a chemical substance, sodium saccharin or Bitrex™ (denatonium benzoate) aerosol, inside the facepiece (**Figure 6.26**). The taste test is the least reliable of the qualitative tests because there is no involuntary response, and individual taste thresholds vary widely. Like the irritant smoke test, sodium saccharin may contain cancer-caus-

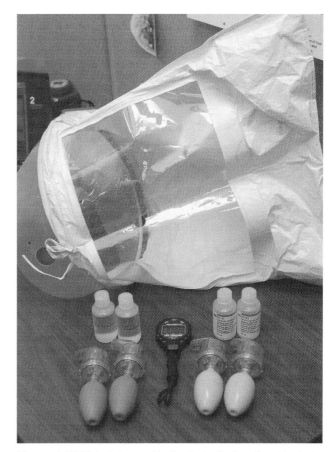

Figure 6.26 Materials used in the taste-test protocol include the hood, two sets of nebulizers, screening and test solutions, and a stopwatch.

ing agents — a situation that should be considered before selecting this method. The following taste test protocol is used for the sodium saccharin solution:

- Explain the screening and test protocol to the test subject prior to the taste threshold screening.

- Use a test apparatus hood that is approximately 12 inches (305 mm) in diameter and 14 inches (356 mm) high with a clear front panel. A ¾-inch (19 mm) hole is located in the front of the hood in the area of the test subject's nose and mouth. This hole accommodates the atomizer (spray) nozzle (**Figure 6.27**). The test subject wears the hood during both the taste threshold screening and the fit test.

- Spray both the taste threshold solution and the fit-test solution into the hood with a De Vilbiss Model 40 Inhalation Medication Nebulizer or equivalent instrument. Use two separate nebulizers for the two functions of screening and fit testing.

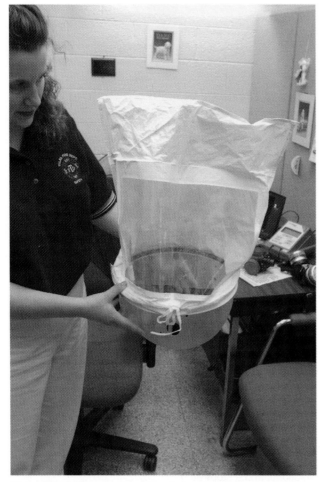

Figure 6.27 The taste-test hood should be large enough to fit over the subject's head while wearing the respirator mask. The tester should inspect the condition of the hood before beginning the test sequence.

— Prepare the threshold solution by dissolving 0.83 gram of sodium saccharin USP (United States Pharmacopeia) in 100 milliliters of warm water.

— Place the test solution in the screen test nebulizer and direct it into the opening in the front of the test hood. Squeeze the bulb 10 times in rapid succession.

— Use approximately 1 milliliter of test solution for the screening test. Rinse and dry the nebulizer each morning and afternoon or at least every 4 hours of the test.

● Have the test subject don the hood for the taste threshold screening without a facepiece in place. Instruct the subject to breathe through the mouth with the tongue slightly extended.

● Instruct the test subject to report if a sweet taste is detected.

NOTE: The screening test may be compromised and give a false reading if the test subject has eaten or drunk something sweet prior to the test. Therefore, instruct test subjects not to eat, drink (except plain water), smoke, or chew gum or tobacco products 15 minutes before the test.

● Note threshold screening test results.

— If the subject reports tasting the sweet taste from the test agent, the test is a success, the taste threshold is noted as 10, and the subject is ready for the fit test.

— If the test subject cannot taste the sweetness, perform a second series of 10 squeezes. If the subject reports tasting the sweet taste from the test agent, the test is a success, the taste threshold is noted as 20, and the subject is ready for the fit test.

— If the test subject cannot taste the sweetness, perform a third series of 10 squeezes. If the subject reports tasting the sweet taste from the test agent, the test is a success, the taste threshold is noted as 30, and the subject is ready for the fit test.

— If the test subject does not report the taste of the saccharin, then the test is a failure. Use another test protocol for the fit testing.

— If the test is successful, ask the test subject to note the taste for reference during the facepiece fit test.

● Prepare to perform the fit test. Have the test subject don the facepiece, make the self-seal check, and then don the test enclosure or hood. Equip the facepiece with a particle filter.

● Fill a second nebulizer (marked for fit testing only) with the fit-test solution of saccharin.

● Instruct the test subject to breath through the mouth with the tongue slightly extended.

● Insert the nebulizer into the hole in the hood and use the same number of squeezes (10, 20, or 30) that was used in the screening test to spray the test agent into the hood (**Figure 6.28**).

● Instruct the test subject to perform the test exercises mentioned earlier.

● Replenish the test agent every 30 seconds by spraying one half the number of original squeezes into the hood.

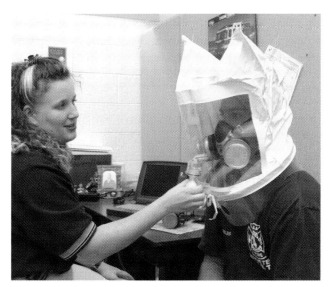

Figure 6.28 During the taste test, the nebulizer is held in front of the hood opening and sprays into the opening with 10 squeezes in rapid succession.

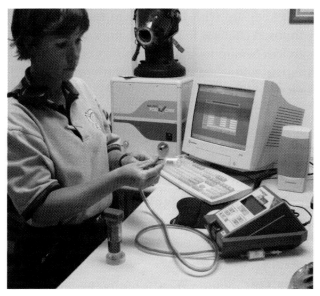

Figure 6.29 Calibration of condensation nuclei counting and controlled negative-pressure fit-test apparatus must be performed by certified technicians following the manufacturer's recommendations.

- Make periodic checks of the nebulizer to ensure that the nozzle does not clog. Clogging invalidates the test.
- Note fit test results.
  — If the test is completed without the test subject tasting the saccharin, the test is a success.
  — If the test subject tastes the saccharin, the test is a failure and a new facepiece is selected and the test repeated.

As mentioned earlier, Bitrex™ may be used in place of saccharin. The taste test may be used for full or half facepiece masks, including particle masks. The screening and fit-test protocol is the same as that used in the saccharin test with the following exceptions:

- Prepare the threshold screening test solution by adding 13.5 milligrams of Bitrex™ to 100 milliliters of 5 percent salt solution in distilled water.
- Prepare the fit-test solution by adding 337.5 milligrams of Bitrex™ to 200 milliliters of a 5 percent salt solution in warm water.

Equipment Calibration

Fit-testing instruments must be calibrated for the type of testing being performed. The units must be checked for proper calibration before each use or according to the manufacturer's recommendations (**Figure 6.29**). The manufacturer may require annual or periodic inspection, calibration, and recertifica-

tion. Records on all maintenance, inspections, and certifications must be maintained on the fit-test instrumentation instruments.

New Testing Technology

Rapid advances in computer technology are affecting the types and designs of fit-test equipment available to fire and emergency services organizations. New equipment designs that have greater particle sensitivity and increased accuracy are currently under development. Concurrently, proposed variations in fit-test protocol are being developed. When changes in fit-test protocol occur, an application for the new protocol must be submitted to OSHA. The application must be supported by a test report from one of the independent government test laboratories, the Lawrence Livermore National Laboratory, the Los Alamos National Laboratory, or the National Institute for Standards and Technology (NIST) stating that the protocol is accurate and reliable. Alternatively, the application may be submitted with an article from a peer-reviewed industrial hygiene professional journal that describes the protocol and explains the tests that support the protocol's accuracy and reliability. When sufficient information is provided, OSHA determines if the protocol should be adopted.

To keep up with advances in technology and proposed changes in protocol, fire and emergency services personnel should monitor OSHA, National Institute for Occupational Safety and Health (NIOSH), ANSI, Canadian Occupational Health and Safety (OH&S) regulations, manufacturer's press releases, and articles in trade journals. Trade shows are also good sources of information on new products.

Testing Types of Respiratory Protection Equipment
[NFPA 1500: 7.12.3]
[NFPA 1404: 6.1.4]

NFPA 1404 requires that fit testing be done on all tight-fitting facepiece respirators that use full facepieces. NFPA 1500 requires fit testing for full and half facepieces. OSHA's fit-testing requirements apply to all types of respiratory protection equipment regardless of facepiece type. The following fit-test procedures are permitted for the specified type of respiratory protection equipment:

- Half-face, negative-pressure air-purifying respirator (less than 100 fit factor): qualitative and quantitative methods

- Full-face, negative-pressure air-purifying respirator (less than 100 fit factor) used in atmospheres up to 10 times the permissible exposure limit (PEL): qualitative and quantitative methods

- Full-face, negative-pressure air-purifying respirator (greater than 100 fit factor): quantitative method only

- Powered air-purifying respirator: qualitative and quantitative methods

- Supplied-air respirators or self-contained breathing apparatus used in negative-pressure (demand) mode (greater than 100 fit factor): quantitative method only

- Supplied-air respirators or self-contained breathing apparatus used in positive-pressure (pressure demand) mode: qualitative and quantitative methods

- Self-contained breathing apparatus used in structural fire fighting, positive-pressure mode: qualitative and quantitative methods

- Self-contained breathing apparatus/supplied-air respirator used in immediately dangerous to life and health (IDLH) atmospheres, positive-pressure mode: qualitative and quantitative methods

- Mouthbit respirator, loose-fitting respirators, and dust masks: fit testing not required

Third-Party or Outside Testing Contractors

Some fire and emergency services organizations may not be able to justify the expense of quantitative fit-testing equipment or the training of personnel to perform fit testing. Considering the potential liability that an improperly fitted facepiece may cause, the fire and emergency service organization may choose to hire a third-party testing laboratory to perform the fit testing. Third-party testing laboratories or outside contractors must meet the same requirements for training, equipment calibration, and safety that the fire and emergency services organization would. Records generated by the third-party testing laboratory are turned over to the fire and emergency services organization following completion of the testing.

Fit testing may also be part of the purchase contract with the respiratory protection equipment vendor. If this situation is the case, the fit testing is limited to the specific product that is being provided. If the fire and emergency services organization uses a variety of respiratory protection equipment, then a contract with a third-party testing laboratory would be preferred for all the respiratory protection equipment the organization uses.

Fit-Test Record Keeping
[NFPA 1500: 7.12.5]

Fit-test records must be maintained in the member's personnel file or in a separate facepiece file and made available to the individual. Fit-test records should include but are not limited to the following information:

- Test subject's name

- Type of fit test performed (quantitative or qualitative)

- Overall fit factor

- Manufacturer of facepiece/respirator

- Model of facepiece/respirator
- Style of facepiece/respirator
- Size of facepiece/respirator
- Date of test
- Test results

Additional information may include any difficulties encountered while giving the test such as interface with protective clothing and equipment or personal fit problems. The name of the person administering the test may also be included in the records. Records on all subsequent retests, whether required annually, due to a change in the work environment, or due to changes in a subject's physical appearance, are also included in this file.

Summary

The individual's medical evaluation and examination and facepiece fit-testing results are important elements of the respiratory protection program. Complete and accurate documentation is essential, and confidentiality is mandatory for the medical records portion. The initial fit test and the annual retesting may use the protocol selected by the authority having jurisdiction as long as tests ensure that the wearer has a tight, comfortable seal with the facepiece. The type of fit test selected does not have to be complicated or expensive to be effective. It does have to be based on an established, documented, and validated protocol meeting NFPA, ANSI, or OSHA requirements.

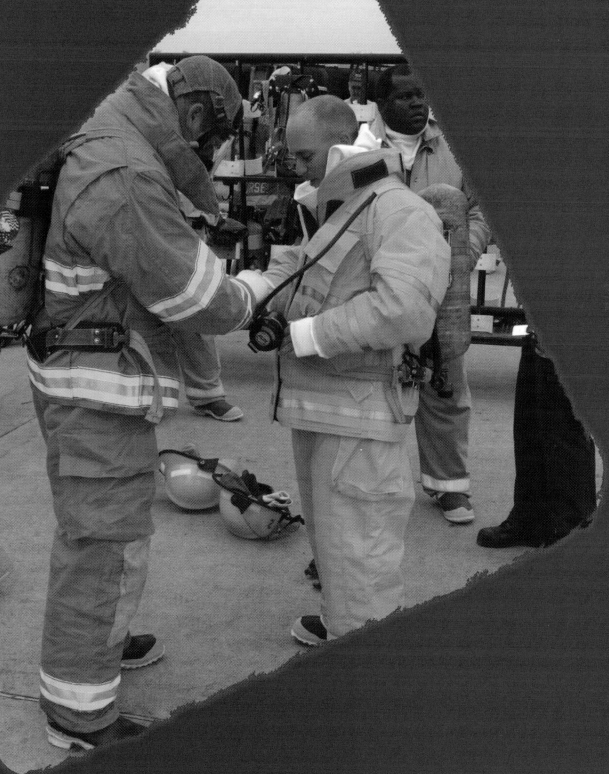

Chapter 7

Training

This chapter provides information that will assist the reader in meeting the following job performance requirements from NFPA 1404, *Standard for Fire Service Respiratory Protection Training*, 2002 Edition, and NFPA 1500, *Standard on Fire Department Occupational Safety and Health Program*, 2002 Edition.

NFPA 1500

4.6.4 The fire department shall maintain training records for each member indicating dates, subjects covered, satisfactory completion, and, if any, certifications achieved.

4.9.1 The health and safety officer shall ensure that training in safety procedures relating to all fire department operations and functions is provided to fire department members.

4.9.3 The health and safety officer shall cause safety supervision to be provided for training activities, including all live burn exercises.

4.9.4 All structural live burn exercises shall be conducted in accordance with NFPA 1403, *Standard on Live Fire Training Evolutions*.

4.9.5 The health and safety officer or qualified designee shall be personally involved in pre-burn inspections of any acquired structures to be utilized for live fire training.

5.1.1 The fire department shall establish and maintain a training and education program with a goal of preventing occupational deaths, injuries, and illnesses.

5.1.2 The fire department shall provide training and education for all department members commensurate with the duties and functions that they are expected to perform.

5.1.3 The fire department shall establish training and education programs that provide new members initial training, proficiency opportunities, and a method of skill and knowledge evaluation for duties assigned to the member prior to engaging in emergency operations.

5.1.8 The fire department shall provide all members with a training and education program that covers the operation, limitation, maintenance, and retirement criteria for all assigned personal protective equipment expected to be utilized by members.

5.1.9 As a duty function, members shall be responsible to maintain proficiency in skills and knowledge provided to the member through department training and education programs.

5.2.1 All members who engage in structural fire fighting shall meet the requirements of NFPA 1001, *Standard for Fire Fighter Professional Qualifications*.

5.2.3 All aircraft rescue fire fighters (ARFF) shall meet the requirements of NFPA 1003, *Standard for Airport Fire Fighter Professional Qualifications*.

5.2.4 All members who are required to perform technical rescue tasks shall meet the requirements of NFPA 1006, *Standard for Rescue Technician Professional Qualifications*.

5.2.7 All members responding to hazardous materials incidents shall meet the operations level as required in NFPA 472, *Standard for Professional Competence of Responders to Hazardous Materials Incidents*.

5.2.9 The fire department shall adopt or develop training and education curriculums that meet the minimum requirements outlined in professional qualification standards covering a member's assigned function.

5.2.10 All live fire training and exercises shall be conducted in accordance with NFPA 1403, *Standard on Live Fire Training Evolutions*.

5.2.11 All training and exercises shall be conducted under the direct supervision of a qualified instructor who meets the equivalency requirements of 1.4.1.

5.2.13 Members shall be fully trained in the care, use, inspection, maintenance, and limitations of the protective clothing and protective equipment assigned to them or available for their use.

5.3.1 Training shall be provided for all members as often as necessary to meet applicable requirements of this chapter.

5.3.2 The fire department shall develop a reoccurring proficiency cycle with the goal of preventing skill degradation and potential for injury and death of members.

5.3.4 The fire department shall provide an annual skills check to verify minimum professional qualifications of its members.

5.3.5 The fire department shall provide training and education events as required to support minimum qualifications and certifications expected of its members.

5.3.6 Members shall practice assigned skill sets on a regular basis but not less than annually.

5.3.7 The fire department shall provide specific training to members when written policies, practices, procedures, or guidelines are changed and/or updated.

5.3.8 The respiratory protection training program shall meet the requirements of NFPA 1404, *Standard for a Fire Department Self-Contained Breathing Apparatus Program*.

5.4.1 The fire department shall provide specific and advanced training to members who engage in special operations as a technician.

5.4.2 The fire department shall provide specific training to members who are likely to respond to special operations incidents in a support role to special operations technicians.

5.4.3 Members expected to perform hazardous materials mitigation activities shall meet the training requirements of a technician as outlined in NFPA 472, *Standard for Professional Competence of Responders to Hazardous Materials Incidents.*

5.4.4 Members expected to perform technical operations as defined in NFPA 1670, *Standard on Operations and Training for Technical Rescue Incidents,* shall meet the training requirements specified in NFPA 1006, *Standard for Rescue Technician Professional Qualifications.*

7.9.3 Members shall be tested and certified at least annually in the safe and proper use of respiratory protection equipment that they are authorized to use.

NFPA 1404

4.2.1 SCBA used by the authority having jurisdiction for training shall meet the requirements of Section 4.3, SCBA Compliance, of NFPA 1852, *Standard on Selection, Care, and Maintenance of Open-Circuit Self-Contained Breathing Apparatus.*

4.2.2 SCBA used in training exercises shall be of the type and manufacture employed by the authority having jurisdiction.

4.2.3 Training policies shall be established by the authority having jurisdiction regulating the use of SCBA equipped with Emergency Breathing Support System (EBSS) commonly known as "buddy" or rescue breathing devices.

4.3 Selection and Use of Supplied-Air Respirators (SAR) in Training. SAR units used in training shall be of the type and manufacture employed by the authority having jurisdiction.

4.4 Selection and Use of Full Facepiece Air-Purifying Respirators (FFAPR) in Training. FFAPR units used in training shall be of the type and manufacture employed by the authority having jurisdiction.

5.1.1 The authority having jurisdiction shall adopt and maintain a respiratory protection program that meets the requirements of Section 7.3 of NFPA 1500, *Standard on Fire Department Occupational Safety and Health Program.*

5.1.2 The authority having jurisdiction shall conduct ongoing respiratory protection training that meets the requirements of this standard.

5.1.3 Respiratory protection training shall be conducted according to written standard operating procedures.

(1) When respiratory protection equipment is to be used

(2) When to exit due to reduced air supply

(3) Emergency evacuation procedures

(4) Procedures for insuring proper facepiece fit

(5) Cleaning of respiratory protection equipment components

5.1.6 The authority having jurisdiction shall establish written training policies for respiratory protection.

5.1.7 Training policies shall include, but shall not be limited to the following:

(1) Identification of the various types of respiratory protection equipment

(2) Responsibilities of members to obtain and maintain proper facepiece fit

(3) Responsibilities of members for proper cleaning and maintenance

(4) Identification of the factors that affect the duration of the air supply

(5) Determination of the point of no return for each member

(6) Responsibilities of members for using respiratory protection equipment in a hazardous atmosphere

(7) Limitations of respiratory protection devices

5.1.8 The members of the authority having jurisdiction shall be trained on the procedures for inspection, maintenance, repair, and testing of respiratory protection equipment in accordance with NFPA 1500, *Standard on Fire Department Occupational Safety and Health Program,* and the manufacturer's recommendations, and NFPA 1852, *Standard on Selection, Care, and Maintenance of Open-Circuit Self-Contained Breathing Apparatus.*

5.2 Requirements of the Respiratory Protection Training Component. The authority having jurisdiction shall ensure that each employee can demonstrate knowledge of the following:

(1) Why the respirator is necessary and how improper fit, usage, or maintenance can compromise the protective effect of the respirator

(2) What are the limitations and capabilities of the respirator

(3) How to use the respirator effectively in emergency situations, including situations in which the respirator malfunctions

(4) How to inspect, don and doff, use, and check the seals of the respirator

(5) What the procedures are for maintenance and storage of the respirator

(6) How to recognize medical signs and symptoms that can limit or prevent the effective use of respirators

(7) General requirements of Section 5.2

6.1.2 Records of all respiratory protection training shall be maintained, including training of personnel involved in maintenance of such equipment, in accordance with Section 4.3 of NFPA 1852 *Standard on Selection, Care, and Maintenance of Open-Circuit Self-Contained Breathing Apparatus.*

6.1.3 Minimum performance standards shall be established by NFPA 1001, *Standard for Fire Fighter Professional Qualifications,* and the authority having jurisdiction for donning respiratory protection equipment.

6.2.1 Re-training shall be administered annually and when the following situations occur:

(1) Changes in the workplace or the type of respirator render the previous training obsolete

(2) Inadequacies in the member's knowledge or use of the respirator indicate that the member has not retained the requisite understanding or skill

(3) Any other situation arises in which re-training appears necessary to ensure safe respirator use

6.2.2 The respiratory protection training program shall provide members with annual training concerning the following:

(1) Safely donning and doffing of SCBA, SAR, and FFAPR

(2) Uses and limitations of respiratory protection equipment

(3) Consequences of an improper fit or poor maintenance impacting the protection being provided

(4) How to perform seal checks

(5) How to recognize medical signs and symptoms that can impact use of respirators

(6) How to inspect the respirator before use

(7) Procedures for maintenance and storage

(8) Individual limitations of members who could be required to use an SCBA, SAR, or FFAPR

6.3.1 Smoke produced from live fire shall be prohibited in SCBA training sessions.

6.3.5 Instruction on the common reasons for the breakdown of procedures or equipment that could cause injuries shall include the following subjects:

(1) Abuse and misuse of equipment

(2) Physiological and psychological factors

(3) Unapproved equipment

(4) Buddy breathing

(5) Information supplied to agencies that collect accident information, where available

6.3.6 Members required to wear respiratory protection equipment in conjunction with specialized protection equipment in training activities (e.g., proximity suits or totally encapsulated suits) shall be evaluated for physical and emotional stresses associated with these specialized applications.

6.3.7 The authority having jurisdiction shall be responsible for establishing a written training component that provides members with training in the use and limitations of respiratory protection equipment and related equipment, the policies and procedures related to the authority having jurisdiction's respiratory protection program, and in those areas outlined by this standard.

6.4.1 The authority having jurisdiction shall provide a means for evaluating a member's ability to don and doff respiratory protection under simulated emergency incidents.

6.4.2 The authority having jurisdiction shall provide a means for evaluating its members in the use and operation of respiratory protection equipment under simulated emergency incidents.

6.4.3 Members shall demonstrate an ability to operate under simulated emergency incident conditions.

6.5.1 Recruit training shall include the identification of SCBA, SAR, and FFAPR components, terminology, and equipment specifications through the following:

(1) Operation of SCBA, SAR units, and FFAPR, and related equipment

(2) Inspection and maintenance of equipment

(3) Donning methods employed by the authority having jurisdiction

(4) Performance of related emergency scene activities, such as advancing hose lines, climbing ladders, crawling through windows and confined spaces, and performing rescues, while wearing respiratory protection

(5) Comprehension of organizational policies and procedures concerning safety procedures, emergency operations, use, inspection, and maintenance

(6) Performance of activities under simulated emergency conditions

(7) Compliance with all performance standards of the authority having jurisdiction

6.5.2 Training shall be conducted in a sequential format with a logical progression towards achieving specific goals, including the following:

(1) Establishing policies by the authority having jurisdiction

(2) Requiring theoretical understanding of respiratory protection

(3) Developing practical skills

6.6.1 The training program of the authority having jurisdiction shall evaluate the ability of personnel to identify the following:

(1) Hazardous environments that require the use of respiratory protection

(2) Primary gases produced by combustion

(3) Primary characteristics of gases that are present or generated by processes other than combustion

(4) Any toxic gases that are unique to the particular authority having jurisdiction resulting from manufacturing or industrial processes

(5) Shipping labels of hazardous materials

6.6.2 Fire department members shall be trained to handle problems related to the following situations that can be encountered during the use of respiratory protection equipment:

(1) Low temperatures

(2) High temperatures

(3) Rapid temperature changes

(4) Communications

(5) Confined spaces

(6) Vision

(7) Facepiece-to-face sealing problems

(8) Absorption through or irritation of the skin

(9) Effects of ionizing radiation on the skin and the entire body

(10) Punctured or ruptured eardrums

(11) Use near water

(12) Overhaul

6.7.1 Understanding the Components of SCBA. The training program of the authority having jurisdiction shall evaluate the ability of members to perform the following skills:

(1) Identify the components of facepieces, regulators, harnesses, and cylinders used by the authority having jurisdiction

(2) Demonstrate the operation of the SCBA used by the authority having jurisdiction

(3) Describe the operation of the SCBA used by the authority having jurisdiction

(4) Describe the potential incompatibility of different makes and models of SCBA

6.7.2 Understanding the Safety Features and Limitations of SCBA. The training program of the authority having jurisdiction shall evaluate the ability of members to perform the following skills:

(1) Describe the operational principles of warning devices required on a SCBA

(2) Identify the limitations of the SCBA used by the authority having jurisdiction

(3) Describe the limitations of the SCBA's ability to protect the body from absorption of toxins through the skin

(4) Describe the procedures to be utilized if unintentionally submerged in water while wearing a SCBA

(5) Demonstrate the possible means of communications when wearing a SCBA

(6) Describe the emergency bypass operation

(7) Describe how to recognize medical signs and symptoms that could prevent the effective use of respirators

6.7.3 Donning and Doffing SCBA. The training program of the authority having jurisdiction shall evaluate the ability of members to demonstrate the following:

(1) Techniques for donning and doffing all types of SCBA used by the authority having jurisdiction while wearing the full protective clothing used by the authority having jurisdiction

(2) That a proper face-to-facepiece seal has been achieved by using the seal check

6.7.4 Practical Application in SCBA Training. The training program of the authority having jurisdiction shall evaluate the ability of members to demonstrate the following:

(1) Knowledge of the components of respiratory protection

(2) Use of all types of SCBA utilized by the authority having jurisdiction under conditions of obscured visibility

(3) Emergency operations that are required when a SCBA fails

(4) Emergency techniques using a SCBA to assist other members, conserve air, and show restrictions in use of bypass valves

(5) Use of a SCBA in limited or confined spaces

(6) Proper cleaning and sanitizing of the facepiece

6.8.1 Understanding the Components of a SAR. The training program of the authority having jurisdiction shall evaluate the ability of members to perform the following skills:

(1) Describe the air source, air hose limitations, and NIOSH-approved inlet pressure gauge range

(2) Identify the components of facepieces, regulators, harnesses, manifold system, and cylinders or compressors used by the authority having jurisdiction

(3) Describe the operation of the SAR used by the authority having jurisdiction

(4) Describe the limitations of the escape cylinder

(5) Describe the potential incompatibility of different makes and models of SAR units

(6) Describe proper procedures for inspection, cleaning, and storage of SAR units

6.8.2 Understanding the Safety Features and Limitations of a SAR. The training program of the authority having jurisdiction shall evaluate the ability of members to perform the following skills:

(1) Describe the operational principles of emergency escape cylinder required on a SAR when used in IDLH atmospheres

(2) Identify the limitations of the SAR used by the authority having jurisdiction

(3) Describe the limitations of the SAR's ability to protect the body from absorption of toxins through the skin

(4) Describe the possible means of communications when wearing a SAR

(5) Describe the prohibition in using compressed oxygen with a SAR system

(6) Describe how to recognize medical signs and symptoms that could prevent the effective use of a SAR

6.8.3 Donning and Doffing SAR. The training program of the authority having jurisdiction shall evaluate the ability of members to demonstrate the following:

(1) Proper techniques for donning and doffing all types of SAR used by the authority having jurisdiction while wearing the full protective clothing

(2) That a proper face-to-facepiece seal has been achieved by using the seal check

(3) Proper methods for tending SAR air hoses

6.8.4 Practical Application in SAR Training. The training program of the authority having jurisdiction shall evaluate the ability of members to perform the following skills:

(1) Demonstrate knowledge of the components of the SAR System

(2) Understand that the use of SAR is prohibited for fire fighting

(3) Demonstrate the use of SAR utilized by the authority having jurisdiction under conditions of obscured visibility

(4) Demonstrate the emergency operations that are required when the SAR fails

(5) Demonstrate the use of SAR when using hazardous materials personal protective equipment if utilized by the authority having jurisdiction

(6) Demonstrate the use of SAR in limited or confined spaces

(7) Demonstrate the proper cleaning and sanitizing of the facepiece

6.9.1 Understanding the Components of FFAPR units. The training program of the authority having jurisdiction shall evaluate the ability of members to perform the following skills:

(1) Identify the components of facepieces, canisters, and cartridges used by the authority having jurisdiction

(2) Describe the operation of the FFAPR used by the authority having jurisdiction

(3) Describe the limitations of the FFAPR

(4) Demonstrate the operation of the FFAPR used by the authority having jurisdiction

(5) Describe how a selected FFAPR must be appropriate for the chemical state and physical form of the contaminate

(6) Determine when to replace canisters and cartridge units

(7) Demonstrate proper procedures for inspection, cleaning, and storage of FFAPR

6.9.2 Understanding the Safety Features and Limitations of FFAPR. The training program of the authority having jurisdiction shall evaluate the ability of members to perform the following skills:

(1) Describe the operational principles of the FFAPR

(2) Identify the limitations of the FFAPR used by the authority having jurisdiction

(3) Describe the limitations of the FFAPR's ability to protect the body from absorption of toxins through the skin

(4) Describe the procedures for determining canister and cartridge selection by color-coded as well as NIOSH-approved labeling

(5) Understand labels are not to be removed from canisters or cartridges

(6) Understand that the use of FFAPR is prohibited for fire fighting

(7) Describe the limitations of FFAPR in fire ground activities

6.9.3 Donning and Doffing FFAPR. The training program of the authority having jurisdiction shall evaluate the ability of members to demonstrate the following:

(1) Proper techniques for donning and doffing all types of FFAPR used by the authority having jurisdiction while wearing the full protective clothing

(2) That a proper face-to-facepiece seal has been achieved

6.9.4 Practical Application in FFAPR Training. The training program of the authority having jurisdiction shall evaluate the ability of members to demonstrate the following:

(1) Knowledge of the components of respiratory protection

(2) Limits of communications when wearing an FFAPR

(3) Use of FFAPR utilized by the authority having jurisdiction under conditions of obscured visibility

(4) Correct selection and installation of canisters and cartridges for a given situation

(5) Proper method of donning and doffing the FFAPR

(6) The positive pressure and the negative pressure facepiece-to face leak test

(7) Use of FFAPR in limited or confined spaces

(8) Proper cleaning and sanitizing

6.10 Training Conditions. Training shall be conducted under simulated stressful circumstances to promote immediate response to emergency operations.

7.1.1 SCBA service checks shall be conducted in accordance with 7.1.2 of NFPA 1852, *Standard on Selection, Care, and Maintenance of Open-Circuit Self-Contained Breathing Apparatus.*

7.1.2 Closed-circuit SCBA used in training shall be inspected at frequencies determined by the authority having jurisdiction in accordance with the manufacturer's recommendations but at no less than weekly intervals.

7.1.3 Closed-circuit SCBA shall be checked before and after each use in accordance with the manufacturer's recommendations.

7.2.1 Inspection, maintenance, and repair records shall be maintained for SAR units used in training as required in Chapter 4 of this standard.

7.2.2 All training SAR units used in emergency situations shall be inspected at least monthly in accordance with the manufacturer's instructions and shall be checked for proper function before and after each use.

7.2.3 All SAR units used in training shall be operated in accordance with the manufacturer's instructions.

7.2.4 The SAR unit shall consist of an emergency-escape air cylinder and a pressure-demand only facepiece when used in an IDLH atmosphere.

7.3.1 Inspection, maintenance, and repair records for FFAPR use in training shall be maintained as required in Chapter 6 of this standard.

7.3.2 The FFAPR used for training shall be thoroughly inspected upon receipt and prior to each use.

7.3.3 The FFAPR used for training shall be tested for leaks prior to each use in accordance with the manufacturer's instructions.

8.1.1 All maintenance and repairs on respiratory protection equipment used for training shall be conducted by qualified persons in accordance with NFPA 1852, *Standard on Selection, Care, and Maintenance of Open-Circuit Self-Contained Breathing Apparatus.*

8.1.2 Annual inspection and servicing of a SCBA and SAR systems used in training shall be conducted by qualified personnel and whenever an operational problem is reported.

8.1.2.1 Inspections and servicing of SCBA shall be performed in accordance with NFPA 1852, *Standard on Selection, Care, and Maintenance of Open-Circuit Self-Contained Breathing Apparatus.* Inspection of SAR units shall be in accordance with manufacturer's instructions for the unit in service.

10.1.1 Members shall be re-evaluated annually in accordance with 6.7.4 to determine their proficiency while using respiratory protection.

Reprinted with permission from NFPA 1404, *Standard for Fire Service Respiratory Protection Training,* and NFPA 1500, *Standard on Fire Department Occupational Safety and Health Program,* Copyright © 2002, National Fire Protection Association, Quincy, MA 02269. This reprinted material is not the complete and official position of the National Fire Protection Association on the referenced subject, which is represented only by the standard in its entirety.

An effective and successful respiratory protection program depends on a thorough respiratory protection training process. This process is designed to reinforce the respiratory protection policies found in the written respiratory protection program. The training process includes information on the types of respiratory protection hazards that emergency personnel face, the psychological and physiological effects caused by the use of respiratory protection equipment, familiarization with the specific types of respiratory protection equipment in use by the fire and emergency services, and drills and evolutions in the use of respiratory protection equipment. This chapter discusses general respiratory protection training requirements, training officer responsibilities, specific training for each type of respiratory equipment, the effects of continuous use on respiratory protection equipment, training-facility design requirements, smoke and live-fire (also called live-burn) training requirements plus specialized training (such as confined space, hazardous materials, etc.), and training record keeping.

General Training Requirements

[NFPA 1500: 5.1.1, 5.1.2, 5.1.3, 5.1.8, 5.1.9, 5.2.9]
[NFPA 1404: 5.1.1, 5.1.2, 5.1.3, 5.1.6, 5.1.7, 5.1.8, 5.2, 6.1.3, 6.3.5, 6.3.7, 6.5.2, 6.6.1, 6.6.2]

Respiratory protection training is fundamental to all emergency-response training programs. Such training begins with entry-level education for firefighters and emergency services personnel. Therefore, it is important that this training include a complete understanding of general hazards and in particular the respiratory protection hazards that emergency services personnel face while perform-

ing their duties (**Figure 7.1**). Emphasis on these hazards, listed in Chapter 1, Introduction to Respiratory Protection, is not intended to scare emergency responders. Rather, it is to educate them and illustrate the importance of the proper use of respiratory protection equipment.

Trainees should be told what to expect from their bodies while wearing various types of facepieces and then have the opportunity to practice with the actual equipment. Emergency responders must be aware of the psychological and physiological effects on themselves when they wear respiratory protection equipment. Psychological effects result from the fear of the unknown danger, claustrophobia caused by the confining effect of the facepiece or protective ensemble, and the excitement of an emergency. Physiological reactions include increased heart rate, increased perspiration, and shallow and increased breathing rates. The user must also be aware of the potential result of misuse or abuse of respiratory protection equipment and

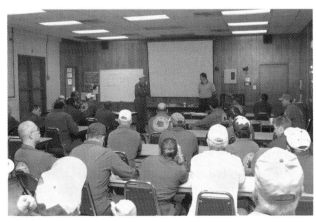

Figure 7.1 Respiratory protection classroom training includes an understanding of the types of respiratory protection hazards that individuals will routinely face while performing their duties.

the use of unapproved equipment or emergency breathing techniques.

Specifically, the respiratory protection training program should ensure that all members have the following knowledge or can demonstrate the following techniques/procedures:

- Know why respiratory protection is necessary.

- Know how improper usage, care, maintenance, and facepiece fit can compromise the protection supplied by a respirator.

- Know the limitations and capabilities of selected respiratory protection equipment.

- Demonstrate proper and effective use of selected respiratory protection equipment during emergency situations.

- Know what limitations are placed on personnel by the use of respiratory protection equipment.

- Demonstrate how to safely and effectively deal with respirator malfunctions.

- Demonstrate proper inspection techniques for selected respiratory protection equipment.

- Demonstrate proper donning and doffing techniques for selected respiratory protection equipment.

- Demonstrate how to check facepiece seal of selected respiratory protection equipment.

- Demonstrate proper service and maintenance procedures for selected respiratory protection equipment.

- Demonstrate proper storage techniques for respiratory protection equipment.

- Know how to recognize medical signs and symptoms that may limit or prevent use of respiratory protection equipment.

- Demonstrate how to use accessories that are part of the respiratory protection equipment.

- Demonstrate emergency escape procedures.

- Know the general requirements of Occupational Safety and Health Administration (OSHA) Title 29 (Labor) *CFR* 1910.134, Respiratory Protection Requirements.

The training program must also evaluate the ability of emergency services personnel to identify the following items:

- Respiratory hazard environments

- Primary gases created by combustion and the characteristics of those gases

- Any toxic gases that may be present in manufacturing, industrial, and transportation within the jurisdiction

- Hazardous materials shipping and storage labels

Incidents requiring respiratory protection may also have additional situations that may affect equipment or personnel as mentioned in Chapter 4, Safety and Risk Management. Training curriculum must provide the participants with an awareness of these situations, the effect they have on respiratory protection equipment and the wearer, and how to overcome the situations. Some of these situations are as follows:

- *Low ambient temperatures* — Affect the user's visibility in the facepiece and may cause exhalation valves to freeze

- *High temperatures* — Affect the ability of personnel to operate for extended periods of time; excessive heat may result in the melting or accelerated degradation of the elastomeric parts of the respirator (**Figure 7.2**)

- *Rapid temperature changes* — Affect the lenses of facepieces and may cause distortions in user vision and leaks around the lens/facepiece seal

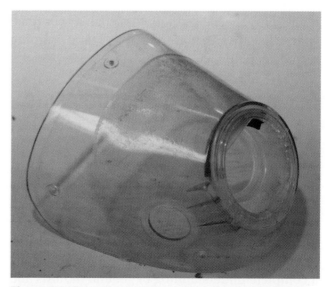

Figure 7.2 High temperatures generated during fire fighting operations can craze and discolor the lenses of SCBA facepieces, requiring them to be replaced after use.

- *Difficult communications*
  - Restricted verbal communications affect and limit voice communications among responders.
  - Ambient noise level affects verbal communication between responders and/or command and safety personnel.
- *Confined-space limitations* — Affect the ability of the user to move when wearing self-contained breathing apparatus (SCBA); the supplied-air respirator (SAR) air-supply hose may be damaged while operating in a confined space
- *Vision defects* — Require corrective lenses because of the restriction on wearing regular glasses with full facepieces; eyeglass kits or contact lenses can be used for this purpose (**Figure 7.3**)
- *Facepiece-to-face seal difficulties* — Compromise the interface, which is prohibited
- *Water submersion* — Not designed for respiratory protection equipment other than self-contained underwater breathing apparatus (SCUBA); include procedures in the event personnel wearing respiratory protection equipment are accidentally submerged in water
- *Overhaul operations* — Sources of gases, vapors, and particulates from fires in harmful concentrations; need for respiratory protection continues

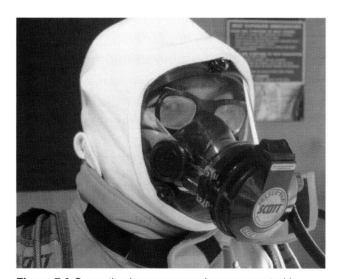

Figure 7.3 Corrective lenses or eyeglasses mounted in facepiece-specific kits can help to improve the wearer's vision.

CAUTION

Fire and emergency services personnel may be exposed to some nonrespiratory hazards. They should be made aware through training that respiratory protection equipment is only effective in protecting the user's respiratory tract and does not provide protection against the following conditions:

- *Absorption through or irritation of the skin* — Be aware of the need for the appropriate types of protective clothing because airborne contaminants such as ammonia and hydrochloric acid can enter the skin.
- *Effects of ionizing radiation on the skin* — Be aware of the proper types of protective clothing for this hazard.
- *Punctured or ruptured eardrums* — Obtain appropriate protection from the organization's physician or comply with medical restrictions because contaminated air can penetrate through the ears.

Training Officer Responsibilities

[NFPA 1500: 5.2.11]

The training officer plays an important part in helping trainees adjust to the use of respiratory protection equipment and understand the importance of safety in the use of the equipment. To be effective, the training program must duplicate the environments that the trainees may experience during actual emergency incidents. This training includes placing physical, physiological, and emotional stress on the individuals (**Figure 7.4**). The training officer must help trainees mitigate or control these various stresses in order to prevent injury or illness.

Training officers should remember that individuals react differently to wearing and working with respiratory protection equipment. This training period is the time to build confidence and not use scare tactics. The training officer should prepare trainees by calming fears, answering questions, telling them what is expected, explaining what is going to happen, and praising them on tasks done well (**Figure 7.5**). Words of encouragement and positive reinforcement go a long way toward building confidence.

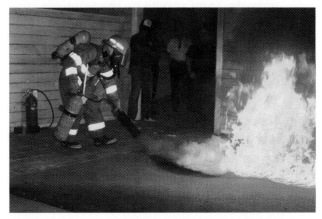

Figure 7.4 Realistic training evolutions while wearing respiratory protection equipment help to reduce the stress that wearing the equipment creates. In this photo a trainee extinguishes a Class B fire with a hand extinguisher while training officers look on. *Courtesy of Chris Mickal.*

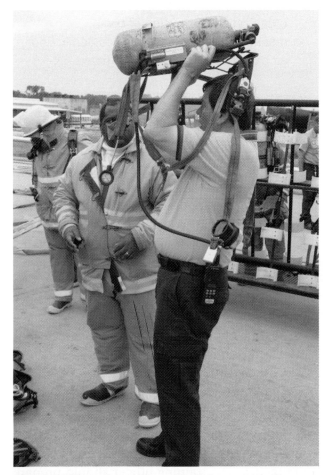

Figure 7.5 The training officer should demonstrate the proper techniques for donning, doffing, and using respiratory protection equipment for trainees.

Most trainees experience at least some physical or mental discomfort when they are learning to use respiratory protection equipment. Training officers should learn to recognize signs of anxiety and claustrophobia so that they can prevent potentially dangerous reactions later in the training sessions or at emergency incidents. The most obvious discomfort signals are apprehensive looks, excessive breathing rates, repeated yawning, heavy perspiration, or even nausea when waiting to enter a smoke room. Other trainees may seem calm, but may indicate their nervousness by constantly readjusting their harness straps, facepieces, or other equipment. The training officer should also watch for trainees who exhibit the following behaviors:

- Ask repeated questions about procedures

- Exhibit nervous chatter

- Participate in excessive horseplay

The training officer must also help emergency responders overcome some of the fears they may have about the respiratory protection equipment itself. Classroom training should include hands-on familiarization with the equipment including donning, doffing, adjusting straps, opening and closing of valves, and determining a suitable breathing rate. Training continues until trainees are thoroughly familiar and comfortable with the new equipment. Trainees must train with the facepieces and equipment for which they have been fit tested and will use during emergency scene operations. In order to enforce correct procedures at the emergency incident scene, the equipment in use at the training center must be the same make and model used by the operational units of the organization.

The training officer should stress that wearing respiratory protection equipment can prevent injury, long-term illness, and even death; it can be a significant factor in keeping emergency services personnel alive under the worst conditions. Training officers may want to stress that all respiratory protection equipment, whether SCBA, SAR, air-purifying respirator (APR), or particulate respirator, is designed to protect the lives of fire and emergency services personnel and allow them to perform their functions of protecting the victims of emergency incidents.

Respiratory Protection Systems Training

[NFPA 1500: 5.2.1, 5.2.13, 5.3.1, 5.3.2, 5.3.4, 5.3.5, 5.3.6, 5.3.8, 7.9.3]

[NFPA 1404: 6.4.1, 6.4.2, 6.4.3, 6.10]

Respiratory protection training is an ongoing and continuous process. Respiratory protection equipment training can occur during the following situations:

- Initial training class
- Annually as required by NFPA and OSHA
- When new equipment is purchased or existing equipment is upgraded
- When personnel display inadequacies in the use of equipment
- When operational protocols are altered
- When other situations arise that indicate retraining is necessary **(Figure 7.6)**

In addition to the entry-level training that new trainees receive, advanced levels of training are available. Advanced-level training provides techniques in specialized types of incidents and gives users an opportunity to gain greater knowledge and confidence in the use of respirators. The respiratory protection equipment training includes all types of equipment in use by the fire and emergency ser-

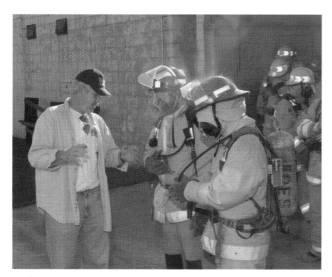

Figure 7.6 When new respiratory protection equipment is purchased, protocol is altered, and when personnel display inadequacies in the use of the equipment, retraining is necessary. This training officer is explaining a search and rescue evolution before sending students into a smoke building.

vices. The training is also specific to each type of equipment used. The following sections outline the training for several types of respiratory protection equipment: SCBA, air-purifying respirator, supplied-air respirator, and emergency breathing support system (EBSS) equipment. In addition to the training program, the fire and emergency services organization must consider the effects of continuous use on the respiratory protection systems used for training. Continuous equipment use results in increased wear that requires frequent cleaning, inspection, maintenance, and repair.

Self-Contained Breathing Apparatus

[NFPA 1404: 4.2.1, 4.2.2, 6.5.2, 6.7.1, 6.7.2, 6.7.3, 6.7.4]

Self-contained breathing apparatus is the only type of respiratory protection equipment that is approved for all types of respiratory protection hazards such as the following:

- Structural and nonstructural fire fighting
- Situations where the combination of particulates and gases or vapors exceeds 2,000 times the permissible exposure limit (PEL) as required by OSHA
- Situations where the oxygen level is less than 19.5 percent
- Situations requiring an emergency entry where the contaminate concentration or oxygen level is unknown

All levels of training should address potential emergency situations such as fire fighting **(Figure 7.7),** confined-space rescue or entry, hazardous materials mitigation and remediation, and postfire loss control operations (salvage and overhaul). The depth of detail depends on the level of training desired, either entry or advanced. Advanced training can be obtained at respiratory protection specialist schools. Annual training and testing or recertification of members who wear SCBA ensure that all personnel remain proficient in the use of the equipment.

Entry-Level Training

The entry-level or initial training includes both classroom theory and simulated emergency scene use of SCBA. NFPA 1404, *Standard for Fire Service Respiratory Protection Training,* recommends three

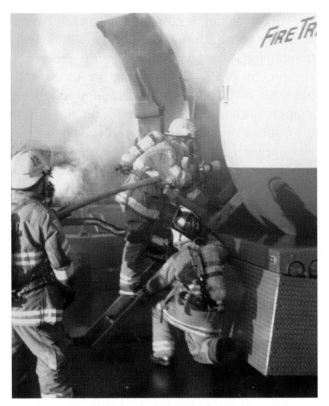

Figure 7.7 Structural fire fighting units that may have to respond to aviation incidents should be thoroughly trained in aircraft fire fighting and rescue. *Courtesy of Maryland Fire and Rescue Institute.*

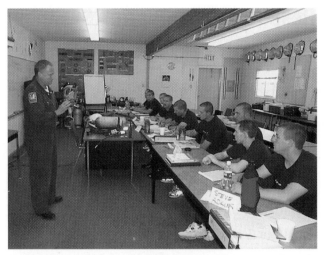

Figure 7.8 Certified training instructors (shown here) or manufacturer's representatives may provide entry-level SCBA training. *Courtesy of Lloyd Lees.*

levels or stages of initial training: classroom instruction, operations within a controlled environment, and operations under simulated emergency conditions.

In the classroom, trainees are taught the reasons SCBAs are worn, when they are worn, and how they are maintained, cared for, and stored. This instruction, developed by the authority having jurisdiction or provided by the SCBA manufacturer, ensures that trainees can meet the basic knowledge listed at the beginning of this chapter and required by NFPA 1404 and OSHA Title 29 *CFR* 1910.134. Certified training officers or manufacturers' representatives, or both, can provide this training (**Figure 7.8**).

Once the theory has been taught, trainees must participate in training exercises or evolutions within a controlled environment that will make them proficient in the use, care, and maintenance of SCBA. The exercises should be divided into stages or steps to allow trainees to learn the skills in easy-to-remember segments. Because the authority having jurisdiction establishes the training program, the following list is only a suggested SCBA training format:

- *Inspection*
  — Familiarization with SCBA components and operation
  — Periodic routine inspection
  — Pre-use inspection
  — Post-use inspection
- *Donning and doffing*
  — Proper methods for donning SCBA
  — Testing for facepiece seal
  — Opening and closing valves
  — Doffing SCBA
- *Use*
  — Proper use at emergency situations
  — Use while performing incident-scene tasks such as setting ladders or advancing hoselines
  — Use of accessories such as integrated personal alert safety system (PASS) devices or quick-fill systems
  — Replacement or refilling of SCBA cylinders (**Figure 7.9**)

CAUTION

Follow the manufacturer's recommendation for the level of SCBA maintenance and repair training requirements. Entry-level personnel will not receive the same level of training that certified maintenance personnel receive.

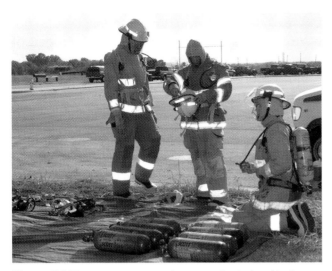

Figure 7.9 Emergency responders must be trained in the proper methods of replacing breathing air cylinders, identifying full and empty cylinders, and refilling cylinders at an incident. *Courtesy of Bob Parker.*

— Emergency escape techniques
— Systems failure troubleshooting
— Use with specialized protective clothing such as hazardous materials or proximity suits

● *Care and cleaning*
— Proper care and handling of SCBAs
— Cleaning techniques for SCBAs
— Facepiece care and cleaning

● *Storage*
— Proper storage of SCBAs
— Familiarization with storage locations on various types of apparatus operated by the jurisdiction (**Figure 7.10**)
— Removal of SCBAs from storage compartments, cases, or brackets
— Replacement of SCBAs in storage compartments, cases, or brackets
— Proper facepiece storage

Specific evolutions should be designed to reinforce these various skills. The organization's training facility should have training equipment to permit the required operations. Suggested types of equipment are described in the Training Facilities section.

Finally, trainees must be given the opportunity to use SCBAs in simulated emergency operations. These simulations involve the use of live-fire structures, flashover simulators, or confined-space and structural-collapse training modules. Live-fire

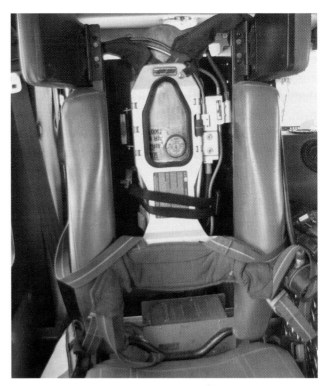

Figure 7.10 Trainees should be instructed in the proper way to store an SCBA (such as in this jump seat) and how to don it from the storage position. *Courtesy of Bob Parker.*

training exercises must conform to the requirements in NFPA 1403, *Standard on Live Fire Training Evolutions.* Training exercises must conform to the actual emergency situations that the organization responds to on a daily basis (**Figure 7.11**). Fire and

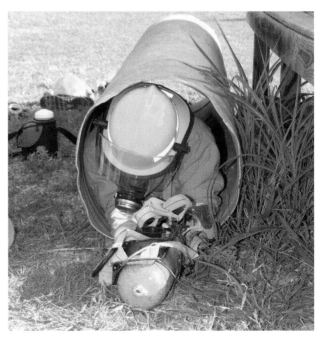

Figure 7.11 Entry-level SCBA training may include the basics of operating in a confined space while wearing respiratory protection. *Courtesy of Bob Parker.*

emergency services personnel must be trained to operate in teams of at least two members and to establish rapid intervention crews (RICs) prior to committing an attack team into any immediately dangerous to life and health (IDLH) situation. Members operating in teams must be able to communicate with each other visually, audibly, physically, by way of a safety rope, through electronic means, or any other method of communication. Safety must be the primary concern during all training evolutions, especially those involving live-fire training.

Training is complete when trainees are able to demonstrate that they have successfully retained the information and skills taught to them. Written and oral examinations and physical skills exercises are used to determine the success of the training. Completion of the testing phase results in the certification of trainees for SCBA system use.

Respiratory Protection Specialist School
[NFPA 1500: 5.4.1, 5.4.2]

The most common advanced training program available to emergency responders is the respiratory protection specialist school (also known as smoke diver school). State fire service training institutions operate many of these schools. However, some manufacturers have mobile training centers that tour the country and can offer training close to an organization's home.

Respiratory protection specialist schools introduce emergency responders gradually to increasingly difficult tasks while wearing SCBA. At these schools, response personnel learn more about their abilities, limitations, and air-consumption rates while using SCBA, and they have more time to perfect their skills with the apparatus (**Figure 7.12**). For instance, trainees intensely practice techniques such as controlled breathing — making repeated and conscious efforts to reduce air consumption by forcing exhalation from the mouth and allowing natural inhalation through the nose. They also learn how to calculate their own points of no return and how to use SCBA in varied, realistic situations.

Typical U.S. respiratory protection specialist schools last between 30 and 60 hours usually spread out over a week or several weekends. The first day's work can include the causes of responder collapse,

physical aspects of breathing and fatigue, and fire environment components — basically a review of what responders learned in the initial training program. Emergency responders then review and practice the basics of using SCBA and become proficient in donning and doffing the apparatus.

Routine training becomes increasingly more difficult as trainees progress in confidence and experience. First, trainees may review how to fit and test their facepieces and how to recharge cylinders. Once they have reviewed the equipment, they are usually given a relatively simple task to perform while wearing the apparatus. As training progresses, trainees practice controlled-breathing techniques and learn how to calculate their individual air-consumption rates. For instance, trainees may be asked to don their breathing apparatus and spend 2 minutes chopping at telephone poles with axes. This exercise allows instructors to measure and evalu-

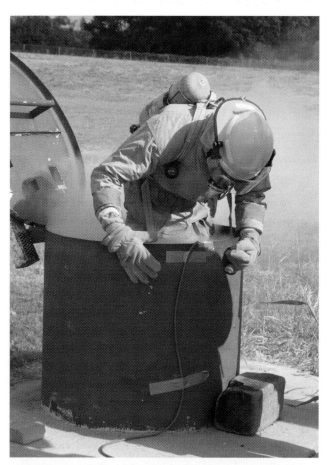

Figure 7.12 Training provided at respiratory protection specialist schools is more advanced and strenuous than entry-level training. In this illustration, a trainee enters a belowground smoke chamber that provides both a confined space and obstructed vision as obstacles. *Courtesy of Bob Parker.*

ate how well trainees can control their breathing while wearing SCBA during strenuous work. Instructors can get the same information by having trainees swing sledgehammers at tire sections anchored to heavy beams. Another exercise to teach controlled-breathing techniques involves having trainees in full personal protective equipment and SCBA walk up and down several stories in a training tower (**Figure 7.13**). Their air-consumption rates are then measured, and the exercise is repeated following controlled-breathing training. Emergency responders can learn to reduce their air consumptions by as much as 50 percent through this training.

At this point trainees may be shown how it feels to depend on their breathing apparatus without being able to see. Instructors put cloth or translucent paper over facepieces so that trainees can see light but nothing else. Then trainees are given another relatively simple task such as following hoselines 100 feet (30 m) through obstacle courses. This exercise allows trainees to practice "seeing" with their hands. They learn to identify objects and obstacles, and by feeling the couplings, they determine which directions they are traveling along hoselines. As trainees become more familiar with their equipment, they learn what to do if the equipment fails or if they run out of air. Participants are

generally given training and practice in team emergency-conditions breathing procedures after classroom instruction in emergency operations (**Figure 7.14**). At some schools this session is done twice — once with machine-generated smoke and once without smoke.

CAUTION

Emergency responders must be familiar with their respective respiratory protection equipment limitations to prevent injury or death.

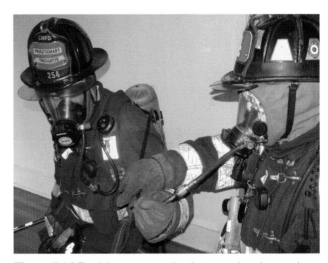

Figure 7.14 Participants operating in teams in advanced training programs are given instruction in the use of buddy-breathing systems. *Courtesy of Kenneth Baum.*

Next, trainees may be taught how to conduct search-and-rescue operations in full protective gear and breathing apparatus. Trainees first hear a classroom lecture on search patterns and rescue techniques. They then spend the rest of the day practicing. Trainees may perform exercises in machine-made smoke wearing clear facepieces; other exercises may be performed with facepieces covered.

The final day of the respiratory protection specialist school may be all practice. Trainees usually perform combined evolutions. They may be shown how it feels to be lowered down narrow shafts to perform rescues while in breathing apparatus. They may be assigned to enter smoky atmospheres, find victims who are "overcome" by smoke or toxic

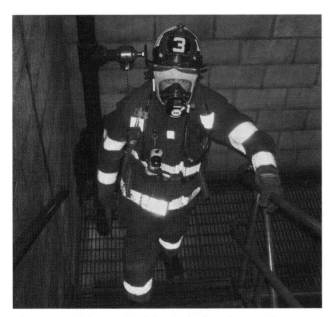

Figure 7.13 Advanced training is designed to test the stamina of participants through various evolutions while wearing SCBA. This firefighter climbs several flights of stairs in a darkened stairwell wearing full protective clothing and SCBA. *Courtesy of Kenneth Baum.*

materials, and bring them outside (**Figure 7.15**). They may be sent into tunnels — such as large culverts blocked at one end — to secure and remove victims in Stokes baskets. In all exercises, trainees are forced to depend on their breathing apparatus in "hazardous" atmospheres. By the end of this intensive course, using SCBA in hazardous atmospheres and emergency situations becomes second nature to trainees.

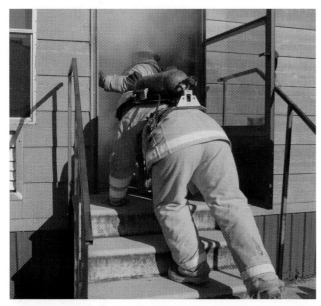

Figure 7.15 Specially designed smoke buildings provide an opportunity for training in search and rescue techniques while working with restricted vision.

Annual Training/Testing

Emergency responders who wear SCBA must be provided with annual training in respiratory protection. They are then required to pass an annual test or recertification requirement to ensure that they remain proficient in the use of the equipment. The authority having jurisdiction establishes the annual training curriculum and testing or recertification criteria. Personnel who fail the tests must be retrained prior to recertification. The retraining focuses on the areas that personnel were unable to pass.

Air-Purifying Respirator and Particulate Mask

[NFPA 1404: 4.4, 6.5.1, 6.5.2, 6.9.1, 6.9.2, 6.9.3, 6.9.4]

Air-purifying respirators may be either full facepiece (also known as FFAPR) units or half facepiece APR

units; both depend on canisters or cartridges to purify the ambient atmospheres. They may also be equipped with blowers to force the ambient air through the respirators. This type of APR is known as a powered air-purifying respirator (PAPR) (**Figure 7.16**). Regardless of the type, the training required must match the type of unit, type of hazard, function being performed, and manufacturer's recommendations. These units are used in hazards involving particulates, known gases and vapors, or combinations of both that are in concentrations of 50 times the permissible exposure limits. Training requirements for all of these units are found in NFPA 1404.

Particulate mask respirators, including both dust types and medical types, are used to protect wearers from large-diameter airborne hazards (**Figure 7.17**). The single-use disposable respirators protect against particulates in concentrations up to five

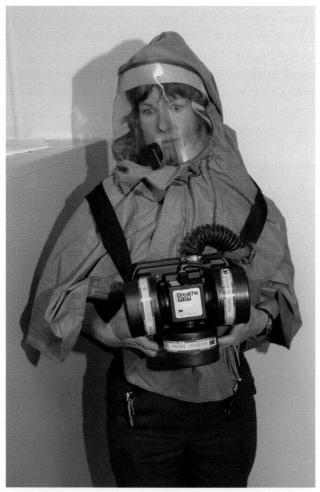

Figure 7.16 This photo shows an example of a powered air-purifying respirator (PAPR). A blower forces ambient air through the filter canister and into the facepiece.

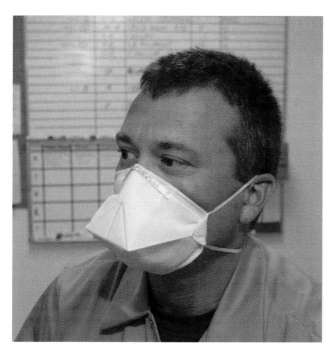

Figure 7.17 Particulate masks such as the one shown are used in a variety of situations from overhaul operations to medical responses to maintenance operations.

- **Inspection**
  - Familiarization with APR or particulate respirator components and operation
  - Periodic routine inspection
  - Pre-use inspection
  - Post-use inspection
- **Donning and doffing**
  - Proper methods for donning APRs or particulate respirators
  - Testing for facepiece seal
  - Doffing APRs or particulate respirators
- **Use**
  - Proper use at emergency situations
  - Selecting the proper level of protection
  - Use of accessories such as eyeglass kits
  - Emergency escape techniques
  - Systems failure troubleshooting
  - Use with specialized protective clothing such as hazardous materials suits
- **Care and cleaning**
  - Proper care and handling of APRs
  - Cleaning techniques for APRs
  - Replacement of filters or cartridges
  - Disposal of filters, cartridges, or contaminated units (**Figure 7.18**)
  - Disposal of single-use particulate respirators

times the PEL of the hazards. Dust respirators protect against any particulate in concentrations up to ten times the PEL. NFPA does not currently specify training requirements for these types of respirators. However, using the manufacturer's instructions and NFPA 1404 as a guide for developing a training protocol makes good sense for the fire and emergency services organization.

Each level of training is based on the types of situations that APRs or particulate masks are used in and the types of hazards they are intended to protect against. Training situations may include structural collapses, postfire investigations, medical responses, or rescues involving grain elevators. The authority having jurisdiction establishes the requirements for annual training, testing, and recertification based on OSHA, NFPA, and manufacturers' recommendations.

Entry-Level Training

Entry-level training is designed for the type of air-purifying respirator or particulate respirator in use, type of hazard that may be encountered, and manufacturer's training and use recommendations. Stages or steps of training may follow the same pattern as those used with SCBA and SAR units. These stages are as follows:

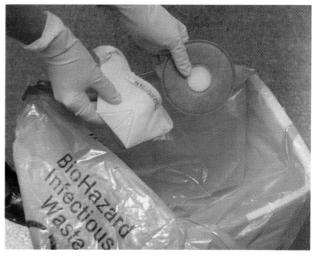

Figure 7.18 Contaminated particulate masks and filters must be disposed of properly such as into a medical waste container.

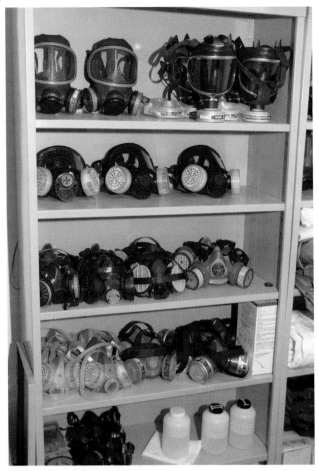

Figure 7.19 This photo shows the organized storage of a variety of models of APRs and replacement parts. APRs are color coded by the type of hazard they are approved to protect against.

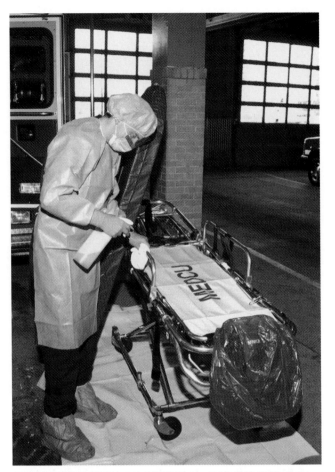

Figure 7.20 EMS personnel are thoroughly trained in the use of respiratory protection equipment. Besides incident use, particulate filter masks may be required when disinfecting medical equipment such as this gurney. *Courtesy of Mike Nixon.*

● *Storage*

— Proper storage of APRs and accessories (**Figure 7.19**)

— Proper storage of particulate respirators

— Familiarization with storage locations on organization-owned apparatus and facilities

— Removal of APRs or particulate respirators from storage compartments or cases

— Replacement of APRs in storage compartments or cases

Entry-level training evolutions depend on the specific type of use the APR or particulate respirator has. Development of these evolutions is the responsibility of the authority having jurisdiction.

Advanced-Level Training

Additional training that qualifies as advanced depends on the specific types of use for APRs. While the entry-level training may be directed toward postincident cleanup or investigation duties, advanced-level training may be provided for emergency medical services (EMS) certified personnel or hazardous materials response teams (**Figure 7.20**). Again, this choice is the responsibility of the authority having jurisdiction. It is unlikely that an advanced level of training would be required for the particulate respirator.

Annual Training/Testing
[NFPA 1404: 6.2.1, 6.2.2, 10.1.1]

Annual training and testing for FFAPR is required in NFPA 1404. This training and testing follows the pattern prescribed in the SCBA section. Annual training and testing is not mandated by NFPA for the other types of APRs. However, it is good practice to establish a program based on NFPA 1404 requirements.

Supplied-Air Respirator and Emergency Breathing Support System

[NFPA 1404: 4.2.3, 4.3, 6.5.1, 6.5.2, 6.7.4, 6.8.1, 6.8.2, 6.8.3, 6.8.4, 7.2.4]

Supplied-air respirators are provided with breathing air through hoselines from breathing-air compressor systems or portable cylinders located outside the work area (**Figure 7.21**). The hoseline is attached to the respirator, and an emergency breathing support system (or emergency escape pack) is required as a safety measure with these units. SARs operated in the pressure mode protect the wearer from particulates or known gas or vapor contaminants in concentrations up to 2,000 times the PEL. When operated in the positive-pressure mode, SARs can be used in environments with particulate or known gas or vapor contaminants in concentrations greater than 2,000 times the PEL.

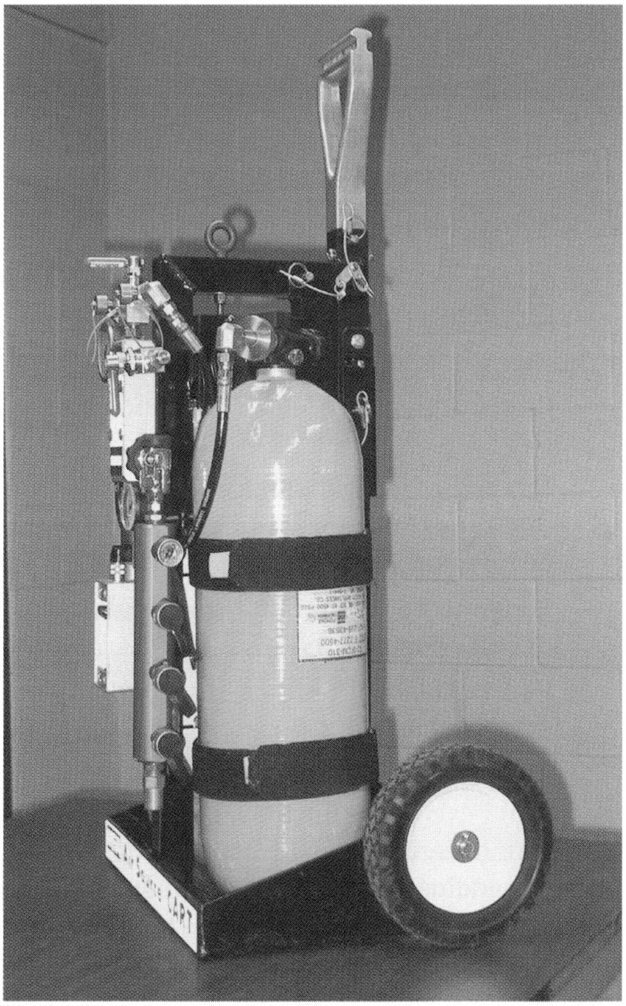

SARs may also be used for unknown contaminants in undetermined concentrations when operated in the positive-pressure mode.

These units may not be used for incidents involving fire or live-fire training. Situations requiring the use of SAR-type respiratory protection include but are not limited to the following:

● Hazardous materials incidents

● Confined-space search and rescue (**Figure 7.22**)

● IDLH incidents when the unit is designed and certified for such use

● Biological and medical incidents

The emergency breathing support system provides a safety factor for both SCBA and SAR units (**Figure 7.23**). All SAR units are required to have

Figure 7.21 Parts of the supplied-air respirator system include the portable breathing air cylinder cart and distribution manifold shown in this photo. *Courtesy of Lloyd Lees.*

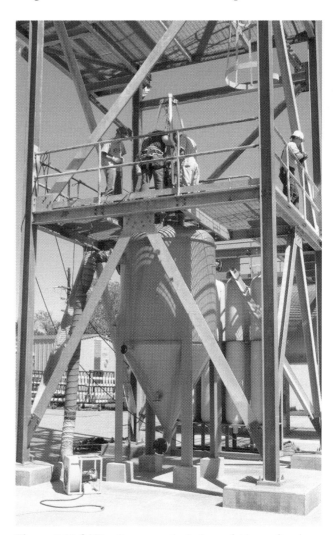

Figure 7.22 SAR units are particularly useful in confined-space operations such as in this aboveground storage tank. The system provides the rescuer with unlimited air supply and very little equipment weight as compared to that normally found with an SCBA.

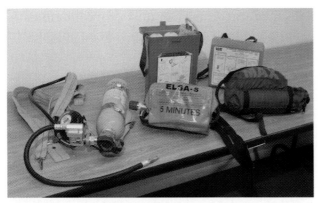

Figure 7.23 This photo shows a variety of emergency breathing support systems (EBSSs). The unit on the left is worn with an SAR system, while the other units are carried in packs and donned when the need arises.

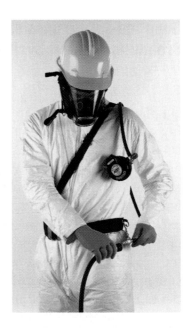

Figure 7.24 Fire and emergency services personnel must be trained in the proper methods of donning and doffing the SAR, connecting the regulator to the facepiece, connecting the air-supply hose, operating the air-supply manifold, and using the EBSS. *Courtesy of Scott Aviation.*

EBSS as part of the system. Entry-level and advanced-level EBSS training follow the criteria established for SCBA and SAR equipment. Annual testing and training are also required.

Entry-Level Training

Initial training should follow the manufacturer's recommendations and the program developed by the authority having jurisdiction. If entry-level personnel will be using this equipment on a regular basis, the training should follow the criteria established for SCBA entry-level training. If specialized rescue teams use SARs, support personnel must be familiar with the equipment to provide effective assistance. The following list gives the minimum requirements that would be required under the latter circumstances:

- *Inspection*
  - Familiarization with SAR and EBSS components and operation
  - Periodic routine inspection
  - Pre-use inspection
  - Post-use inspection
- *Donning and doffing*
  - Proper methods for donning SARs (**Figure 7.24**)
  - Testing for facepiece seal
  - Doffing SARs
- *Use*
  - Proper use at emergency situations
  - Use of accessories such as eyeglass kits and PASS devices

- Emergency escape techniques, including the use of an EBSS
- Systems failure troubleshooting
- Use with specialized protective clothing such as confined-space clothing
- Understanding the potential incompatibility of different makes and models of SARs

- *Care and cleaning*
  - Proper care and handling of SARs and EBSSs
  - Cleaning techniques for SARs and EBSSs
- *Storage*
  - Proper storage of SARs, EBSSs, and accessories
  - Familiarization with storage locations on various types of apparatus operated by the jurisdiction
  - Removal of SARs from storage compartments or cases (**Figure 7.25**)
  - Replacement of SARs in storage compartments or cases

Training evolutions would include entry into and search and exit of confined-space environments, hazardous materials incidents, and obscured-vision mazes. In addition, entry-level personnel should be trained in support functions such as monitoring or supervising air-supplying hoselines, general operation of the breathing-air compressor or supply cylinders, and the responsibilities of the RIC of which they are a part. Air supplies should be moni-

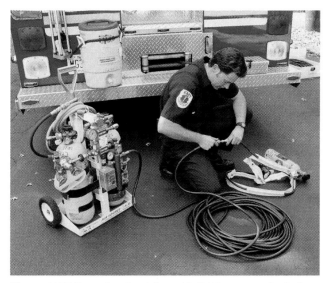

Figure 7.25 Entry-level training with SAR systems includes the proper method for removing the system from its storage compartment, inspecting it, and placing it into service. *Courtesy of Kenneth Baum.*

tored at all times to ensure that adequate supplies are available. Trainees must also be aware that the air-supply hose must be protected from snags, kinks, or sharp objects.

Trainees must understand that the EBSS cylinder valve must not be opened until the SAR air supply is depleted. If the valve is opened during normal operations, the EBSS cylinder will be depleted first. The EBSS cylinder valve does not operate automatically; it must be activated manually. Depending on the size of the cylinder, the duration of operation will be only 5 to 10 minutes (7 cubic feet [0.198 cm] of air is equivalent to 5 minutes duration while 15 cubic feet [0.425 cm] is approximately 10 minutes).

Advanced-Level Training

The advanced level of training would be designed for specialized rescue, confined-space rescue, or hazardous materials team members. This training would help members perfect the skills needed to operate in situations involving structural collapse, trench rescue, subway or subterranean passages rescue, maritime fire fighting, hazardous materials leaks or spills, or other IDLH situations that require long-duration breathing-air supplies (**Figure 7.26**). The manufacturer, a state or regional training center, or a national training center that has expertise in these types of operations may provide this training.

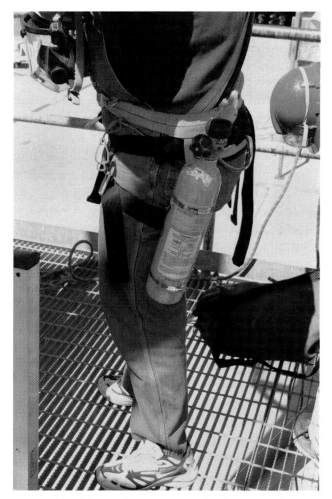

Figure 7.26 Advanced-level training with SAR and EBSS respiratory protection equipment increases the trainee's proficiency while working in confined spaces. An EBSS (shown in use during a training exercise) must be worn with all SARs used in potentially IDLH situations.

Advanced-level training for emergency escape packs should follow the advanced-level training provided for the particular SCBA or SAR it is used with. Advanced training can stress various types of emergency situations involving loss of primary air supply.

Annual Training/Testing
[NFPA 1404: 6.2.1, 6.2.2, 10.1.1]

Because these units are designed for use in IDLH situations, annual training, testing, and recertification of members are mandatory requirements. This training and testing should follow the guidelines given for SCBA plus any recommendations given by manufacturers. Requirements for training and testing are found in NFPA 1404 and OSHA Title 29 *CFR* 1910.134.

Effects of Continuous Use on Equipment

[NFPA 1404: 7.1.1, 7.1.2, 7.1.3, 7.2.1, 7.2.2, 7.2.3, 7.3.1, 7.3.2, 7.3.3, 8.1.1, 8.1.2, 8.1.2.1]

Personal protective equipment, respiratory protection equipment, tools, hose, and other equipment used in training receive far more wear than other equipment assigned to emergency response units. Because the equipment used in training should be the same as the equipment used by operational units, the fire and emergency services organization may choose any of a number of methods to meet this requirement. First, operational units may be required to use their own equipment during training exercises, which allows the operational units to use equipment that they work with daily. It also allows the training division and health and safety officer opportunities to inspect the equipment periodically to ensure its safe condition. Second, equipment used for training may be used or reserve equipment that has been removed from first-line service, which allows for the replacement of older equipment with newer equipment and still provides useful service to the organization. Finally, the organization may purchase all new equipment to support the operational and training functions **(Figure 7.27)**. This method ensures that all equipment is similar and that reserve units are available in the event of a major incident. Regardless of the method of supplying training respiratory protection equipment, the organization must be aware of the effects of continuous use on the equipment.

Continuous operation results in more frequent need for inspection, cleaning, and maintenance. Inspections occur as part of the training program and should be made prior to and after each use and periodically as required. Cleaning should occur following each use. Full facepieces, if shared, should be cleaned prior to storage. Personally assigned facepieces should be cleaned prior to returning them to service. Preventive maintenance should occur in accordance with NFPA 1852, *Standard on Selection, Care, and Maintenance of Open-Circuit Self-Contained Breathing Apparatus*, and manufacturers' recommendations. Some manufacturers have developed air-flow-test schedules based on the frequency of use that can be used to determine the required maintenance of units in continuous operation. Manufacture-certified technicians must perform all maintenance, preventive service, or unscheduled repairs **(Figure 7.28)**. Continuous operation of respiratory protection equipment requires an inventory of additional parts, additional spare units, units with increased breathing-air capacities, and additional repair labor time. These additions must be taken into consideration during the budgeting and purchasing phases when acquiring new or replacement equipment (see Chapter 5, Respiratory Protection Equipment Selection and Procurement). Additional information on maintenance requirements may be found in Chapter 9, Inspection, Care, and Maintenance.

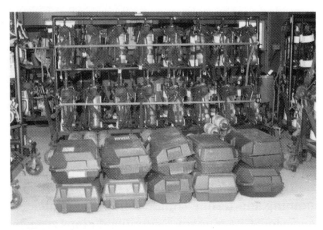

Figure 7.27 SCBAs used at this training facility were purchased specifically for training functions. They are stored on easily moved carts that are taken to the various training sites required by the daily training schedule.

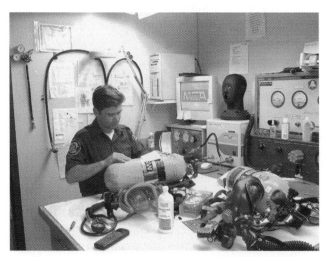

Figure 7.28 SCBAs used specifically for training receive more wear than units assigned to operational units. Continuous use, therefore, requires continuous maintenance by certified technicians like the one shown. *Courtesy of Lloyd Lees.*

Training Facilities

Respiratory protection training facilities can range from elaborate structures costing hundreds of thousands of dollars to buildings that are about to be torn down for community improvement projects. All buildings used for respiratory protection training should be inspected so that safe conditions are ensured. NFPA 1403 and NFPA 1404 should be referenced when applicable. NFPA 1500, *Standard on Fire Department Occupational Safety and Health Program*, and NFPA 1521, *Standard for Fire Department Safety Officer*, must also be used to determine the safety of individuals when using breathing apparatus in training situations and actual emergencies. Fire and emergency services organizations throughout the United States and Canada have effectively used many types of facilities to train their personnel to use respiratory protection equipment. Fixed and mobile training centers/laboratories (including mazes and makeshift facilities) are as varied as the number of agencies using respiratory protection equipment.

Permanent Training Centers

Departments/organizations that are financially capable can construct ideal permanent training centers to train fire and emergency services personnel in all types of incidents. Many centers, for example, have an academic building for classroom work and a fire building and training tower for more practical exercises. In the fire building are layouts using practically every feature an emergency responder might find in a building — a variety of roofs, steps, ramps, fire escapes, and balconies. Simulated store basements or utility vaults, rooms and hallways like those found in high-rise apartments, residential attics with attic ladders and scuttle holes, garden apartments, and elevator doors and shafts are also found. A multilevel tower may also be used for stairwell and high-rise building evolutions. Many training centers include smoke rooms and mazes for special respiratory protection training (**Figure 7.29**).

Mazes

Mazes are designed to help responders recognize their personal limitations. Facilities — permanent and mobile — commonly have mazes to train personnel to use respiratory protection equipment. Mazes can be operated with or without machine-produced smoke to give responders experience in overcoming some of the obstacles they commonly find at emergency incidents. Smokeless mazes generally use darkened facilities that have black walls (**Figure 7.30**). All facilities need to allow maximum instructor/trainee contact to enhance the training. Typical maze components include the following:

- Tunnels
- Drops
- Small spaces
- Dead ends

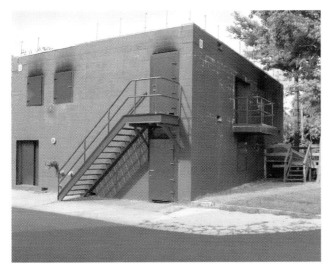

Figure 7.29 Permanent respiratory training structures may include one- and two-story smoke buildings such as this one. *Courtesy of Kenneth Baum.*

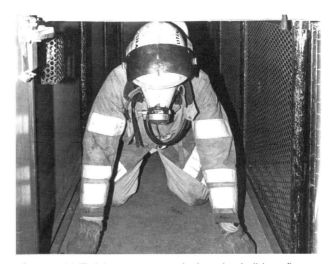

Figure 7.30 Training mazes are designed to build confidence and train personnel in techniques for moving through darkened areas without becoming disoriented.

Trainees without hand lights have to feel their way through these mazes. Generally mazes are monitored by two instructors who are posted inside in case a trainee encounters difficulties. Once inside a maze, trainees crawl through tunnels, climb down a drop, and then crawl up an incline to more small tunnels on the second level. They leave the maze after navigating more drops and tunnels.

Mobile Training Laboratories

Although some emergency responders may travel to train at a permanent regional facility, training officers in a variety of states and provinces take their facilities to the organizations within their jurisdiction. The permanent facility may be supplemented with mobile training laboratories complete with mazes and smoke rooms. State and provincial fire schools often use these mobile mazes to provide practical breathing apparatus equipment training on location (**Figure 7.31**). Personnel train by navigating a maze in pairs through realistic scenarios while wearing full personal protective clothing and respiratory protection. The amount of air that participants use when going through a maze can be measured, thus giving them an idea of their individual consumption rates when under exertion.

A typical mobile maze may be a 45-foot (14 m) trailer, containing a three-level maze that can be arranged in numerous ways. The maze can have crawl spaces, hatchways, tunnels, various openings, and dead ends. Barriers in the maze may be made of fences or movable partitions. Trainees encounter many obstacles in a mobile maze, and they must decide which way to go when they come to a barrier. The maze may also have a series of radiant heaters in the walls to simulate the high temperatures encountered in live-fire conditions. Ambient noises and distractions may also be added to the maze.

Before trainees are allowed to enter a mobile training facility, they must first exercise to raise their heart rates to 60 percent of their maximum aerobic states. A heart-monitoring machine can be incorporated into a ladder climb exercise and monitored from the command module. The trainees then negotiate these obstacles while their senses are besieged by heat, actual fireground sounds, and simulated radio traffic. The training officer con-

stantly monitors trainees using the mobile training facility from the command module via closed circuit television monitors and infrared cameras (**Figure 7.32**). Additionally, a safety officer is in constant attendance inside the training area when the unit is in use.

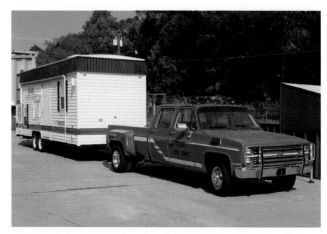

Figure 7.31 Some jurisdictions own and operate portable training structures that provide the same maze-like interiors that permanent structures do.

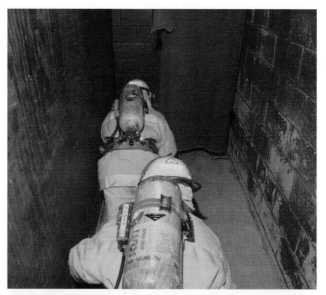

Figure 7.32 Training personnel must continuously monitor the progress of trainees within the maze to ensure that they do not become disoriented, panic, and accidentally injure themselves. Monitoring may be accomplished by listening to the progress of the trainees, following them into the maze (as indicated from the perspective of the camera), or stationing training personnel at intervals within the maze.

Makeshift Facilities

Fire and emergency services organizations without money for expensive, permanent training facilities have often found ingenious ways to use the equipment and facilities at hand to provide realistic respiratory protection training for their personnel. For instance, an emptied apparatus bay provides a large, open area that can depict the layout of a typical one-floor ranch-style residence. Walls, furniture, entrances, and confined spaces can be constructed with ordinary equipment owned by the organization (**Figure 7.33**). Typical materials used in the construction of makeshift facilities are as follows:

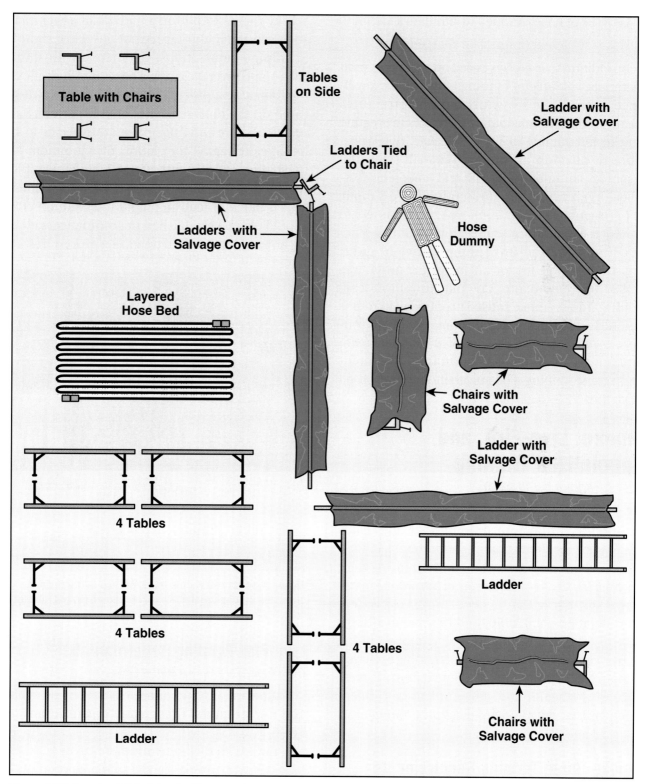

Figure 7.33 A makeshift training facility uses the resources that are locally available to provide SCBA training when a mobile or permanent facility is not available.

- Ladders
- Salvage covers or tarps
- Tables
- Chairs and sofas
- Empty SCBA boxes
- Lengths of hose wrapped to simulate a victim
- Hoses stretched to simulate charged lines

In addition to exercises based on these common materials, resourceful training officers have developed other exercises with common structures locally available. Imagination is the key to creating a makeshift training facility. With creativity, it is possible to develop an innovative drill from the resources common to the fire and emergency services organization or community. For example, departments/organizations have used motels to conduct search-and-rescue training. Training officers simply waited until the number of guest registrations was low or a wing of the motel was closed for remodeling. The machine-produced, nonhazardous smoke caused no damage to rooms and furnishings. One organization put its personnel into full protective gear and SCBA and sent them into a high-rise university dormitory for search-and-rescue training. The university students posed as victims.

Smoke, Live-Fire, and Specialized Training

[NFPA 1500: 4.9.1, 5.2.10]
[NFPA 1404: 6.3.1]

Respiratory protection training that duplicates emergency incidents requires additional facilities. Smoke-room, live-fire, and specialized-incident training (such as confined space, hazardous materials, shipboard, etc.) need increased safety considerations. NFPA 1500 and 1521 require the involvement of the health and safety officer during the development of these types of training exercises. Although all of these exercises benefit from the presence of the health and safety officer or incident safety officer, only live-fire incident training exercises require their presence.

Smoke-Room Training Requirements

Smoke rooms are training rooms or areas that can be filled with smoke to simulate emergency condi-

tions requiring respiratory protection (**Figure 7.34**). Because NFPA 1500 prohibits hazardous or live-fire smoke in SCBA training sessions, smoke-generating devices fill the rooms with nonhazardous smoke. Usually, trainees are grouped into teams of three or four members each and sent into the dark, smoky rooms to perform individual assignments such as search and rescues or gas valve shutoffs. Standpipe connections, gas meters with shutoff valves, and several electrical boxes may be built into the rooms. Equipment in the smoke room is duplicated on the outside of the room for briefing and practice before entering. Teams are expected to systematically search for victims or equipment and finish their assignments after reaching their objectives. Furniture and room partitions provide an added touch of realism. Rapid intervention crews should also be established in accordance with the organization's standard operating procedures.

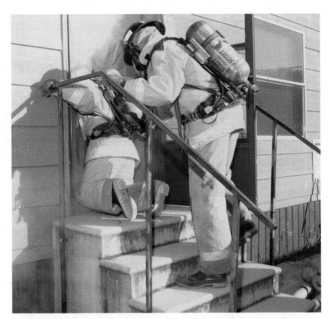

Figure 7.34 Smoke rooms used for respiratory training exercises can be created from portable buildings, mobile homes, or other inexpensive structures.

Live-Fire Training Requirements

[NFPA 1500: 4.9.3, 4.9.4, 4.9.5]

To duplicate the environments found at structural and nonstructural fires, many organizations use live-fire exercises to familiarize trainees and current members with these environments. NFPA 1403 establishes the criteria for the safe operation of live burns. Live-burn training exercises include the following components:

- *Structures*
  — Specially designated burn buildings (**Figure 7.35**)
  — Acquired structures located at remote sites (**Figure 7.36**)
- *Gas-fired permanent training structures*
- *Nongas-fired permanent training structures*
- *Exterior props*
  — Flashover simulators (**Figure 7.37**)
  — Vehicles
  — Trailers
  — Railroad tank cars
  — Class A combustibles
- *Exterior Class B fires*
  — Liquefied petroleum gas
  — Flammable/combustible liquids

NOTE: Regardless of the type of live burn, NFPA 1500 and 1521 require the involvement of the health and safety officer and an incident safety officer. The health and safety officer is responsible for preventing unsafe acts from occurring and for eliminating any unsafe conditions. This responsibility extends to the safety of all participants, training personnel, visitors, and spectators. The health and safety officer works closely with members of the training division to ensure that all live-burn structures and equipment meet the requirements of NFPA 1403.

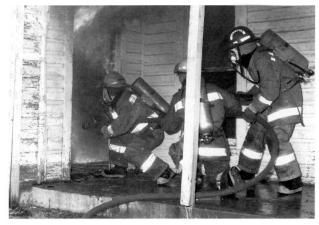

Figure 7.36 Some jurisdictions acquire old buildings that have been abandoned or donated and use them for live-fire exercises.

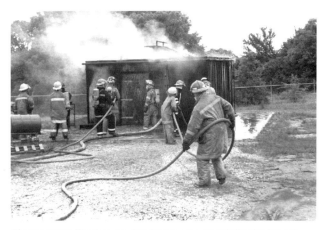

Figure 7.37 Flashover simulators are specially designed gas-fired, metal structures that simulate the extremely high temperatures generated during such events.

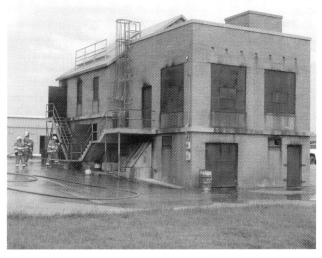

Figure 7.35 Live-fire burn buildings are constructed from masonry or concrete materials with steel covers over openings. The buildings are intended to withstand high heat and repeated exposure to fire.

Specialized-Training Requirements

Specialized training, which may be provided as advanced-level training, includes but is not limited to the following topics:

- Confined-space (tanks, vessels, silos, etc.) rescue
- Hazardous materials incidents
- Shipboard or maritime fire fighting
- Aircraft rescue and fire fighting
- High-angle rescue

Each of these areas of specialized training requires specific training modules and equipment. The general safety and operational concerns regarding protective clothing and equipment, weather conditions, water supply, and RIC personnel remain the same as those in other training exercises.

Confined-Space Rescue

[NFPA 1500: 5.2.4, 5.4.4]

Confined-space rescue training requires trench cave-in modules, underground passages, and simulated building collapse sites. The main consideration is to create a realistic yet structurally sound training environment (**Figure 7.38**). Personnel engaged in these types of training must not be placed at risk during the exercises. SCBA, APR, and SAR units may be used as appropriate. Guidelines (tag lines), communications, and safety harnesses are also required, depending on the organization's protocol for confined-space operations.

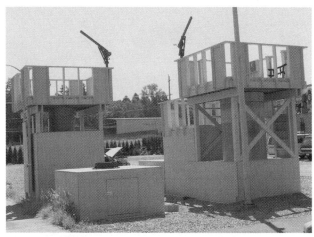

Figure 7.38 Confined-space training structures can take many forms, including the all-wood construction buildings shown. *Courtesy of Lloyd Lees.*

Hazardous Materials Incidents

[NFPA 1500: 5.2.7, 5.4.3]
[NFPA 1404: 6.3.6]

Hazardous materials incident training involves both the flammable/combustible liquids and liquefied petroleum gas training mentioned with Class B training plus chemical spills and chemical vapor leaks. Training should meet the requirements of NFPA 472, *Standard on Professional Competence of Responders to Hazardous Materials Incidents.* Due to the inherent hazard of nonburning hazardous materials, these incidents have to be simulated. The training division designates personal protective clothing based on the type of hazard involved. Nonburning exterior props such as railroad tank cars, bulk tanks, and tank trailers provide the hazard scene. The training objectives are as follows:

- Train personnel in the handling of hazardous materials spills or leaks.
- Familiarize personnel in the use of hazardous materials protective clothing.
- Familiarize personnel in the use of respiratory protection equipment while wearing hazardous materials protective clothing (**Figure 7.39**).

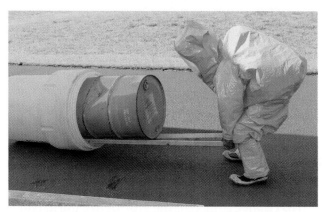

Figure 7.39 Hazardous materials training is very specialized and requires participants to perform various activities while fully encapsulated and wearing respiratory protection equipment. This emergency responder is placing a damaged drum into an overpack container. *Courtesy of Kenneth Baum.*

Shipboard Fire Fighting

Shipboard or maritime fire fighting has some similarities to both high-rise and confined-space operations on shore. Operations may be long duration, involve unventilated spaces, and lack emergency site access/egress. Respiratory protection training for these types of operations should focus on efficient use of limited air supplies, communication difficulties, access/escape procedures, and the use of search and rescue teams in addition to fire fighting training. Training facilities such as mazes, makeshift facilities, confined-space modules, and smoke rooms can be used to simulate the conditions found on a ship. When possible, however, a shipboard training facility or a real ship should be used for training (**Figure 7.40**). See IFSTA's **Marine Fire Fighting** and **Marine Fire Fighting for Land-Based Firefighters** manuals for details.

Aircraft Rescue and Fire Fighting

[NFPA 1500: 5.2.3]

Aircraft rescue and fire fighting is similar to vehicle rescue and flammable liquids incidents. Respiratory

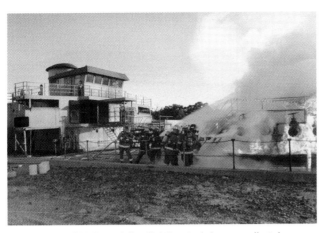

Figure 7.40 Shipboard fire fighting training usually takes place at simulated facilities on dry land. These trainees are attacking a controlled petroleum-based fire on a tanker simulation unit.

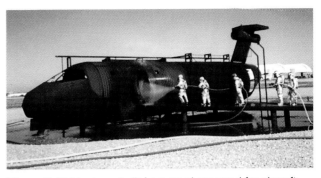

Figure 7.41 Mockups built from steel are used for aircraft fire fighting training. This one is situated over a pit that will contain the contaminated runoff from the exercise.

protection equipment is worn under entry-level suits that are similar to hazardous materials suits but designed for high temperatures and direct flame contact. Respiratory protection equipment is worn on the outside of proximity suits, which consist of structural personal protective clothing with increased thermal protection and a metallic reflective outer shell. SCBA may have additional protection in the form of a shroud for the air cylinder. Respiratory protection training would coincide with aircraft rescue and fire fighting training. Training objectives are as follows:

- Familiarize personnel with the use of respiratory protection equipment with entry-level and proximity protective clothing.
- Familiarize personnel with aircraft rescue and fire fighting protocols.
- Train personnel in the use of power extrication tools.

Simulated aircraft rescue modules can be specially built or created within a classroom as a temporary facility (**Figure 7.41**). A live-burn aircraft fuselage can be constructed and piped with propane or natural gas fire simulators. Training with the live-burn simulator is the same as using the specifically designed live-burn structure already mentioned. Derelict aircraft fuselages may be used for rescue training but should not be used for live burns due to the high amount of fuel loading and the damaging effects to the atmosphere. See IFSTA's **Aircraft Rescue and Fire Fighting** manual for more information.

High-Angle Rescue
[NFPA 1500: 5.2.4, 5.4.4]

High-angle rescue training usually requires a training tower or elevated area. Most high-angle rescues occur out of doors and away from respiratory protection hazards. It may be necessary, however, to enter a cave, a basement, or an underground tunnel by way of high-angle rescue systems. In these cases, respiratory protection may be required, so training in this type of incident is necessary. If the area to be entered has unknown oxygen content, SCBA or SAR is required. Training in rope descent and ascent while wearing this equipment is mandatory. If the oxygen content is sufficient, then APR equipment may be all that is needed. High-angle training is advanced-level training and may only be required for a select number of members of the organization (**Figure 7.42**).

Training Record Keeping
[NFPA 1500: 4.6.4, 5.3.7]
[NFPA 1404: 6.1.2]

Regardless of the type of training a member completes, an accurate training record must be kept by the fire and emergency services organization. Members should be allowed to review these records to check for accuracy. Record keeping can range from a simple handmade sheet kept by the training officer to computer records and data files. These records are in addition to the medical, equipment, and air-quality records discussed elsewhere in this manual. Accurate respiratory protection training records include information on many elements of the respiratory protection program. The following training records should be maintained by the fire and emergency services organization:

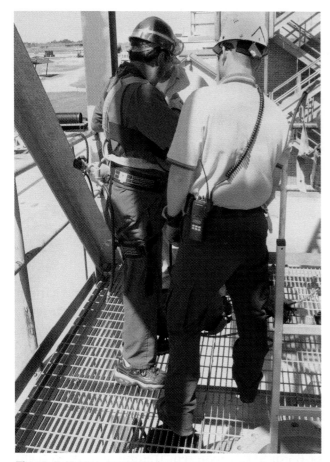

Figure 7.42 High-angle rescue training requires tall training towers made of open-steel construction (such as the one shown) or concrete multilevel buildings. Training may include rescues that require wearing SARs or SCBAs.

- *Fit testing and medical certifications* — This information is covered in Chapter 6, Medical Requirements and Facepiece Fit Testing.

- *Air-consumption data* — As fire and emergency services personnel progress through the stages of respiratory protection training, instructors should collect data on each member's breathing and air-consumption rates. These air-consumption records allow members to compare the amount of air they used at the beginning and end of the training course. They learn how to decrease their air intakes as they learn controlled-breathing techniques, and they learn to use the air-consumption statistics to calculate their points of no return. Not only do the members learn to conserve air but they also gain more confidence in their equipment and their personal skills.

- *Levels of training obtained* — These records reflect the levels of skills and knowledge held by individual members (**Figure 7.43**). Levels include

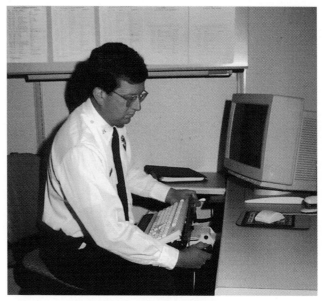

Figure 7.43 Respiratory protection training records are maintained by the organization's training staff. The records may be compiled on a computer (as shown here) or in manually compiled files.

entry- or initial-level training, advanced-level training, annual testing, or specialized training such as high-angle or confined-space rescue or hazardous materials incident training. By documenting the level of training attained by the organization as a whole, the organization may be able to obtain changes in insurance ratings or access to various governmental grants.

- *Individual and unit training records* — These records confirm the hours of training each member of the organization has completed and the amount of training that each unit has completed. These records are mandated by OSHA and must be available upon request by the U.S. Department of Labor either at the federal or state level.

Summary

Respiratory protection training is based on the fire and emergency services organization's written respiratory protection program. The authority having jurisdiction establishes the goals and objectives of the training program within the guidelines provided by NFPA 1404 and OSHA Title 29 *CFR* 1910.134. The resulting training program should be thorough, effective, and realistic for the participants. Personnel completing the program will have the knowledge and skills necessary to perform their duties safely while wearing respiratory protection equipment.

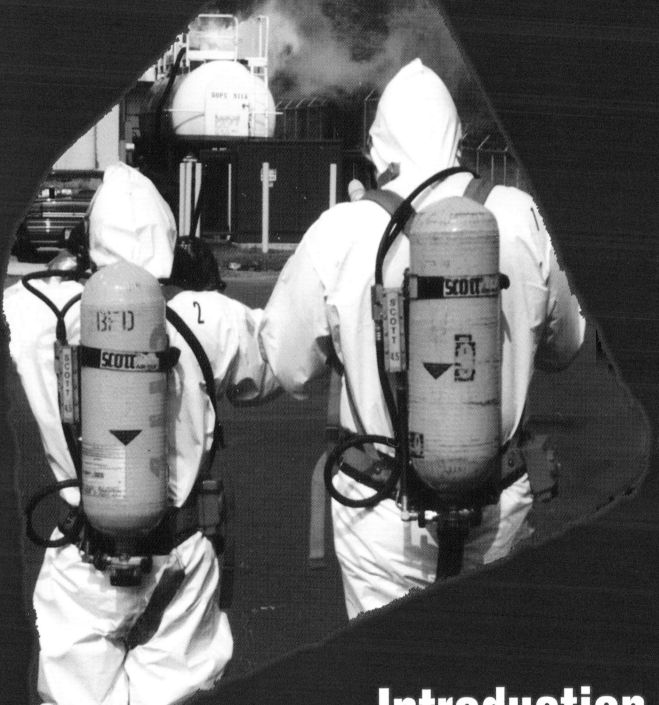

Chapter 8

Introduction to Operational Issues

This chapter provides information that will assist the reader in meeting the following job performance requirements from NFPA 1500, *Standard on Fire Department Occupational Safety and Health Program*, 2002 Edition.

NFPA 1500

5.1.11 All members who are likely to be involved in emergency operations shall be trained in the incident management and accountability system used by the fire department.

7.1.2 Protective clothing and protective equipment shall be used whenever the member is exposed or potentially exposed to the hazards for which it is provided.

7.1.3 Structural fire-fighting protective clothing shall be cleaned at least every 6 months as specified in NFPA 1581, *Standard on Fire Department Infection Control Program*.

7.2.1 Members who engage in or are exposed to the hazards of structural fire fighting shall be provided with and shall use a protective ensemble that shall meet the applicable requirements of NFPA 1971, *Standard on Protective Ensemble for Structural Fire Fighting*.

7.2.6 The fire department shall require all members to wear all the protective ensemble specific to the operation as required in Chapter 8.

7.3.1 Members whose primary responsibility is proximity fire fighting and members who participate in proximity fire-fighting training shall be provided with and shall use both proximity protective coats and proximity protective trousers, or a proximity protective coverall, for limb/torso protection.

7.4.1 Members who perform emergency medical care or are otherwise likely to be exposed to blood or other body fluids shall be provided with emergency medical garments, emergency medical face protection devices, and emergency medical gloves that meet the applicable requirements of NFPA 1999, *Standard on Protective Clothing for Emergency Medical Operations*.

7.5.1.1 Members who engage in operations during hazardous materials emergencies that will expose them to known chemicals in vapor form or to unknown chemicals shall be provided with and shall use vapor-protective suits.

7.5.2.1 Members who engage in operations during hazardous chemical emergencies that will expose them to known chemicals in liquid-splash form shall be provided with and shall use liquid splash-protective suits.

7.8.1 The fire department shall establish standard operating procedures for the use of wildland protective clothing and equipment.

7.8.2 Members who engage in or are exposed to the hazards of wildland fire-fighting operations shall be provided with and use protective garments that meet the requirements of NFPA 1977, *Standard on Protective Clothing and Equipment for Wildland Fire Fighting*.

7.14.1 PASS devices shall meet the requirements of NFPA 1982, *Standard on Personal Alert Safety Systems (PASS)*.

7.14.2 Each member shall be provided with, use, and activate their PASS device in all of the following situations:

(1) Fire suppression

(2) Rescue

(3) Other hazardous duty

7.14.3 Each PASS device shall be tested at least weekly and prior to each use, and shall be maintained in accordance with the manufacturer's instructions.

8.1.2 An incident management system that meets the requirements of NFPA 1561, *Standard on Emergency Services Incident Management System*, shall be established with written standard operating procedures applying to all members involved in emergency operations.

8.1.3 The incident management system shall be utilized at all emergency incidents.

8.1.5 At an emergency incident, the incident commander shall be responsible for the overall management of the incident and the safety of all members involved at the scene.

8.1.6 As incidents escalate in size and complexity, the incident commander shall divide the incident into tactical-level management components and assign an incident safety officer to assess the incident scene for hazards or potential hazards.

8.1.9 The fire department shall establish and ensure the maintenance of a fire dispatch and incident communications system that meets the requirements of NFPA 1561, *Standard on Emergency Services Incident Management System*, and NFPA 1221, *Standard for the Installation, Maintenance, and Use of Emergency Services Communications Systems*.

8.1.10 The fire department standard operating procedures shall provide direction in the use of clear text radio messages for emergency incidents.

8.3.1 The fire department shall establish written standard operating procedures for a personnel accountability system that is in accordance with NFPA 1561, *Standard on Emergency Services Incident Management System*.

8.3.2 The fire department shall consider local conditions and characteristics in establishing the requirements of the personnel accountability system.

8.3.3 It shall be the responsibility of all members operating at an emergency incident to actively participate in the personnel accountability system.

8.3.4 The incident commander shall maintain an awareness of the location and function of all companies or crews at the scene of the incident.

8.3.5 Officers assigned the responsibility for a specific tactical level management component at an incident shall directly supervise and account for the companies and/or crews operating in their specific area of responsibility.

8.3.6 Company officers shall maintain an ongoing awareness of the location and condition of all company members.

8.3.7 Where assigned as a company, members shall be responsible to remain under the supervision of their assigned company officer.

8.3.8 Members shall be responsible for following personnel accountability system procedures.

8.3.9 The personnel accountability system shall be used at all incidents.

8.3.10 The fire department shall develop the system components required to make the personnel accountability system effective.

8.3.11 The standard operating procedures shall provide the use of additional accountability officers based on the size, complexity, or needs of the incident.

8.3.12 The incident commander and members who are assigned a supervisory responsibility for a tactical level management component that involves multiple companies or crews under their command shall have assigned a member(s) to facilitate the ongoing tracking and accountability of assigned companies and crews.

8.4.4 Members operating in hazardous areas at emergency incidents shall operate in crews of two or more.

8.4.5 Crew members operating in hazardous areas shall be in communication with each other through visual, audible, or physical means or safety guide rope, in order to coordinate their activities.

8.4.6 Crew members shall be in proximity to each other to provide assistance in case of emergency.

8.4.9 The standby members shall remain in radio, visual, voice, or signal line communication with the crew.

8.5.1 The fire department shall provide personnel for the rescue of members operating at emergency incidents.

8.5.2 A rapid intervention crew/company shall consist of at least two members and shall be available for rescue of a member or a crew.

8.5.2.1 Rapid intervention crews/company shall be fully equipped with the appropriate protective clothing, protective equipment, SCBA, and any specialized rescue equipment that could be needed given the specifics of the operation underway.

8.5.7 At least one dedicated rapid intervention crew/company shall be standing by with equipment to provide for the rescue of members that are performing special operations or for members that are in positions that present an immediate danger of injury in the event of equipment failure or collapse.

8.6.1 The fire department shall develop standard operating procedures that outline a systematic approach for the rehabilitation of members operating at incidents.

8.6.2 The incident commander shall consider the circumstances of each incident and initiate rest and rehabilitation in accordance with the standard operating procedures and with NFPA 1561, *Standard on Emergency Services Incident Management System*.

8.6.3 Such on-scene rehabilitation shall include at least basic life support care.

8.6.4 Each member operating at an incident shall be responsible to communicate rehabilitation and rest needs to their supervisor.

Chapter 8
Introduction to Operational Issues

Respiratory protection policy and equipment are provided by the fire and emergency services organization for the safety and protection of individual employees. During emergency incidents, the application of the respiratory protection policy and the use of equipment are the responsibilities of the individual emergency responder, the incident commander (IC), and the incident command staff. This chapter introduces the various components of emergency scene operational issues as they relate to respiratory protection from the standpoints of both the individual responder's responsibilities and the incident commander's responsibilities.

Individual Responder's Responsibilities

The individual emergency responder's responsibilities in following respiratory protection operational and safety policies include wearing the proper level of personal protective clothing and respiratory protection equipment, using an accountability system, using a personal alert safety system (PASS) device, and maintaining communications while in immediately dangerous to life and health (IDLH) areas. While some of these issues may apply to only one type of emergency response, they must all be understood and adhered to by emergency responders. Emergency responders can ensure their own safety at an emergency scene by taking the following steps:

- Follow the organization's operational and safety policies.
  — Wear personal protective equipment.
  — Use an accountability system.
  — Use a PASS device.
  — Maintain communications in dangerous areas.

- Follow the instructions and orders of the incident commander, incident safety officer, or immediate supervisor.

- Apply the knowledge and skills learned in training.

- Inspect and use respiratory protection equipment according to established and written protocols.

- Take responsibility for own actions.

Personal Protective Equipment
[NFPA 1500: 7.1.2, 7.1.3, 7.2.1, 7.2.6, 7.3.1, 7.4.1, 7.5.1.1, 7.5.2.1, 7.8.1, 7.8.2]

The emergency responder is responsible for the care, cleaning, storage, and use of the personal protective equipment that the organization provides. At the beginning of each work shift, the equipment must be inspected and placed in service (**Figure 8.1**). Repairs or replacement of damaged equipment should be *addressed immediately* once the need is recognized. Damaged equipment of any kind, especially respiratory protection equipment, must never be used in an emergency situation. Damaged or faulty equipment increases the likelihood that an emergency responder may become a victim.

When emergency responders arrive at an incident, time is critical. Proper protective equipment must be donned, tested, and activated in a minimum amount of time. Training and practice help reduce this preparation time. Once responders are properly equipped, they are ready to employ the accountability system (**Figure 8.2**).

NOTE: When emergency service personnel use respiratory protection equipment, they are predominately working in hazardous environments.

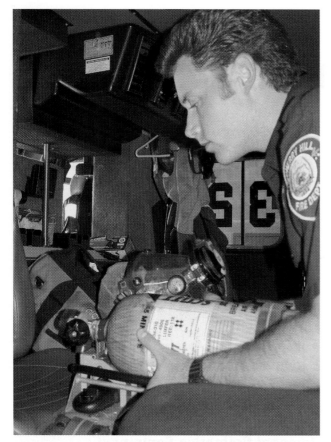

Figure 8.1 At the beginning of each work period, fire and emergency response personnel must inspect their personnel protective equipment. *Courtesy of Kenneth Baum.*

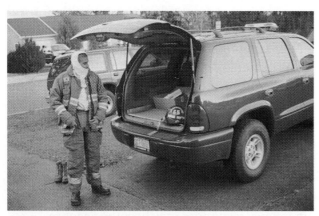

Figure 8.2 Volunteer fire and emergency responders usually carry their personal protective equipment and sometimes their respiratory protection equipment with them in their personal vehicles. Periodic inspection of this equipment ensures that it is ready for immediate use.

Emergency service responders must have confidence using respiratory protection in these environments under both normal and emergency conditions. This level of proficiency only comes through continuous training with respiratory protection equipment available for their use.

Accountability System

[NFPA 1500: 5.1.11, 8.3.1, 8.3.2, 8.3.3, 8.3.4, 8.3.5, 8.3.6, 8.3.7, 8.3.8, 8.3.9, 8.3.10, 8.3.11, 8.3.12]

The accountability system is like a life insurance policy for the individual emergency responder. It provides a level of security in the event that a responder becomes trapped, lost, or incapacitated. The accountability system is part of the Incident Management System (IMS) and is intended to help the incident commander maintain a rapid accounting of all personnel, manage the resources at the scene, and safeguard emergency response personnel engaged in the operation. The use of IMS and an accountability system is a requirement of NFPA 1500, *Standard on Fire Department Occupational Safety and Health Program*, and NFPA 1561, *Standard on Emergency Services Incident Management System*. While the fire and emergency services organization establishes the protocol for the accountability system and the incident commander applies it, the individual responder is responsible for adhering to the policy. How an individual adheres to the accountability system depends on the specific protocol developed by the fire and emergency services organization. In general, the requirements are as follows:

- Use the accountability system as established in the written policy.

- Check in with the accountability officer or incident safety officer when arriving at a scene (**Figure 8.3**).

- Never operate alone.

- Check out when leaving the hot zone or an incident scene.

- Maintain communications when operating in the hot zone.

Personal Alert Safety System Device

[NFPA 1500: 7.14.1, 7.14.2, 7.14.3]

A second element of the accountability "insurance policy" is the personal alert safety system device. The PASS device is a battery-operated motion detector that emits a loud noise and flashing light when the wearer is motionless for 30 seconds or longer (**Figure 8.4**). This noise/light allows rescuers to rapidly locate victims and provide assistance.

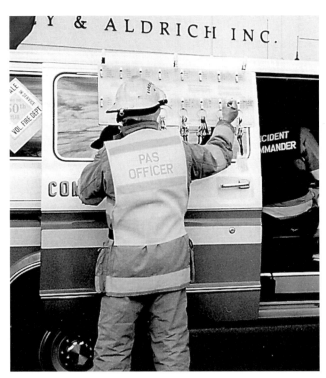

Figure 8.3 The incident commander, incident safety officer, or the accountability officer collects accountability tags from all personnel at the incident and posts them on the accountability board at the command post. *Courtesy of Clemens Industries, Inc.*

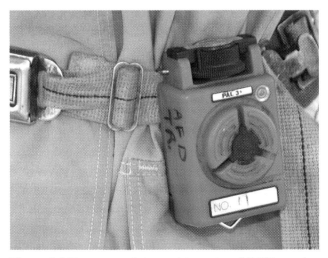

Figure 8.4 The personal alert safety system (PASS) may be attached to the SCBA harness (as shown), attached to the protective clothing, or integrated into the SCBA itself. In any case, it must be worn and activated to be effective. *Courtesy of Bob Parker.*

PASS devices may be single units worn on the protective clothing or integrated within the self-contained breathing apparatus (SCBA) unit.

Regardless of its design, the PASS device is only beneficial if it is worn and activated. The unit must be tested prior to every work shift and repaired or

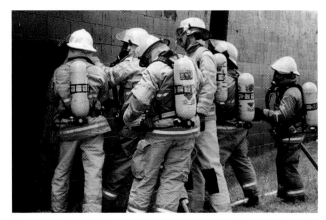

Figure 8.5 PASS devices must be worn and activated at all incidents. In this photo, PASS devices are visible on the SCBA waist straps of three of the responders. *Courtesy of Chris Mickal.*

replaced immediately if it fails to function. It is the emergency responder's responsibility to wear the unit, turn the unit on, and test the unit before entering the hot zone. The unit should be worn at all incidents, whether interior or exterior (**Figure 8.5**).

Communication Methods

[NFPA 1500: 8.1.10, 8.4.4, 8.4.5, 8.4.6, 8.4.9]

Communication is the element of the accountability system and IMS that connects the individual emergency responder to both rescue personnel nearby and the incident command post. It provides reassurance, information, and safety for the responders and the command officers. Emergency responders must be familiar with the various communication methods and adhere to their uses. The individual responder is responsible for ensuring that the particular communications system is working and that communication protocol is fully understood before entering the hot zone. Emergency scene communications takes many forms including the following:

- Direct/verbal
  - Voice amplification
  - Radio
- Visual
- Physical
  - Physical contact
  - Tag lines
- Combined systems (confined space)

Direct/Verbal

Direct communication between individuals is the most effect means of transmitting information (**Figure 8.6**). At an emergency incident, especially one involving smoke or contaminated atmospheres, direct communication is not always possible. The use of respiratory protection equipment decreases the ability to speak clearly and articulate properly. The facepiece reduces the volume of the voice while the incident scene noise level reduces the ability to hear (**Figure 8.7**). The emergency responder must practice speaking while wearing respiratory protection equipment during training to develop the most effective means of communication. If available, two methods for voice enhancement may be used: voice amplification and radio systems.

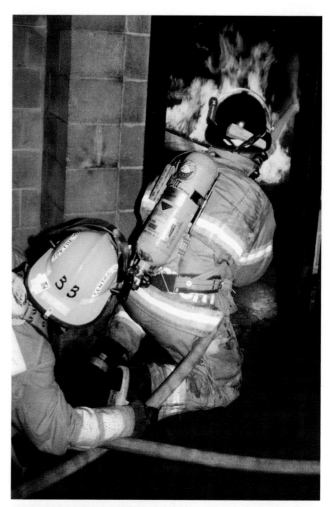

Figure 8.7 Ambient noise created by the incident, apparatus noises, and the fire itself add to the difficulty of communicating while wearing respiratory protection equipment. *Courtesy of Joe Marino.*

Voice amplification. Voice amplification can be mechanical or electronic. The mechanical speaking diaphragm is commonly found on SCBA and supplied-air respirator (SAR) facepieces and allows the wearer to be heard at close range (**Figure 8.8**). Because the mechanical speaking diaphragm does not always permit clear and concise communication, some manufacturers are providing an electronic voice amplification system. This lightweight, battery-operated device fits onto the facepiece exhalation diaphragm. It amplifies the volume of the speaker to permit audible communication (**Figure 8.9**).

Radio systems. SCBA and SAR manufacturers working with telecommunications manufacturers have developed radio communications systems that permit the use of handheld or portable radios while wearing full facepieces. Depending on the

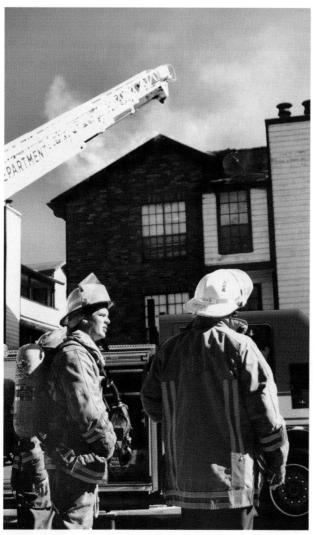

Figure 8.6 The most effective means of communication is direct or verbal between two individuals. Instructions can be understood and questions/answers clarified. *Courtesy of Chris Mickal.*

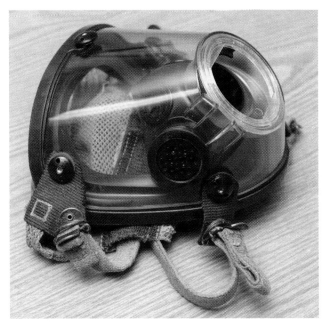

Figure 8.8 The majority of full facepieces are equipped with mechanical speaking diaphragms that provide a limited ability to be understood when speaking.

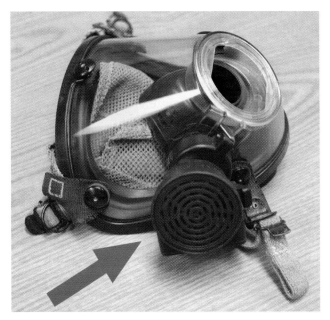

Figure 8.9 An improvement over the mechanical speaking diaphragm is the voice amplifier that is provided as an option by respirator manufacturers.

design, the system may include a facepiece-mounted microphone, throat microphone, bone-conduction microphone attached to the wearer's head, nonintegrated microphone worn on the harness, or simply a handheld radio separate from the respiratory protection system (**Figure 8.10**). To comply with National Institute for Occupational Safety and Health (NIOSH) certification, communications systems that are integrated with

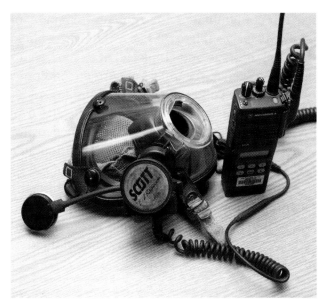

Figure 8.10 One method of improving radio communications while wearing a respiratory protection facepiece is with an integrated radio system.

the facepiece must be tested and approved as part of the respiratory protection system. Field modifications void all certification and must not be made.

> # WARNING!
>
> **All communications devices that attach to or penetrate the facepiece must meet NIOSH approval. Field modifications are not permitted.**

Visual

During fire-suppression operations, search and rescues, and confined-space operations, emergency responders must remain in visual contact with one another. Some of the things that can affect or reduce the ability to remain in visual contact are as follows:

- Smoke or contaminants in the atmosphere
- Low-light conditions
- Structural members
- Wreckage or debris
- Confined space
- Protective equipment

The emergency responder has control over only a few of the aforementioned factors. First, intrinsically safe portable radios and hand lights should be used in contaminated atmospheres, darkness, or confined spaces (**Figure 8.11**). Hand lights should be standard issue and employed at all emergency operation scenes, regardless of current conditions because these conditions may deteriorate and require the use of hand lights. Second, reflective trim on protective clothing should be maintained to provide the greatest reflectivity. This maintenance includes the proper cleaning and repair of reflective trim on coats, trousers, and helmets. Third, the facepieces of respiratory protection equipment, helmet-mounted faceshields, and hazardous materials suits must be cleaned and maintained to provide the best visibility.

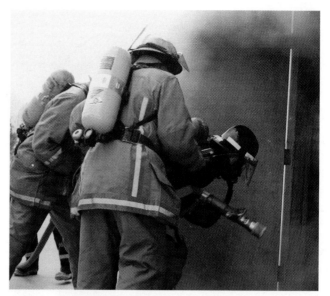

Figure 8.12 Physical contact provides reassurance that responders are not alone in dark, contaminated atmospheres. *Courtesy of Chris Mickal.*

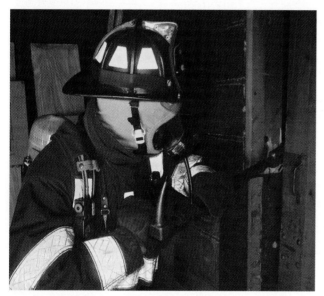

Figure 8.11 The use of handheld lights in dark or smoky areas helps to maintain visual contact between responders by illuminating the reflective trim (as shown) on personal protective clothing. *Courtesy of Kenneth Baum.*

Physical

Physical communication includes both physical contact and the use of tag lines. Physical contact in a stressful situation can provide reassurance as well as communication. The emergency responder is responsible for understanding the use of physical contact and tag lines and the communication code employed with both.

Physical contact. Physical contact between team members is essential during interior emergency and confined-space operations. Physical contact is reassuring to members in reminding them that they are not alone (**Figure 8.12**). The emergency responder must maintain contact, if at all possible,

throughout an interior or confined-space operation. A prearranged code should be used for passing limited information by touch when visibility is restricted and vocal communication is difficult. Depending on local protocol, this code may take the form of taps such as one tap for okay, two for advance, three for withdraw, etc.

Tag lines. Tag lines are used in confined-space, hazardous materials, and interior emergency operations. The tag line is a lifeline that is secured to the waist, rescue harness, or SCBA harness of the first member of a team entering a structure or confined space (**Figure 8.13**). Subsequent team members hold onto the line. At least one member of the rapid intervention crew must monitor the tag line at all times. All members of the rapid intervention crew are fully equipped and ready for immediate response. A prearranged system of communication should be established between the interior team and the RIC. A traditional method is called the *O-A-T-H* method. Each letter and its corresponding tug on the line has specific meaning: *O* — one tug means *okay, A* — two tugs mean *advance, T* — three tugs mean *take-up,* and *H* — four tug means *help.* Any signal given on the line should be acknowledged by the same signal from the other end. Care, storage, and maintenance of tag lines are the responsibilities of individual responders. Training improves skills and prepares responders for the potential use of tag lines.

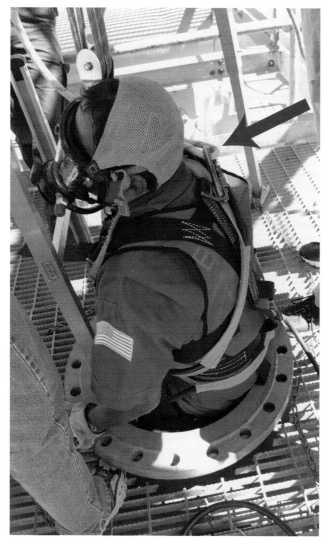

Figure 8.13 Tag lines are attached to rescue harnesses, protective clothing, or respiratory protection harnesses to provide both a means of physical communication and rescue when working in a confined space.

Combined Systems (Confined Space)

Confined-space entry is one of the most dangerous procedures performed by emergency responders. Therefore, only persons trained in confined-space entry techniques should attempt such operations. SAR equipment should be used instead of SCBA due to limited air supply and tight-fitting spaces. Trained personnel who undertake confined-space operations are responsible for following established protocols and maintaining communications with other team members and personnel outside the space (**Figure 8.14**). Emergency responders are responsible for maintaining their skill levels and the equipment. They must also realize their limitations and never enter a confined space if they are not trained to do so.

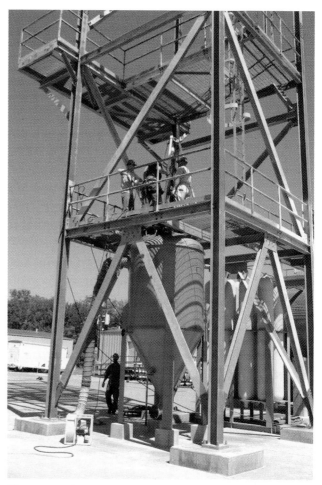

Figure 8.14 Personnel who are assigned to confined-space rescue teams must undergo extensive training in all types of confined-space operations.

Due to the risks involved to responders, communications within a confined space use redundant or backup systems. Tag lines are always used followed by handheld radios. Because the confined space may restrict the number of responders to only one person at a time, visual, physical contact, and voice enhancement may not be possible, depending on the situation. Use of an accountability system and deployment of a rapid intervention crew are also mandatory before entry into a space.

> # WARNING!
> Confined-space entry is one of the most dangerous procedures performed by emergency responders. Therefore, only persons trained in confined-space entry techniques should attempt such operations.

Incident Commander's Responsibilities

[NFPA 1500: 8.1.2, 8.1.3, 8.1.5]

The incident commander has the ultimate responsibility for the emergency operation and the safety of involved personnel. If an incident is small, the incident commander may have to directly supervise all aspects of the incident. If it is large, then the incident commander can delegate duties to other members of the incident command staff such as an incident safety officer. The incident commander is responsible for having a thorough knowledge of the Incident Management System and employing it at an incident (**Figure 8.15**). Detailed information on the use of the Incident Management System can be found in NFPA 1561 and the Fire Protection Publications (FPP) IMS Consortium series of publications. IMS elements that affect the use of respiratory protection include the rapid intervention crew, rehabilitation section, accountability system monitoring, communications monitoring, and mutual aid coordination.

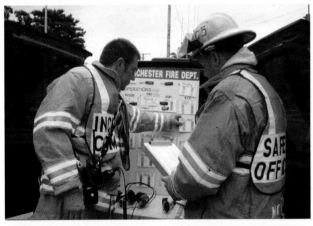

Figure 8.15 The incident commander (IC) is responsible for implementing the Incident Management System (IMS). If the incident is large, the IC delegates IMS functions to various members of the command staff. In this illustration, the incident safety officer is given responsibility for the accountability system.

Incident Management System

[NFPA 1500: 8.1.3, 8.1.6]

The Incident Management System is designed to be applicable to incidents of all sizes and types. It applies to small, single-unit incidents that may last a few minutes and to complex, large-scale incidents that can possibly last for days or weeks and involve several agencies and many mutual aid units. When applied to an emergency incident, the IMS provides clear communication and effective and efficient use of resources. The incident commander must be able to apply the elements of the IMS to provide a near-safe working environment for responding personnel. That application includes delegating the duties of the incident safety officer to a qualified member of the command staff. This individual then has responsibility for the accountability system function, the rapid intervention crew, rehabilitation section, and monitoring of communications.

Accountability System Monitoring

[NFPA 1500: 8.3.9, 8.3.10, 8.3.11, 8.3.12]

Accountability begins the moment the first responding unit arrives at an incident. During single-unit emergencies, the member remaining with the apparatus manages the accountability system and tracks the remaining members of the crew. As the incident develops and additional personnel arrive on the scene, the incident commander or incident safety officer monitors the accountability function. Depending on the system in use by the organization, this accountability may take the form of a regular tag system or an SCBA tag system (**Figure 8.16**).

In the regular tag system, the incident commander or incident safety officer monitors the individual by removing a clip-on or Velcro®-attached name tag from the individual's protective clothing and placing it on a control board at the command post. This system allows the incident commander and the staff to assign personnel to specific divisions, branches, or sections based on need and to follow their progress. The incident commander is responsible for keeping track of personnel as they enter or leave an incident. It also allows the incident commander or incident safety officer to ensure that personnel checking in are completely equipped with personal protective clothing and respiratory protection.

The SCBA tag system provides an additional level of accountability (**Figure 8.17**). A tracking tag that contains the user's name and the air pressure of the cylinder is attached to each SCBA. This tag is placed on the control board. This system allows the incident commander or incident safety officer to

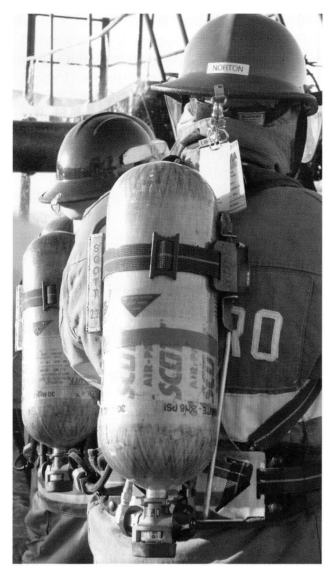

Figure 8.16 Accountability tags may be attached to personal protective clothing such as the helmet before a responder enters the hot zone.

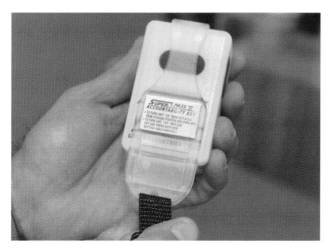

Figure 8.17 A recent innovation in electronic accountability tags combines the tag with the PASS device. The PASS is activated when the tag is removed and cannot be deactivated until the tag is clipped back on.

estimate the time that a crew or individual will be able to operate on supplied air and dispatch relief crews before an operating team's cylinder air levels become too low for members to withdraw safely.

Rapid Intervention Crew

[NFPA 1500: 8.5.1, 8.5.2, 8.5.2.1, 8.5.7]

The incident commander or the designated incident safety officer is responsible for establishing the rapid intervention crew before any interior fire-suppression, confined-space, or hazardous materials operations occur. Rapid intervention crews are required by NFPA 1500 and the *two-in two-out* provision in OSHA Title 29 (Labor) *CFR* 1910.134, Respiratory Protection Requirements. Any rapid intervention crew should have necessary tools and equipment in addition to personal protective clothing and respiratory protection equipment. Rapid intervention crews must monitor tag lines and communications with interior teams. One member of a crew may be assigned other duties as long as that person is ready to respond when needed. It is the incident commander's duty to establish this crew in accordance with the local IMS protocol. See Chapter 4, Safety and Risk Management, and Chapter 10, Emergency Scene Use, for details on rapid intervention crews (**Figure 8.18**).

Rehabilitation Section

[NFPA 1500: 8.6.1, 8.6.2, 8.6.3, 8.6.4]

Because of the inherent hazards that emergency responders face, providing rehabilitation facilities is an important function of the IMS. The incident commander is responsible for establishing a rehabilitation section although the duty may be delegated to the incident safety officer. Rehabilitation provides an opportunity for personnel to rest, cool down, get nutrition, or obtain medical aid. It also provides the incident safety officer an opportunity to monitor the conditions of emergency responders. In addition, rehabilitation provides time to refill SCBA cylinders, exchange batteries, and attend to other equipment needs (**Figure 8.19**). See the IFSTA/Brady *Emergency Incident Rehabilitation* book for more information.

No specific time is scheduled when rehabilitation should occur. However, the incident safety officer may want to check the conditions of personnel

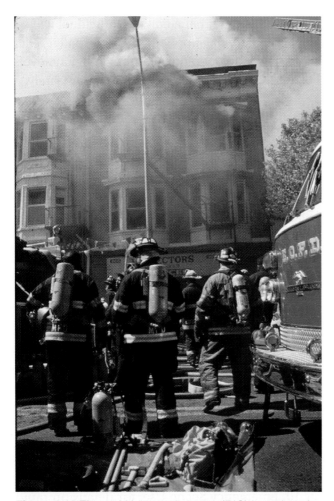

Figure 8.18 The rapid intervention crew (RIC) is equipped with all the tools that may be needed to locate and remove trapped responders at an emergency incident. *Courtesy of Ron Jeffers.*

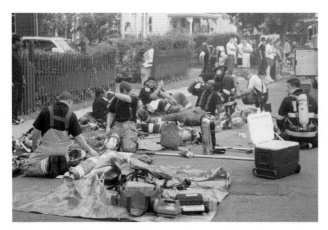

Figure 8.19 The rehabilitation section provides rest, nutrition, water, and medical aid to fire and emergency responders. *Courtesy of Bill Tompkins.*

when they have each used one cylinder of air. The amount of air consumed depends on the amount of energy exerted by the wearer and environmental conditions. Some personnel may require rehabili-

tation more quickly or more often than others. It is the responsibility of the incident safety officer to monitor personnel and direct them to the rehabilitation site as needed. Local protocol should establish the number of cylinders personnel can use before assigning them to other duties at an incident.

Communications Monitoring

[NFPA 1500: 8.1.9, 8.1.10]

Communications are an essential part of the IMS. However, the incident commander and the incident safety officer are only able to monitor two types: tag lines and radio systems. The incident commander delegates monitoring tag-line communications to rapid intervention crews. However, the incident commander must remain in contact with rapid intervention crews in the event they receive messages from interior or confined-space teams.

The incident commander assigns the incident safety officer the task of monitoring radio system communications to ensure that barriers or obstacles to clear communication are overcome. As learned earlier, the use of respiratory protection equipment can interfere with communications. Closely monitoring radio traffic is essential to the safety of personnel operating out of a supervisor's sight. The incident safety officer must work to eliminate the following radio-communication barriers:

- Low-charge batteries
- Background noise
- Static
- Bleed-over transmissions
- More than one microphone keyed at the same time

The incident safety officer must also listen for signs of distress from fatigued personnel who are having difficulty speaking, personnel who are reporting trouble situations, or crews that are operating in the wrong area. This information must be made available to the incident commander immediately.

Mutual Aid Coordination

The incident commander is responsible for all personnel assigned to the emergency incident, including units provided through mutual aid agreements. The original agreements must formally establish authority, cooperation, training, and compatibility of equipment, which ensure a firm groundwork for the cooperative effort. Responding mutual aid units are responsible for complying with the IMS and the orders of the incident commander (**Figure 8.20**). The incident commander is responsible for applying all elements of the IMS to the mutual aid units including monitoring personnel accountability systems, establishing rapid intervention crews, requiring personal protective equipment (including respiratory protection) and PASS devices, monitoring communications, and establishing rehabilitation sites. If respiratory protection equipment is not compatible, the incident commander must ensure that the mutual aid unit provides sufficient spare air cylinders and facepieces for its own personnel. If the radio communication systems equipment is not compatible, spare radios from the command post need to be assigned to the mutual aid unit.

Summary

Operational issues vary from incident to incident and are covered in greater detail in Chapter 10, Emergency Scene Use. Emergency responders must be able to apply the basic elements of respiratory protection and IMS to each emergency event based on the specific requirement. If this application is performed, then fire and emergency services personnel can perform their duties effectively and efficiently. In addition, emergency personnel must understand the basics of inspection, care, and maintenance of respiratory protection equipment, which is the topic of Chapter 9, Inspection, Care, and Maintenance.

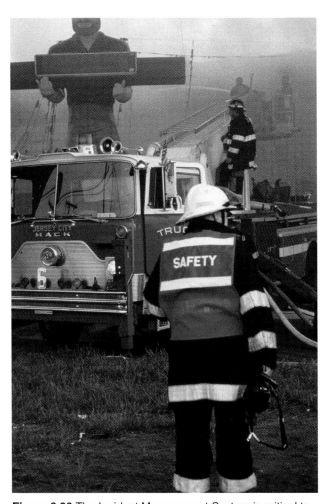

Figure 8.20 The Incident Management System is critical to the success of operations that involve many organizations and mutual aid assignments. The incident commander must keep track of all responding units and their locations. *Courtesy of Mike Nixon.*

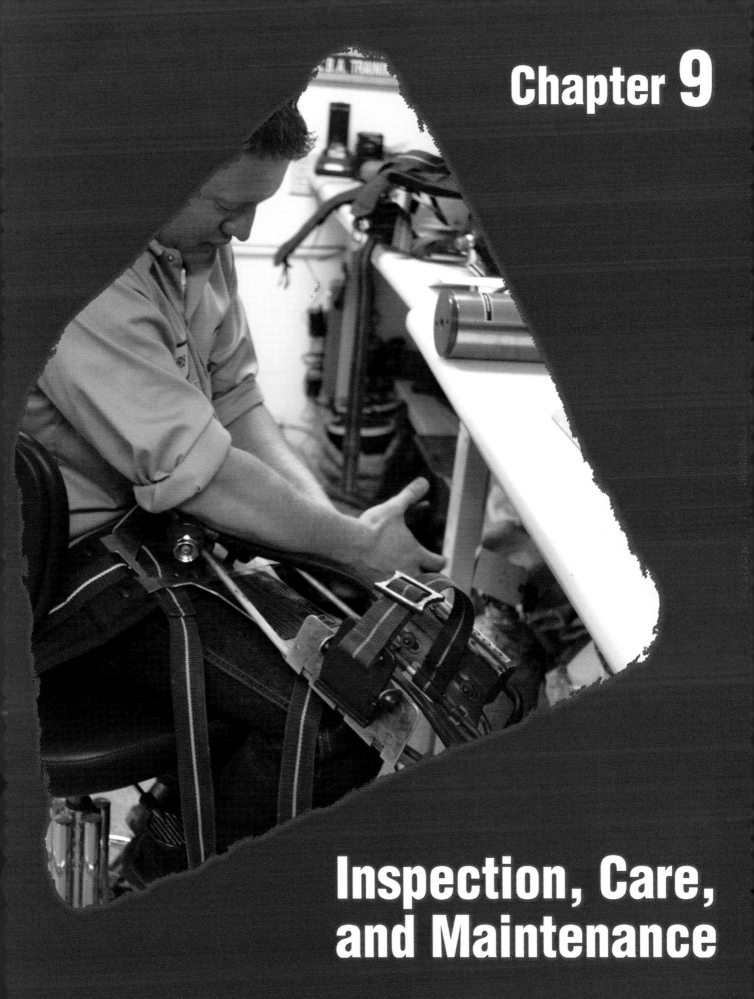

Chapter 9

Inspection, Care, and Maintenance

This chapter provides information that will assist the reader in meeting the following job performance requirements from NFPA 1404, *Standard for Fire Service Respiratory Protection Training*, 2002 Edition; NFPA 1852, *Standard on Selection, Care, and Maintenance of Open-Circuit Self-Contained Breathing Apparatus*, 2002 Edition; and NFPA 1500, *Standard on Fire Department Occupational Safety and Health Program*, 2002 Edition.

NFPA 1500

7.2.1 Members who engage in or are exposed to the hazards of structural fire fighting shall be provided with and shall use a protective ensemble that shall meet the applicable requirements of NFPA 1971, *Standard on Protective Ensemble for Structural Fire Fighting.*

7.3.1 Members whose primary responsibility is proximity fire fighting and members who participate in proximity fire-fighting training shall be provided with and shall use both proximity protective coats and proximity protective trousers, or a proximity protective coverall, for limb/torso protection.

7.9.1 The fire department shall adopt and maintain a respiratory protection program that addresses the selection, care, maintenance, and safe use of respiratory protection equipment, training in its use, and the assurance of air quality.

7.10.1 Breathing air used to fill SCBA cylinders shall comply with the requirements of ANSI/CGA G7.1, *Commodity Specification for Air*, with a minimum air quality of Grade D, a moisture content of no more than 24 parts per million, and a maximum particulate level of 5 mg/m^3 air.

7.10.2 When a fire department purchases compressed breathing air in a vendor-supplied SCBA cylinder, the fire department shall require the vendor to provide documentation that a sample of the breathing air obtained directly at the point of transfer from the vendor's filling system to the SCBA cylinder has been tested at least quarterly and that the air is compliant with the requirements of 7.10.1 of this section.

7.10.3 When a fire department compresses its own breathing air, the fire department shall be required to provide documentation that a sample of the breathing air obtained directly from the point of transfer from the filling system to the SCBA cylinder has been tested at least quarterly and that it is compliant with the requirements of 7.10.1 of this section.

7.10.4 When a fire department obtains compressed breathing air from a supplier and transfers it to other storage cylinders, cascade system cylinders, storage receivers, and other such storage equipment used for filling SCBA, the supplier shall be required to provide documentation that a sample of the breathing air obtained directly at the point of transfer from the filling system to the storage cylinders, cascade system cylinders, storage receivers, and other such storage equipment has been tested at least quarterly and that it is compliant with the requirements of 7.10.1 of this section.

7.10.5 The fire department shall obtain documentation that a sample of the breathing air obtained directly from the point of transfer from the storage cylinders, cascade system cylinders, storage receivers, and other such storage equipment to the SCBA cylinder has been tested at least quarterly and that it is compliant with the requirements of 7.10.1 of this section.

7.13.1 Cylinders made of alloy 6351-T6 shall not be used with SCBA.

7.13.2 SCBA cylinders shall be hydrostatically tested as required by the manufacturers and applicable governmental agencies.

7.13.3 In-service SCBA cylinders shall be stored fully charged.

7.13.4 In-service SCBA cylinders shall be inspected weekly, monthly, and prior to filling according to NIOSH requirements, CGA standards, and manufacturer's recommendations.

7.13.5 During filling of SCBA cylinders, all personnel and operators shall be protected from catastrophic failure of the cylinder.

7.13.6 Due to the possibility of catastrophic failure of SCBA cylinders during filling, cylinders shall not be filled while being worn by the user.

7.14.3 Each PASS device shall be tested at least weekly and prior to each use, and shall be maintained in accordance with the manufacturer's instructions.

NFPA 1404

4.1.4 All respiratory protection equipment shall be stored in accordance with Section 6.3 of NFPA 1852, *Standard on Selection, Care, and Maintenance of Open-Circuit Self-Contained Breathing Apparatus.*

6.11 Maintenance and Testing. Training in the maintenance and testing of respiratory protection equipment shall be in accordance with the provisions of Chapter 7 of NFPA 1852, *Standard on Selection, Care, and Maintenance of Open-Circuit Self-Contained Breathing Apparatus.*

6.12 Manufacturer's Instructions. Training for maintenance and testing of SAR and FFAPR shall be in accordance with the manufacturer's instructions for the units provided.

7.1.1 SCBA service checks shall be conducted in accordance with 7.1.2 of NFPA 1852, *Standard on Selection, Care, and Maintenance of Open-Circuit Self-Contained Breathing Apparatus.*

7.1.2 Closed-circuit SCBA used in training shall be inspected at frequencies determined by the authority having jurisdiction in accordance with the manufacturer's recommendations but at no less than weekly intervals.

7.1.3 Closed-circuit SCBA shall be checked before and after each use in accordance with the manufacturer's recommendations.

8.1.1 All maintenance and repairs on respiratory protection equipment used for training shall be conducted by qualified persons in accordance with NFPA 1852, *Standard on Selection, Care, and Maintenance of Open-Circuit Self-Contained Breathing Apparatus.*

8.1.2 Annual inspection and servicing of a SCBA and SAR systems used in training shall be conducted by qualified personnel and whenever an operational problem is reported.

8.1.2.1 Inspections and servicing of SCBA shall be performed in accordance with NFPA 1852, *Standard on Selection, Care, and Maintenance of Open-Circuit Self-Contained Breathing Apparatus.* Inspection of SAR units shall be in accordance with manufacturer's instructions for the unit in service.

8.1.3 Cleaning and sanitizing of SCBA training units shall be conducted in accordance with Section 6.1 of NFPA 1852, *Standard on Selection, Care, and Maintenance of Open-Circuit Self-Contained Breathing Apparatus.*

8.1.4 SAR units and FFAPR training units shall be cleaned and sanitized as specified in the manufacturer's instructions.

8.1.5 Fire fighters, or other designated and trained personnel, shall clean and sanitize each SCBA, SAR unit, and FFAPR after each training session use or upon their return to the fire station.

8.1.5.1 SCBA units shall be cleaned and disinfected in accordance with Chapter 6 of NFPA 1852, *Standard on Selection, Care, and Maintenance of Open-Circuit Self-Contained Breathing Apparatus.*

8.1.5.2 SAR and FFAPR units shall be cleaned and disinfected in accordance with the manufacturer's instructions.

8.1.5.3 The entire device shall be cleaned, filter cartridges replaced if appropriate, and the facepiece and breathing tube shall be sanitized.

9.1 **Air Quality Control.** Air for respiratory protection training taken from the regular production of a compressor and storage system shall meet the testing and quality requirements of NFPA 1500, *Standard on Fire Department Occupational Safety and Health Program.*

9.2.1 Air cylinders used in training shall be inspected and filled in accordance with the provisions of Chapter 7 of NFPA 1500, *Standard on Fire Department Occupational Safety and Health Program.*

9.2.2 Air cylinders shall be filled only by personnel who have been trained on the procedures and equipment.

9.2.3 The operating procedures and safety precautions shall be posted in a conspicuous location at the fill station.

NFPA 1852

4.4.8 The organization shall create, maintain, and disseminate the following as required:

(1) Written instructions for care, maintenance, and repair that correspond to those provided by the manufacturer

(2) Written instructions for checks while donning SCBA

(3) Written instructions for inspection, including procedures to be followed if defects are found

(4) Forms to document the findings during inspection

(5) Forms to record and to report defects, found during inspection, and to track the SCBA or cylinder as it is repaired

(6) Forms to document inspections, tests, and repairs by SCBA users and technicians that shall include the following:

    a. SCBA make, model, and serial number and other information to identify components.

    b. Documentation of the date, result of the inspection or test, and all actions taken as well as who acted.

(7) Written instructions for filling and for testing cylinders

(8) Written policy and procedure concerning training and authorization of SCBA technicians as well as documentation of that training and authorization

(9) Written procedures for the inspection of cylinders by technicians

(10) Written procedures for recording information about the inspection and repair of cylinders

(11) Stickers, tags, or other similarly effective means to alert users and technicians to defects, to document inspections, and to certify that tests, repairs, and other actions have been completed

(12) Written procedures for periodic tests and comprehensive inspections that comply with the SCBA manufacturer's instructions

(13) Documentation of the tests to verify SCBA performance

(14) Schedule for retention, disposition, and disposal of each report, record, and document

(15) Methods of identifying all SCBAs, cylinders, parts, and components so that these can be identified and tracked from initial receipt by the organization until removed from the possession and control of the organization

(16) Documentation when a defective or obsolete SCBA or component part is removed from service in accordance with the following:

    a. Until retirement and disposal of a defective or obsolete SCBA or component as specified in 4.6.3, a tag shall be conspicuously placed on the SCBA or component.

    b. The tag shall indicate the date and time the SCBA or component was removed from service, by whom, and for what reason.

    c. SCBA and components that are removed from service shall be stored separately from other SCBA and components and secured, as necessary.

    d. Access to tagged SCBA and components shall be limited, and only authorized persons shall remove tags after repair or service.

(17) Records for maintenance of each individual SCBA regulator, reducer, harness, cylinder including valve

assembly, and facepiece including the following information:

a. The manufacturer's serial number or other unique identifier

b. Date of manufacture, receipt, service, inspection, test, maintenance, and repair

c. Inspections, service, repairs, and tests

d. Who performed the work

e. Other comments

(18) Records of training provided to each user showing date(s) and subject(s) covered

(19) Such other reports, records, and documents including forms, tags, stickers, and other means necessary to effectuate the purposes of record keeping and the intent of this standard.

4.6.1 Retired SCBA shall be destroyed, or altered in a manner assuring that they will not be used for respiratory protection and shall be rendered unable to hold pressure, or the ownership of the SCBA shall be transferred to the manufacturer or the manufacturer's agent.

4.6.2 Where SCBA or SCBA components are contaminated beyond the ability to decontaminate so the SCBA or components can be returned to service, such SCBA or component shall be disposed of.

4.6.2.1 Contaminated SCBA or components as identified according to 4.6.2 shall be segregated from other equipment and personnel, and disposed of in a manner consistent with the type of contamination and any governmental regulations governing contaminated items.

4.6.2.2 Prior to disposal, contaminated SCBA or components shall be altered in a manner assuring that they cannot be used for any purpose.

4.6.3 Defective or obsolete SCBA components or defective or obsolete SCBA that have been removed from service and can not be repaired or upgraded shall be destroyed, or altered in a manner assuring that they will not be used in any fire fighting or other emergency activities including training, or the ownership of the SCBA shall be transferred to the manufacturer or the manufacturer's agent.

4.6.4 SCBA elastomeric components, including but not limited to facepieces, O-rings, and hose, shall be destroyed or altered in a manner assuring that they can not be used for any purpose when the component reaches the SCBA manufacturer's specified component service life.

4.6.5 SCBA composite cylinders shall be removed from service and retired when they reach the end of the service life specified by the SCBA manufacturer. Such composite cylinders shall be destroyed, or altered in a manner assuring that they will not be used for respiratory protection and shall be rendered unable to hold pressure, or the ownership of the composite cylinder shall be transferred to the manufacturer or the manufacturer's agent.

4.6.6 Any SCBA cylinders that are beyond repair shall be destroyed, or altered in a manner assuring that they are marked and identified that they are no longer a breathing air cylinder and shall be rendered unable to hold pressure.

4.8.1 Where the portion of the respiratory protection program component that addresses the maintenance of SCBA, as specified in 4.2.6, includes SCBA technicians that are members of the organization, such technicians shall be qualified and authorized by the SCBA manufacturer to perform specified allowable maintenance.

4.8.1.1 Allowable maintenance shall include periodic inspection, repair, and overhaul of all SCBA components and assemblies.

4.8.1.2 Technicians shall also be qualified and authorized in the use of all special tools and equipment required to test and maintain the SCBA.

4.8.2 The program component shall establish policies and procedures for qualification and selection of personnel for SCBA technician training and authorization.

4.8.3 The organization shall maintain evidence that all SCBA technicians that are members of the organization have current authorization by the SCBA manufacturer and have maintained their level of competency.

6.1.1 The external surfaces of the SCBA shall be cleaned and disinfected according to the manufacturer's instructions using only those agents indicated by the manufacturer.

6.1.2 The facepiece shall be thoroughly cleaned after each use and disinfected as needed. Facepiece cleaning and disinfecting shall be performed according to the manufacturer's instructions using only those agents indicated by the manufacturer.

6.1.2.1 The exhalation valve shall be cleaned and flushed.

6.1.2.2 The facepiece shall be dried, and drying shall not be done in direct sunlight or in high heat.

6.1.2.3 The exhalation valve shall be cycled to assure proper operation.

6.1.3 The second stage regulator shall be thoroughly cleaned and disinfected if the internal components have been exposed to bodily fluids, exhaled breath, dirt, or debris. The cleaning and disinfecting shall be performed according to the manufacturer's instructions using only those agents indicated by the manufacturer.

6.1.4 SCBA straps and harness assemblies shall be cleaned and disinfected when required according to manufacturer's instructions. Straps and harness assembly cleaning and disinfecting shall be performed according to the manufacturer's instructions using only those agents indicated by the manufacturer.

6.1.4.1 Under no circumstances shall a chlorine bleach ever be used to clean straps and harness assemblies.

6.1.4.2 The straps and harness assemblies shall be dried, and drying shall not be done in direct sunlight or in high heat.

6.1.5 SCBA cylinder valve assemblies shall be cleaned and disinfected according to the manufacturer's instructions using only those agents indicated by the manufacturer.

6.1.5.1 Care shall be taken to ensure that the valve is free of debris.

6.1.5.2 The burst disc outlet shall be inspected and, if debris is present, the cylinder shall be removed from service.

6.1.6 Caution shall be taken to prevent water or cleaning materials from entering the connection between the cylinder valve and the mating SCBA inlet connector.

6.1.7 Pneumatic component cleaning and disinfecting shall be performed according to the manufacturer's instructions using only those agents indicated by the manufacturer.

6.1.7.1 All pneumatic components shall be thoroughly dried after cleaning.

6.1.7.2 Drying of pneumatic components shall not be done in direct sunlight or in high heat.

6.1.8 All other SCBA components shall be thoroughly air-dried prior to storage in a compartment that does not allow for air circulation.

6.1.9 Appropriate inspections according to 7.1.2 shall be performed after cleaning.

6.2.1 Where SCBA is suspected of being contaminated, it shall be tagged out-of-service and segregated from other equipment and personnel. Tags shall include details of the incident including known and suspected contaminants.

6.2.2 The SCBA manufacturer shall be contacted to determine if any additional special procedures can be used to decontaminate the SCBA.

6.2.3 In all cases, decontamination shall be conducted in accordance with the SCBA manufacturer's instructions.

6.2.4 Where it is determined, in accordance with 4.2.3.1, that the SCBA is contaminated beyond the ability to decontaminate it and return it to service, the SCBA shall be disposed of in accordance with 4.6.3.

6.3.1 SCBA shall be stored in their original carrying or storage cases, or in a wall or apparatus bracket/rack, designed for quick removal and for protection of the SCBA. Brackets/racks shall protect the SCBA and shall be adjusted so they do not cause physical damage to cylinders, hoses, regulator, or straps.

6.3.2 Fire apparatus with brackets for securing SCBA shall meet the requirements of 10.1.6 of NFPA 1901, *Standard for Automotive Fire Apparatus.*

6.3.3 SCBA shall be stored with the cylinder valves closed. Other valves or controls shall be positioned according to manufacturer's specifications.

6.3.4 The facepieces of all SCBA shall be positioned to avoid distortion of parts during storage.

6.3.5 All harness straps shall be adjusted to their maximum length during storage.

6.3.6 In all instances the SCBA shall be stored in a manner to control and minimize exposure to shock, vibration, sunlight, heat, extreme cold, excessive moisture, damaging chemicals, and environmental elements.

6.3.7 All in-service SCBA cylinders shall be stored fully charged.

6.3.7.1 Cylinders shall be filled when the pressure falls to 90 percent of the manufacturer's specified pressure level.

6.3.7.2 A positive pressure shall be maintained in depleted SCBA cylinders by keeping the valve closed until they are filled to keep external contamination and condensation out of the cylinder.

6.3.8 SCBA cylinders shall be stored in a manner that prevents damage to the valve and cylinder.

7.1.1.1 Where SCBA is assigned to an individual user for a duty period, the inspection specified in 7.1.2 shall be performed by the individual user at the beginning of each duty period.

7.1.1.2 Where additional SCBA are available for use on response vehicles but not assigned to individual users, the inspection specified in 7.1.2 shall be performed on such additional SCBA at least once each duty period.

7.1.1.3 Where SCBA are not assigned to an individual user for a duty period, the inspection specified in 7.1.2 shall be performed at least once per week on all SCBA that are available for use.

7.1.1.4 In all cases, the interval between the inspections specified in 7.1.2 shall not exceed one week.

7.1.2.1 All of the following SCBA components shall be present:

(1) Facepiece

(2) Backframe and harness assembly

(3) Cylinder

(4) Hose

(5) End-of-service-time indicator(s)

(6) Regulators

(7) Accessories

7.1.2.2 Facepiece inspection shall include the following:

(1) Checking the material for deterioration, dirt, cracks, tears, holes, pliability, and tackiness

(2) Checking the head-harness buckles, strap, and webbing for breaks, loss of elasticity, or wear

(3) Checking the lens for holes, cracks, scratches, heat-damaged areas, and a proper seal with the facepiece material

(4) Checking the exhalation valve, where present, for valve seat, springs, and covers for proper operation and for cleanliness

(5) Checking the regulator connection(s) for proper operation and damage

(6) Checking the speaking diaphragm where present for damage

7.1.2.3 Backframe and harness assembly inspection shall include the following:

(1) Checking the harness straps and backframe for cuts, tears, abrasion, indications of heat damage, and indications of chemical-related damage

(2) Checking all buckles, fasteners, and adjustments for proper operation

(3) Checking the cylinder retention system for damage, and proper operation, and checking that the cylinder is securely attached to the backframe

(4) Checking that the harness straps are fully extended

7.1.2.4 Cylinder assembly inspection shall include the following:

(1) Checking that the hydrostatic test date on the cylinder is current

(2) Checking the gauge for damage

(3) Checking the cylinder body for cracks, dents, weakened areas, indications of heat damage, and indications of chemical damage

(4) Checking the composite portion of the cylinder for cuts, gouges, loose composite materials, and the absence of resin

(5) Checking the cylinder valve outlet sealing surface and threads for damage

(6) Checking the valve hand wheel for damage, proper alignment, serviceability and secure attachment

(7) Checking the burst disc outlet area for debris

(8) Checking that the cylinder is fully charged

7.1.2.5 Hose inspection shall include the following:

(1) Checking for cuts, abrasions, bubbling, cracks, heat damage, and chemical damage

(2) Checking external fittings for visual signs of damage

(3) Checking for tight connections

7.1.2.6 End-of-service-time indicator(s) inspection shall include the following:

(1) Checking the alarm and mounting hardware for damage, secure attachment, dirt, and debris

(2) Checking the end-of-service-time indicator(s) for proper activation at 20 to 25 percent of rated cylinder pressure

7.1.2.7 Regulators inspection shall include the following:

(1) Checking regulator controls, where present, for damage and proper function

(2) Checking pressure relief devices visually for damage

(3) Checking housing and components for damage

(4) Checking the regulator for any unusual sounds such as whistling, chattering, clicking, or rattling during operation

(5) Checking the regulator and bypass for proper function when each is operated. Where this is accomplished by donning the facepiece and contamination between users is a possibility, the regulator, facepiece, or both shall be cleaned and disinfected.

7.1.2.8 Pressure indicator inspection shall include the following:

(1) Checking the pressure indicator for damage

(2) Checking that the cylinder pressure gauge and the remote gauge read within 10 percent of each other

7.1.2.9 Where SCBA has an integrated PASS, the SCBA-Integrated-PASS inspection shall include the following:

(1) Checking for wear and damage

(2) Checking covers/compartments for secure attachment

(3) Checking all operating modes for proper function

(4) Checking for the low battery warning signal

7.1.2.10 Where other accessories are attached to the SCBA, such accessories shall be inspected for signs of wear, damage, secure attachment, and proper operation.

7.1.2.11 As the final inspection item, the entire SCBA shall be checked for pressure retention by closing all regulator valves, opening the cylinder valve thereby pressuring the SCBA, and then closing the cylinder valve. The SCBA shall hold system pressure, in accordance with the manufacturer's specifications, after the cylinder valve is closed. Following the pressure check, the system pressure shall be released.

7.2.1.3 The SCBA shall be tested on a breathing machine specified in 7.4.6 in accordance with the organization's SOPs or in accordance with the SCBA manufacturer's instructions, whichever is more frequent, but in all cases at least annually.

7.2.2.1 Technicians shall perform the level of inspection for which they have been trained and have been qualified to conduct by the SCBA manufacturer.

7.2.2.2 Where an SCBA is removed from service in accordance with 7.1.4, the technician shall verify the user-reported condition. Where the user-reported condition is verified by the technician, the technician then shall determine the appropriate action to be taken to repair, return to service, or retire the SCBA or SCBA component(s).

7.2.2.3 Where the user-reported condition cannot be substantiated, the technician shall perform a complete SCBA inspection in accordance with the manufacturer's instructions.

7.2.3.1 Technicians shall perform the level of repair or the rebuild for which they have been qualified and are authorized to conduct by the SCBA manufacturer.

7.2.3.2 The technician shall verify that all parts and tools used in the maintenance, repair, and rebuild of SCBA are specified by the SCBA manufacturer for the specific SCBA model being repaired.

7.2.4.1 Any SCBA or SCBA component that is damaged and cannot be repaired shall be removed from service and retired as specified in Section 4.6.

7.2.4.2 Any SCBA or SCBA components that have been exposed or are suspected of having been exposed to a chemical, biological, or nuclear agent(s), and where such exposure can not be remedied by a decontamination process authorized by the SCBA manufacturer, such SCBA or component shall be retired as specified in Section 4.6.

7.2.4.3 Any SCBA cylinder that is beyond repair shall be removed from service and retired as specified in Section 4.6.

7.2.4.4 Composite cylinders shall be removed from service and retired as specified in Section 4.6 when they reach the end of the SCBA manufacturer's specified service life.

7.2.4.5 Any elastomeric component, including but not limited to facepieces, O-rings, and hose, shall be removed from service and retired as specified in Section 4.6, when they reach the end of the SCBA manufacturer's specified service life.

7.3.1 Prior to filling SCBA cylinders, the cylinder inspection specified in 7.1.2.4 shall be performed.

7.3.2 SCBA cylinders shall be filled as soon as possible after use. Breathing air shall meet the requirements stated in 5.3.6 of NFPA 1500, *Standard on Fire Department Occupational Safety and Health Program.*

7.3.3 The SCBA manufacturer's specified fill rate shall not be exceeded.

7.3.4 During filling of SCBA cylinders, all operators and personnel shall be protected from catastrophic failure of the cylinder.

7.3.5 SCBA cylinders shall be requalified as specified by the SCBA manufacturer.

7.4.4.1 Calibration shall be performed periodically in accordance with the test equipment manufacturer's instructions but shall be calibrated at least annually.

Inspection, Care, and Maintenance

To ensure the safe use of respiratory protection equipment during emergency operations, a complete and thorough inspection, care, and maintenance program must be established. The authority having jurisdiction must include the inspection, care, and maintenance requirements in the written respiratory protection program. The specific inspection, care, and maintenance protocol should be included in the organization's standard operating procedures (SOPs) manual.

The responsibility for performing inspection and maintenance functions is divided between various personnel and/or organizations, depending on the type of inspection and maintenance required. At the operational level, daily inspections, routine care, and cleaning rest with the user. Manufacturer-trained and certified specialists/technicians must perform annual inspections, testing, and maintenance that require disassembly of the units. These specialists/technicians may be internal to the organization or under contract from another agency or commercial vendor. Some maintenance may only be performed by the manufacturer at an authorized service center. Regardless of the level of inspection and maintenance, all repaired equipment must be tested and results recorded before returning the equipment to service. The decision to retire or dispose of respiratory protection equipment may be the responsibility of the specialist/technician based on guidelines established by the jurisdiction. All equipment that is retired or disposed of must be recorded in the appropriate data file. Breathing-air cylinders must be tested, inspected, maintained, and disposed of according to standards developed by the Compressed Gas Association (CGA). This chapter provides guidelines for the inspection, care,

maintenance, disposal and retirement of respiratory protection equipment and breathing-air cylinders.

NOTE: Always follow the inspection, care, cleaning, storage, maintenance, and disposal instructions provided by the manufacturer.

Respiratory Protection Equipment Inspection Schedules

[NFPA 1500: 7.9.1, 7.13.4, 7.14.3]
[NFPA 1852: 7.1.1.1, 7.1.1.2, 7.1.1.3, 7.1.1.4, 7.2.2.1, 7.2.2.2, 7.2.2.3]

As indicated in Chapter 5, Respiratory Protection Equipment Selection and Procurement, respiratory protection equipment is initially inspected when it is purchased (**Figure 9.1**). Once the equipment is placed into service, periodic inspections are performed by the organization's members. Operational inspections of respiratory protection equipment occur after each use, daily or weekly, monthly, and annually. NFPA 1404, *Standard for Fire Service Respiratory Protection Training*, NFPA 1500, *Standard on Fire Department Occupational Safety and Health Program*, and NFPA 1852, *Standard on Selection, Care, and Maintenance of Open-Circuit Self-Contained Breathing Apparatus*, require daily/weekly and annual inspection schedules and provide the inspection requirements for those organizations that adhere to the standards. The Canadian Standards Association (CSA) standard CAN/CSA Z94.4, *Selection, Use, and Care of Respirators*, has similar requirements as well. Occupational Safety and Health Association (OSHA) requires inspections before and after each use and *at least monthly* for units not in continuous service.

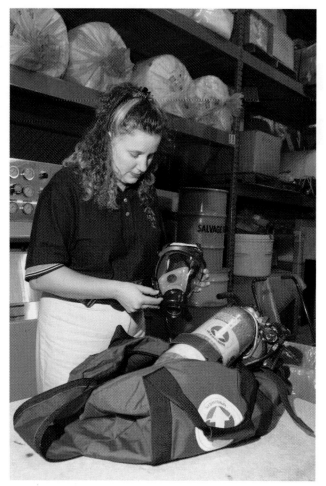

Figure 9.1 New respiratory protection equipment is inspected when it arrives from the vendor for condition and completeness. The health and safety officer (shown) may be responsible for the acceptance inspection.

National Institute for Occupational Safety and Health (NIOSH) recommends that all stored units be inspected weekly.

The organization must define the frequency and type of inspection in the respiratory protection policy. Depending on the manufacturer's recommendation, severity of the operating environment, amount of use, and specific work-site issues, the frequency of inspections may be increased and additional weekly or monthly inspections required by the authority having jurisdiction (**Figure 9.2**). Equipment instruction, training, and evaluation must also be provided to ensure that personnel who use or maintain the equipment meet the skills level required by the policy and manufacturer. Records of inspections performed are kept for each piece of respiratory protection equipment.

Respiratory protection equipment that is assigned to an individual for a specific duty period must be inspected at the beginning of that duty period. Spare equipment that is carried on the apparatus but not assigned to an individual must be inspected daily. Units that are not assigned to an individual or apparatus must be inspected weekly. The interval between inspections must never be greater than 1 week. Individually assigned facepieces are also inspected before each duty period. Units that are in long-term storage and are

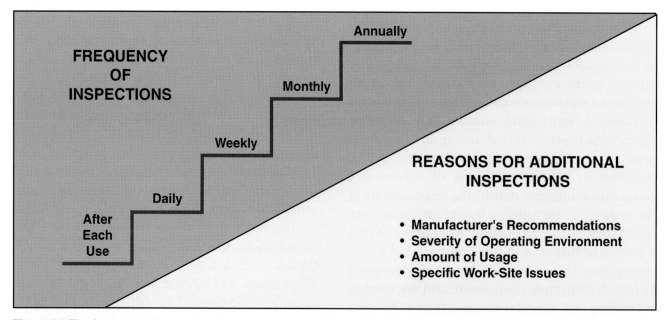

Figure 9.2 The frequency of inspections for respiratory protection equipment may increase based on various conditions as indicated in this illustration.

not intended for immediate use do not require periodic inspections but must be inspected before being placed in service. Units that have been repaired must be inspected before placing them back in service.

WARNING!

Under no circumstances use or store a respiratory protection device that is known to be defective. Remove such units from service and replace or repair immediately.

Postincident Inspections

Respiratory protection equipment units must be inspected during cleaning and following use before being placed back in service or into storage (**Figure 9.3**). The inspection steps are the same as those performed for the daily or weekly inspections that are outlined in the following section.

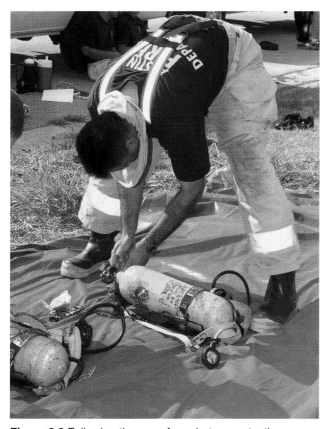

Figure 9.3 Following the use of respiratory protection equipment at an incident, the equipment must be inspected and cleaned before being placed into storage or back in service. *Courtesy of Bob Parker.*

Daily or Weekly Inspections

The specific inspection steps for respiratory protection equipment vary depending on the type of equipment in use. Daily or weekly inspection procedures for self-contained breathing apparatus (SCBA), supplied-air respirators (SARs), and air-purifying respirators (APRs) are listed separately in the sections that follow.

Self-Contained Breathing Apparatus

[NFPA 1404: 7.1.1, 7.1.2, 7.1.3]
[NFPA 1852: 7.1.2.1, 7.1.2.2, 7.1.2.3, 7.1.2.4, 7.1.2.5, 7.1.2.6, 7.1.2.7, 7.1.2.8, 7.1.2.9, 7.1.2.10, 7.1.2.11]

The following components of the self-contained breathing apparatus that need to be inspected are listed with the inspection requirements for each:

- *Facepiece* — Inspect for the following items:
  — Deterioration, pliability, and tackiness of the facepiece skirt; also cracks, tears, and holes in the skirt and dirt
  — Breaks, wear, or loss of elasticity in head-harness buckles, straps, and webbing
  — Full extension of head-harness straps
  — Holes, cracks, scratches, and heat damage to the lens and a proper seal with the facepiece material (**Figure 9.4**)
  — Cleanliness and proper operation of valve seat, springs, and covers for the exhalation valve where present
  — Proper operation of and damage to regulator connection(s)
  — Damage to and cleanliness of the speaking diaphragm where present
  — Operation of inhalation valve on the nose cup
- *Backframe and harness assembly* — Inspect for the following items:
  — Cuts, tears, abrasion, heat damage, and chemical-related damage
  — Proper operation of buckles, fasteners, and adjustments (**Figure 9.5**)
  — Damage to and proper operation of the cylinder retention system (cylinder should be securely attached to the backframe)

— Full extension of harness straps

— Cylinder's original manufacturer date (ensure that the cylinder's service life has not expired)

- *Cylinder assembly* — Inspect for the following items:

— Current hydrostatic test date on the cylinder (**Figure 9.6**)

— Damage to the cylinder pressure gauge

— Cracks, dents, weakened areas, indications of heat damage, and indications of chemical damage in the cylinder body

— Cuts, gouges, loose composite materials, and the absence of resin in the composite portion of the cylinder

— Damage to cylinder valve outlet sealing surface and threads

— Damage to and proper alignment, serviceability, and secure attachment of valve hand wheel

— Debris in and cleanliness of burst disc outlet area

— Cylinder fully charged to within 90 percent of rated capacity

- *Hose* — Inspect for the following items:

— Cuts, abrasions, bubbling, cracks, and heat or chemical damage (**Figure 9.7**)

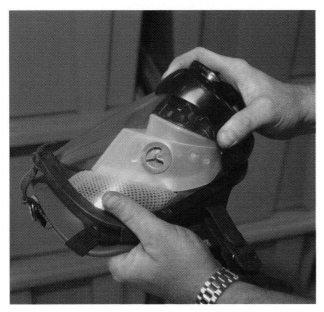

Figure 9.4 During any inspection of the SCBA facepiece, the condition of the facepiece lens and the seal between the lens and facepiece material must be inspected for damage or separation.

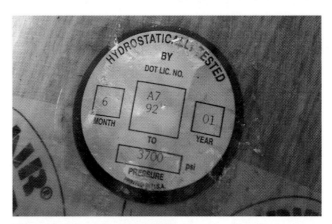

Figure 9.6 The inspection of the breathing air cylinder includes checking to make certain that the hydrostatic test date is visible and current. If there is any doubt, the cylinder must be removed from service and tested.

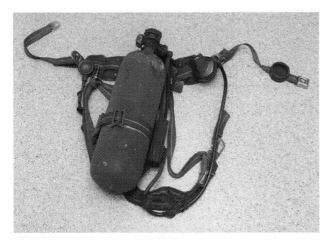

Figure 9.5 To thoroughly inspect an SCBA backpack harness assembly, it may first be necessary to clean and decontaminated it. A thick coating of smoke prevents any visual inspection of the unit shown.

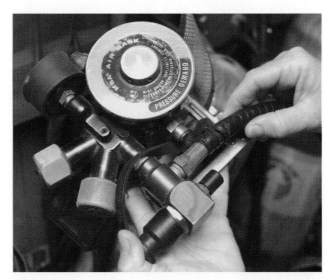

Figure 9.7 The high-pressure hose and connections must be inspected for cracks, cuts, heat and chemical damage, abrasions, and bubbling.

— Visual signs of damage to external fittings

— Tight connections with regulator, cylinder, and facepiece fittings

— Condition of protective sleeves

• *End-of-service-time indicator(s)* — Inspect for the following items:

— Damage to, cleanliness, and secure attachment of the alarm and mounting hardware

— Proper activation at 20 to 25 percent of the rated cylinder pressure

• *Regulator* — Inspect for the following items:

— Damage to and proper operation of regulator controls where present

— Visual damage to pressure relief devices (**Figure 9.8**)

— Damage to housing and components

— Any unusual sounds such as whistling, chattering, clicking, or rattling during operation

— Proper function of regulator and bypass during operation

• *Pressure indicator* — Inspect for the following items:

— Damage

— Cylinder pressure gauge and the remote gauge read within 10 percent of each other (**Figure 9.9**)

Accessories such as communications devices that are attached to the SCBA are inspected for wear, damage, security, cleanliness, and proper operation. Quick-fill male and female connections, voice amplifiers, and so forth should be maintained in accordance with manufacturer guidelines. The alarm should sound once when the unit is initially pressurized. During inspection, the dual alarm should be checked as well. Personal alert safety system (PASS) devices that are integrated into the SCBA system are inspected for the following items:

• Wear and damage

• Secure attachment of covers and compartments

• Proper operation of all modes (**Figure 9.10**)

• Operation of the low-battery warning signal

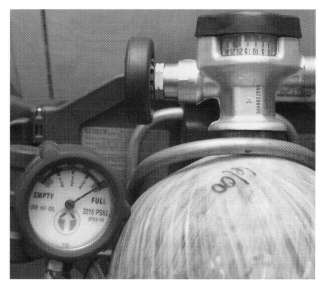

Figure 9.9 The air pressure indicators on the regulator and the breathing-air cylinder must be inspected with pressure on the system. The two gauges should register within 10 percent of each other.

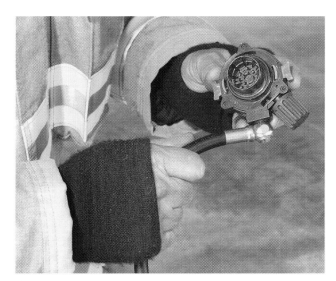

Figure 9.8 The regulator (such as this facepiece-mounted unit) must be inspected for proper operation and cleanliness.

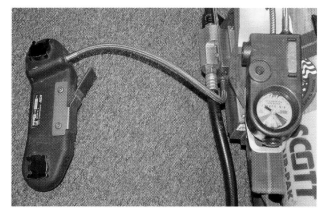

Figure 9.10 Integrated PASS devices must be inspected visually for damage and cleanliness and then operated in all modes to ensure proper operation.

After each component of the system is inspected, the entire SCBA is checked for pressure retention by closing all regulator valves, opening the cylinder valve thereby pressuring the SCBA, and then closing the cylinder valve. The SCBA shall hold the system pressure (per the manufacturer's specifications) after the cylinder valve is closed. Following the pressure check, the system pressure is released. The unit is then cleaned, placed in service or storage, or submitted for repairs depending on the outcome of the inspections.

Supplied-Air Respirator

The components of the SAR system that need to be inspected are as follows:

- Facepiece
- Harness assembly
- Air source
- Hose
- End-of-service-time indicator(s)
- Regulator
- Accessories
- Emergency breathing support system (EBSS) **(Figure 9.11)**

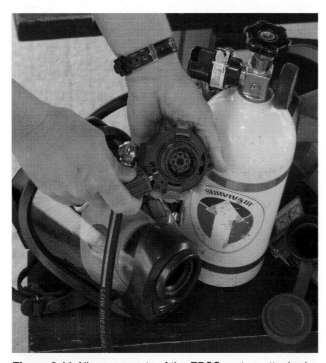

Figure 9.11 All components of the EBSS system attached to an SAR must be inspected, including the valves, hoses, cylinder, harness, and regulator connections shown in this photo.

In addition to the inspection steps used for the SCBA, combination SCBA/SAR units should be inspected for the condition and operation of the airline connection and control valve. SAR units equipped with EBSS should follow the same outline as the SCBA with the following addition: SCBA/SAR units that are intended for use with fully encapsulating hazardous materials suits must include the inspection of the air-supply line fittings on the suit.

Air-Purifying Respirator

Visual inspections provide assurance that an APR is ready to be placed into service and will provide its designed level of protection. The inspection process recommended by NIOSH for APRs includes the following components and inspection items:

- *Facepiece* — Inspect for the following items:
  — Excessive dirt
  — Cracks, tears, holes, or distortion from improper storage
  — Inflexibility (stretch and massage the material to restore flexibility)
  — Cracked or badly scratched lenses in facepieces **(Figure 9.12)**
  — Incorrectly mounted lens or broken or missing mounting clips
  — Cracked or broken air-purifying element holders, badly worn threads, or missing gaskets

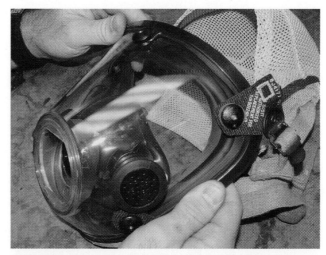

Figure 9.12 Facepiece lenses should be inspected for physical, chemical, or heat damage that may obscure the user's vision.

- *Head straps or head harness* — Inspect for the following items:
  - Breaks
  - Loss of elasticity
  - Broken or malfunctioning buckles and attachments
  - Excessively worn serration on the head harness that might permit slippage
- *Exhalation valve* — Inspect for the following items:
  - Debris in and around the valve seat (**Figure 9.13**)
  - Cracks, tears, or distortions in the valve material
  - Improper insertion of the valve body in the facepiece
  - Cracks, breaks, or chips in the valve body, particularly in the sealing surface
  - Missing or defective valve cover
  - Improper installation of the valve in the valve body

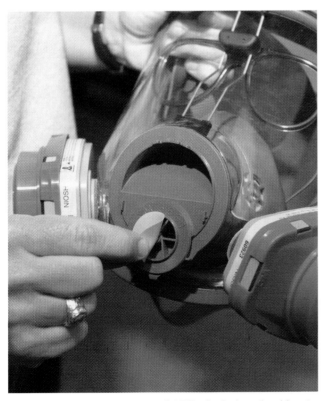

Figure 9.13 The inspection of APRs includes checking to ensure that no debris is lodged around the exhalation valve that would prevent it from closing and sealing completely.

- *Egress or escape unit* — Inspect the breathing-air cylinder following the items listed under Self-Contained Breathing Apparatus section given earlier.
- *Air-purifying element* — Inspect for the following items:
  - Incorrect cartridge, canister, or filter for the assigned hazard
  - Incorrect installation, loose connections, missing or worn gaskets, or cross-threading in the holder (**Figure 9.14**)
  - Expired shelf-life date on the cartridge or filter
  - Cracks or dents in outside case of filter, cartridge, or canister
  - Evidence of prior use of sorbent cartridge or canister (indicated by absence of sealing material, tape, or foil over the inlet)

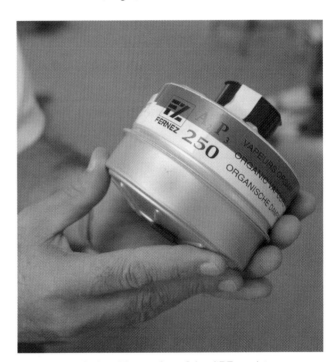

Figure 9.14 A visual inspection of the APR canister, cartridge, or filter includes looking at its cleanliness, condition, and use-by or expiration date.

- *Corrugated breathing tube* (if part of APR) — Inspect for the following items:
  - Broken or missing end connectors, gaskets, or O-rings
  - Missing or loose hose clamps
  - Deterioration (determined by stretching the tube and looking for cracks) (**Figure 9.15**)

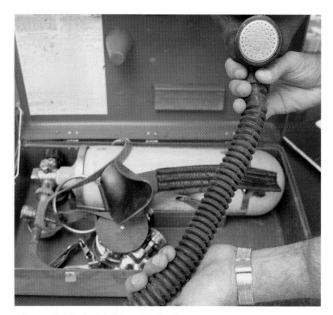

Figure 9.15 Respiratory protection equipment (such as this old model APR) that are equipped with low-pressure hoses require additional care during inspection. The hose should be stretched to determine if pinholes or cracks exist in the depths of the folds and around the clamps used at connection points.

- *Front- or back-mounted gas mask harness* — Inspect for the following items:

   — Damage or wear to the canister holder that may prevent its being held securely in place

   — Broken harness straps or fastenings (**Figure 9.16**)

   — Cleanliness

   — Absorbent type and condition

Filters intended for the removal of gases and vapors may be equipped with NIOSH-approved

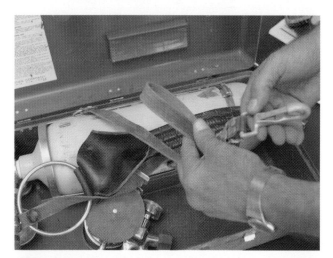

Figure 9.16 APR harness assemblies must be inspected for condition of the straps, buckles, slides, and fittings.

end-of-service-life indicators (ESLI). These ESLIs warn the user that the sorbent is approaching saturation and is no longer effective (**Figure 9.17**). The remaining usefulness of the filter should be determined and the filter replaced as needed. For filters without ESLIs, a sorbent change schedule must be established. This schedule is based on the manufacturer's recommendation for filter use. The manufacturer may also provide information about the chemical hazard the filter is designed to protect against.

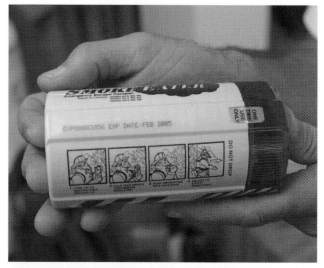

Figure 9.17 Some APR canisters and cartridges are marked with end-of-service-life or use-by dates. Note these dates during periodic inspections, and remove units that are out of date from the inventory.

Annual Inspections

[NFPA 1404: 8.1.2]
[NFPA 1852: 7.2.1.3, 7.4.4.1]

Respiratory protection equipment must be inspected and tested in accordance with the manufacturer's recommendations or the organization's SOP (whichever is more frequent) but in all cases at least annually. These inspections and tests are performed by manufacturer-trained and certified technicians. Respiratory protection maintenance technicians must be certified for the specific make and model of equipment that the organization owns. Contract vendors must also meet these requirements. Depending on the type of respiratory protection equipment, the annual inspection and testing includes the following procedures:

- Disassemble and inspect the facepiece exhalation valve (**Figure 9.18**).

- Disassemble and inspect the regulator housing and end-of-service-time indicator(s).

- Inspect breathing-air cylinder interior and valve assembly.

- Test regulator on an approved breathing machine.

- Perform leak check after cleaning and reassembly of components.

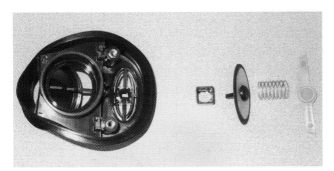

Figure 9.18 Annual inspections by manufacturer-trained and certified technicians include the complete disassembly of facepiece exhalation valves. *Courtesy of Lloyd Lees.*

Record Keeping

[NFPA 1500: 7.2.1, 7.3.1]
[NFPA 1852: 4.4.8]

Records should be maintained in accordance with departmental/organizational policy and the manufacturer recommendations. All nondisposable respiratory protection equipment, breathing-air compressor systems, cascade systems, and fill stations must be inventoried and assigned tracking numbers. NFPA 1500 and 1852 require that records on SCBA, SAR, and SCBA/SAR combination units must be maintained in a database either on a computer or in hard-copy files. General record-keeping requirements have already been covered in Chapter 5, Respiratory Protection Equipment Selection and Procurement. Inspection, testing, and maintenance records should include the following items:

- *Record of daily/weekly inspections*
  - Date and time
  - Name of person performing inspection
  - Unit serial and/or inventory number
  - General condition of unit

- Repairs requested
- If unit is placed out of service, record the following items:
  † Date and time
  † When repairs are made
  † When the unit is placed back in service

- *Annual inspection, maintenance, and testing*
  - Date and time
  - Name of technician performing inspection, maintenance, and testing
  - Unit serial and/or inventory number
  - General condition of unit
  - Breathing machine test results
  - Maintenance performed
  - Date and time unit returned to service

Respiratory Protection Equipment Care and Maintenance

[NFPA 1404: 6.12, 8.1.1, 8.1.2, 8.1.2.1]

Three levels of maintenance are defined by NFPA: operational or user level, field/specialist level, and technician level. Operational-level maintenance is performed daily and following each use by operational personnel. It includes care, cleaning, storage, and disposal of respiratory equipment. Specialist maintenance is performed by personnel who have received training beyond that of operational personnel. These personnel can perform basic repairs. Technician-level maintenance is performed by manufacturer-trained personnel who are certified to work on the specific units. These personnel can disassemble and test specific respiratory equipment models.

Operational-Level Maintenance

Operational-level maintenance consists of the care, decontamination, cleaning, disinfecting, storage, and disposal of respiratory protection materials. See Respiratory Protection Equipment Disposal and Retirement section for details on disposal procedures. Operational-level maintenance and cleaning is usually performed along with the daily/ weekly and postincident inspections. Personnel should always consult manufacturer's recommendations for how to conduct inspections and cleaning as well as frequency of these procedures. The only requirement is that the units be cleaned and disinfected as necessary and following each use. Training in the care, cleaning, disinfecting, and storing of respirators ensures that the equipment will be ready for immediate use and provide an adequate level of protection. In addition, proper care and storage decrease damage and maintenance costs.

Frequency of Maintenance

The local authority having jurisdiction should establish the care, cleaning, and maintenance schedules based on the manufacturer's recommendation, NFPA standards, or OSHA requirements. The minimum requirements are as follows:

- Clean respiratory protection equipment as needed during the daily/weekly inspections at the beginning of the work period.

- Inspect, clean, and disinfect respiratory protection equipment following use before placing it back into service (**Figure 9.19**).

- Clean respiratory protection equipment units that are used infrequently during the weekly inspection when required. Clean units that are to be stored before placing them into storage. When the units are removed from storage, clean as needed.

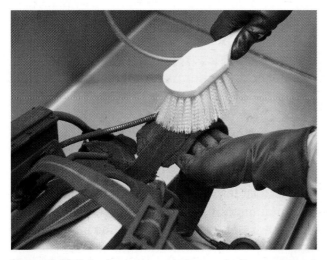

Figure 9.19 Following use, respiratory protection equipment (such as this SCBA backpack harness) should be cleaned to remove dirt, grime, and contaminants. Personnel should wear protective gloves and other garments to protect themselves from exposure to any unknown contaminants.

Part of the postincident care and cleaning process is to replace used filters, cartridges, and canisters. Because these items may have been contaminated with potentially hazardous materials, care must be taken and protocols followed. The manufacturer's recommendations should be followed along with the authority's policy. Other recommendations may include the following:

- Wear respiratory, eye, and hand protection.

- Dispose of the contaminated material with other biological or hazardous waste.

Proper procedures are especially important when disposing of oxygen-generating canisters from closed-circuit SCBA. The Chemox™-type canister can pose the threat of a violent explosion if not disposed of properly (**Figure 9.20**). While these types of canisters are rare and outdated, they can still be found in military use. Further information on disposal procedures is included in the Respiratory Protection Equipment Disposal and Retirement section later in this chapter.

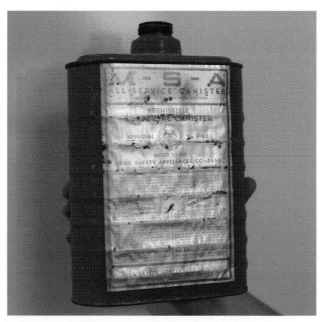

Figure 9.20 Oxygen-generating canisters such as this Chemox™ canister must be disposed of according to the manufacturer's recommendations.

Decontamination of Respirators

Before cleaning and disinfecting respiratory equipment, inspect for possible contamination from chemical, biological, or nuclear contaminants. Decontamination is accomplished by following normal protocols or referring to appropriate material safety data sheets (MSDSs) to neutralize the hazard. The United States Centers for Disease Control (CDC) can also provide guidelines for decontamination. Full protective clothing, eye protection, and respiratory protection must be worn during the decontamination process.

Cleaning and Disinfecting Procedures

[NFPA 1404: 8.1.3, 8.1.4, 8.1.5, 8.1.5.1, 8.1.5.2, 8.1.5.3]
[NFPA 1852: 6.1.1, 6.1.2, 6.1.2.1, 6.1.2.2, 6.1.2.3, 6.1.3, 6.1.4, 6.1.4.1, 6.1.4.2, 6.1.5, 6.1.5.1, 6.1.5.2, 6.1.6, 6.1.7, 6.1.7.1, 6.1.7.2, 6.1.8, 6.1.9, 6.2.1, 6.2.2, 6.2.3, 6.2.4]

Cleaning and disinfecting procedures should follow the manufacturer's recommendations. Because equipment is made from various types of materials, some cleaning solutions may have a detrimental effect on parts of the equipment. Cleaning and disinfecting procedures should be established as part of the respiratory protection program and should be coordinated with the infection control program of the organization. Infection control procedures are outlined in NFPA 1581, *Standard on Fire Department Infection Control Program*. The organization's health and safety officer may be responsible for this program and should be consulted.

Both NFPA 1581 and OSHA Title 29 (Labor) *CFR* 1910.1030, Bloodborne Pathogens, require that the cleaning and disinfecting areas of the facility be separate from the living quarters and from each other. Contaminated equipment must never be cleaned in the kitchen or bathroom area. The separate cleaning and disinfecting areas must be designated and equipped for the specific purpose.

Normally, respiratory protection equipment is cleaned in a wash sink in the cleaning area (**Figure 9.21**). The cleaning area is equipped with a wash

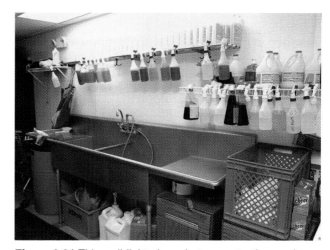

Figure 9.21 This well-lighted respiratory protection equipment cleaning area includes two sinks, shelves, drain boards, and storage for cleaning supplies.

Generic Cleaning Procedures for Respiratory Protection Equipment

The methods used for cleaning and disinfecting respiratory protection equipment must not cause damage to the equipment or harm to the user. Generic cleaning procedures are as follows:

Step 1: Remove filters, cartridges, or canisters. Disassemble the facepiece to the extent instructed by the manufacturer. Discard or repair defective parts.

Step 2: Wash components in warm (maximum 110°F [43°C]) water with a mild detergent or with a cleaner recommended by the manufacturer. Use a stiff bristle (not wire) brush to facilitate the removal of dirt or grime.

Step 3: Rinse components *thoroughly* in clean, warm, preferably running water. Drain.

NOTE: The importance of thorough rinsing cannot be overemphasized. Detergents or disinfectants that dry on facepieces may cause dermatitis. In addition, some disinfectants may cause deterioration of rubber parts or corrosion of metal parts if they are not completely removed.

Step 4: Immerse the respirator components in one of the disinfectants listed below for at least 2 minutes if the cleaner does not contain a disinfecting agent:

- Hypochlorite solution (50 ppm chlorine)
- Aqueous solution of iodine (50 ppm)
- Other disinfectants approved by the manufacturer that are equally potent

Step 5: Repeat Step 3 if Step 4 was implemented.

Step 6: Air-dry or hand-dry components with a clean, lint-free cloth.

Step 7: Reassemble the facepiece, replacing the filtering elements.

Step 8: Test the respirator to verify that all components work properly.

sink, a drain board, fresh hot- and cold-water faucets, a drain (filtered or contained, depending on local water protection codes), a ventilation area, and a drying area. Drains must not open onto the floor causing a slipping and contamination hazard. Cleaning solutions, brushes, sponges, wash gloves, and other cleaning materials are stored in this area.

Disinfecting areas are normally used for removing contamination from biological and hazardous materials. Stainless steel two-bay sinks and drain boards are provided along with paddle-handle faucets, stainless steel shelves, and drying racks (**Figure 9.22**). Respiratory, eye, and splash protections are provided in this area along with the approved cleaning materials and solutions. Written protocols should also be posted in the area. Disinfecting of respiratory protection equipment takes place in this area only when a known biological or hazardous material has contaminated the equipment.

Respiratory protection equipment that does not require the removal of biological or hazardous contaminates is maintained in the cleaning area and cleaned by hand with detergent and water. This cleaning removes debris and grime from facepieces, harnesses, and regulator bodies. Use damp cloths, sponges, or brushes (natural or synthetic bristles, *not* wire) to clean the outside of regulators with connection caps in place. Following the washing process, facepieces are disinfected separately with a bactericide (**Figure 9.23**). If only one person uses a facepiece, disinfecting is not absolutely necessary. However, it is especially important if the facepiece is shared between personnel. Facepieces should be immersed in disinfecting solutions in accordance with manufacturer instructions. Commercial disinfecting solutions are readily available and should be supplied by the organization. Examples of sources for producing disinfecting solutions are as follows:

- *Hypochlorite solution* (50 ppm of chloride) — Make solution by adding approximately 2 milliliter (ml) of hypochlorite (laundry) bleach to 1 liter of water.

- *Aqueous solution of iodine* (50 ppm of iodine) — Make solution by adding approximately 0.8 milliliter (ml) tincture of iodine per liter of water. The iodine is approximately 7 percent ammonium and potassium iodide, 45 percent alcohol, and 48 percent water.

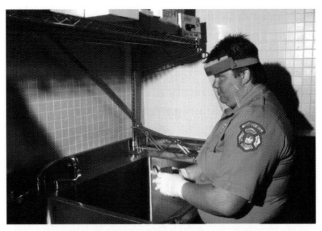
Figure 9.22 Areas used for disinfecting equipment should include stainless steel sinks, shelves, and drain boards.

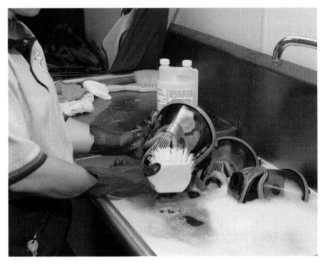
Figure 9.23 Soft bristle brushes (like the one shown in use) can clean and disinfect facepieces without scratching the lens surface.

To avoid damaging the rubber and plastic that is used in the construction of the respiratory protection equipment, the water, cleanser, and disinfectant must not exceed 110°F (43°C). However, to ensure adequate cleaning, it must not be less than 110°F (43°). When the equipment is thoroughly washed and disinfected, it must be rinsed to remove any traces of cleaning solution or disinfectant. OSHA Title 29 *CFR* 1910.134 (Respiratory Protection), Appendix B-2, Respiratory Cleaning Procedures (Mandatory) recommends using 110°F (43°C) temperature water for washing and rinsing. In all cases, consult the manufacturer's instructions.

The respiratory protection equipment may be allowed to dry on a clean surface after rinsing or hand-dried with a lint-free towel. It may also be hung to dry in a well-ventilated area (**Figure 9.24**). Commercial drying cabinets are also available that decrease the drying time by using a heating element and recirculating fan. While drying, the equipment should be protected from dust or other airborne contaminates, damaging chemicals, direct sunlight, and temperature extremes. Before storing, inspect the equipment to ensure that all moisture has evaporated from crevices and porous materials.

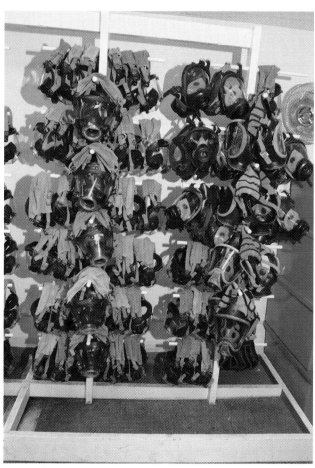

Figure 9.24 Following cleaning, facepieces are hung in well-ventilated spaces to completely dry.

Storage

[NFPA 1404: 4.1.4]
[NFPA 1852: 6.3.1, 6.3.2, 6.3.3, 6.3.4, 6.3.5, 6.3.6, 6.3.7, 6.3.7.1, 6.3.7.2, 6.3.8]

Respiratory protection equipment is stored in many locations and by several methods such as the following:

- In seat brackets on apparatus (**Figure 9.25**)

- In brackets or cases in apparatus compartments (**Figure 9.26**)

- In specially designed storage compartments on apparatus

- On wall brackets in facilities

- In cabinets, on shelves, or in cases in facilities

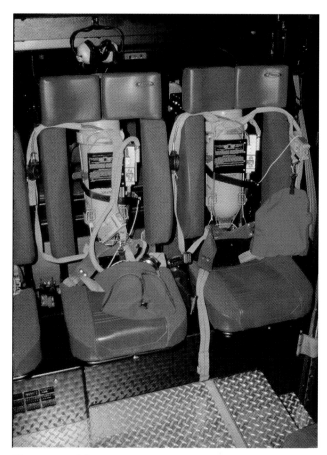

Figure 9.25 SCBA may be stored in apparatus seat backs in ready-to-use condition. Clamps must be strong enough to prevent the units from becoming dislodged in the event of an accident. A release handle allows the wearer to release the tension and pull the unit free when needed.

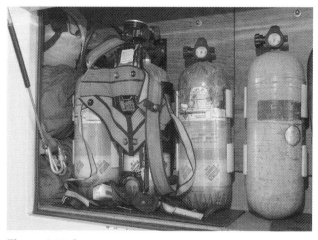

Figure 9.26 Compartment brackets may be used to store either complete SCBA systems or spare breathing-air cylinders (shown in this photo).

Regardless of the storage location or method, respiratory protection equipment must be protected from the following elements:

- Dust and contamination
- Direct sunlight
- Temperature extremes
- Excessive moisture
- Exposure to chemicals
- Mechanical damage or abrasion

NIOSH strongly recommends that freshly cleaned SCBA/SAR facepieces and APRs be placed in reusable plastic bags for storage. They should be stored in a clean, dry location that is out of direct sunlight. The ultraviolet (UV) rays of the sun can deteriorate and destroy the material of the respirator. Moisture can form inside the plastic bag causing mildew and mold to grow. The respirator should be stored with the exhalation valve in a normal position to prevent the rubber or plastic from distorting. Other equipment should not be allowed to rest on top of the respirator or to press against it.

If facepieces or respirators are individually assigned, facepiece bags should be issued with them (**Figure 9.27**). These bags may be either disposable or reusable. Not only will bags prevent damage to the facepiece lens, straps, and body, but they will also provide a means for marking the name of the unit or individual to whom the facepiece is assigned.

Replacement filters, cartridges, and canisters should be labeled for type of hazard and color-coded with the NIOSH-approval label, segregated by type, and stored in a closed cabinet to prevent the collection of dust and exposure to light that might deteriorate the units. Do not permit the interchange of filters, cartridges, or canisters between different brands of respirators. Not only can this mixing be dangerous, but it can also void the NIOSH approval and certification of the system.

Field/Specialist-Level Maintenance
[NFPA 1404: 6.11]

Personnel who have received specialized training in the maintenance of respiratory protection equipment beyond the level of operational maintenance are at the field/specialist level. These individuals are trained to make basic repairs on the equipment without taking the unit out of service. Depending on the manufacturer's training, these repairs may include but are not limited to the following:

- Replacement of facepiece harness straps
- Installation of nose cups and eyeglass kits (**Figure 9.28**)
- Replacement of backpack harness components
- Replacement of complete regulators
- Replacement of low-pressure breathing hoses
- Replacement of filters, cartridges, or canisters
- Replacement of PASS device or communications system batteries

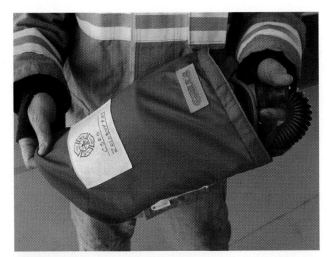

Figure 9.27 To protect the facepiece from wear and filth, accessories such as facepiece storage bags may be purchased from the manufacturer or from after-market vendors.

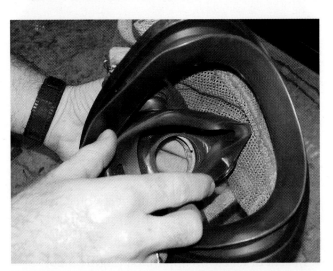

Figure 9.28 Specialist-level maintenance personnel should be trained to install and replace eyeglass kits, harness assemblies, and nose cups on facepieces.

Field/specialist personnel can be trained and certified to perform maintenance that requires the disassembly of the facepiece, regulator, or any valves. More complicated repairs, however, are the responsibility of the respiratory protection equipment technician.

Technician-Level Maintenance

[NFPA 1852: 4.8.1, 4.8.1.1, 4.8.1.2, 4.8.2, 4.8.3, 7.2.3.1, 7.2.3.2]

The respiratory protection equipment technician is an individual who has been trained and certified by the manufacturer of the equipment in use by the organization. This person is authorized to disassemble, inspect, clean, repair, reassemble, and test specific brands and models of respiratory protection equipment. The manufacturer usually requires periodic recertification. This level of maintenance can take two forms: in-house and contract. The decision on which form to use is part of the selection process mentioned in Chapter 5, Respiratory Protection Equipment Selection and Procurement. The maintenance level is based on the cost, efficiency, and personnel requirements of each form. Regardless of the form that technician-level maintenance takes, close supervision and accurate and complete records are vital.

In-House Maintenance

Depending on the size of the emergency services organization, in-house maintenance may include the use of a self-contained, fully staffed internal repair function or a repair function that is part of another agency within the jurisdiction **(Figure 9.29)**. Either way, the maintenance personnel must be trained and certified. In addition, a repair facility including a workspace in a clean room, parts inventory storage, and a breathing-air supply must be provided. The clean room ensures that the workspace is free of contaminants that might be trapped in the equipment's regulators or valves during repair.

Contract Maintenance

Some organizations may find that it is cost-effective to contract this level of maintenance **(Figure 9.30)**. The manufacturer's representative can provide a list of certified repair facilities in the area. The fire and emergency service organization should thoroughly investigate the ability of the repair facility to provide the necessary level of support. Areas of concern include the following:

- Certification for specific model of equipment
- Parts inventory
- Maintenance time
- Test documentation
- Pickup and delivery services
- Loaner equipment
- Cost
- Agreements with manufacturers (consult local legal department for limitations)

These items must be clarified and included in the service contract. The organization should

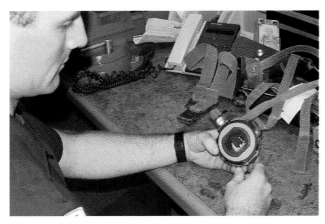

Figure 9.29 Only manufacturer-trained and certified personnel should attempt to disassemble, clean, repair, and test the regulators of SCBA and SAR systems. *Courtesy of Kenneth Baum.*

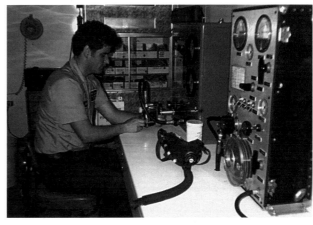

Figure 9.30 Some respiratory protection equipment manufacturers or their vendors may provide mobile maintenance centers to serve organizations that do not have internal maintenance facilities or personnel. *Courtesy of Weis Fire Equipment Company.*

periodically verify that the facility and its technicians are still certified and authorized by the manufacturer. This certification can be done annually when the contract is renewed.

Air and Oxygen Cylinder Inspections and Maintenance

Cylinders used in respiratory protection contain either breathing air or oxygen under pressure. A damaged cylinder can cause a catastrophic incident during filling, use, or storage (**Figure 9.31**). The potential exists to send metal shrapnel in all directions, injuring or killing personnel in the area. To prevent such an occurrence, cylinders must be inspected, filled, tested, and stored with care. Because air-supplied respirators represent the sole source of protection in hazardous environments, breathing-air and oxygen supplies must meet established quality standards.

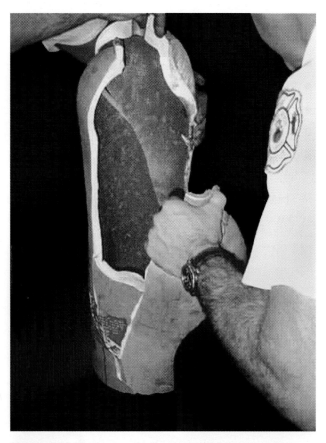

Figure 9.31 Damage and injury can result from a catastrophic failure of a breathing-air cylinder such as the one shown. *Courtesy of Dennis Hawkins.*

Inspecting Cylinders

[NFPA 1500: 7.13.1, 7.13.2, 7.13.3, 7.13.4]

Breathing-air cylinders are parts of the SCBA, SCBA/SAR, and EBSS respiratory protection systems. They are also used to provide bulk breathing air in cascade systems. Oxygen cylinders are part of the closed-circuit SCBA system. All compressed air and oxygen cylinders must meet the requirements of OSHA, U.S. Department of Transportation (DOT), and CGA C-6.2, Guidelines for Visual Inspection and Requalification of Fiber Reinforced High Pressure Cylinders. Inspection requirements are found in Title 29 *CFR* 1910.134, Respiratory Protection, and NFPA 1852.

The daily/weekly inspection requirements were included earlier in this chapter under the Respiratory Protection Equipment Inspection Schedules section. Daily/weekly visual inspections are important because they can catch the early signs of damage to a cylinder (**Figure 9.32**). Cylinders must also be inspected before filling to prevent ruptures in the fill process. Damage may be caused by the following elements:

- Exposure to heat
- Direct flame contact
- Exposure to chemicals
- Mechanical damage caused by dropping, impact, or improper storage
- Misthreaded valve in cylinder neck

In addition to the presence of damage, the visual inspection should also confirm that the cylinder has been identified with the date of manufacture and the date of the last hydrostatic test. Steel and aluminum cylinders must be tested every 5 years while composite cylinders must be tested every 3 years (**Figure 9.33**). Currently, composite cylinders must be removed from service after 15 years. After July 1, 2001, the U.S. DOT permitted carbon fiber composite cylinders to be hydrotested every 5 years. Kevlar® aramid fiber and fiberglass composite cylinders maintain hydrostatic testing requirements every 3 years.

Respiratory protection equipment technicians are responsible for removing the cylinder valve and inspecting the threads for damage and the cylinder neck for stress fractures and cracks (**Figure 9.34**). An outside vendor who is under contract and certi-

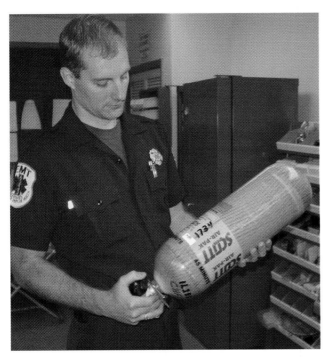

Figure 9.32 Early signs of damage to breathing-air cylinders can be discovered during the weekly inspection. Damage may be caused by abuse, abrasion, heat or chemical exposure, or metal fatigue. *Courtesy of Kenneth Baum.*

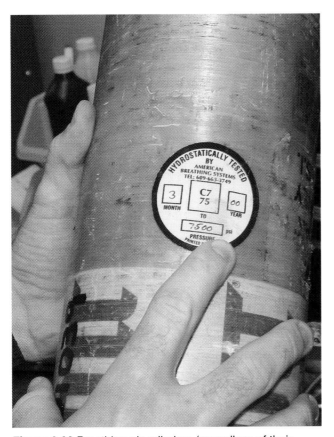

Figure 9.33 Breathing-air cylinders (regardless of their construction materials) must have a current hydrostatic test date displayed on the cylinder. This cylinder was last tested in March, 2000. *Courtesy of Kenneth Baum.*

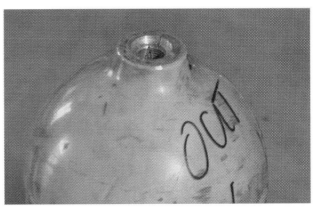

Figure 9.34 The breathing-air cylinder neck must be inspected for damage to the threads and for hairline stress fractures that are only visible when the pressure valve is removed.

fied to perform hydrostatic testing usually provides the testing service. Cylinders that are out of date for hydrostatic testing must not be filled and must be removed from service until the test is performed and the cylinder certified.

The technician responsible for respiratory protection equipment maintenance must monitor NIOSH and manufacturer product notices on cylinder failures. Because cylinders are manufactured by companies that are specialists in this area, product notices concerning cylinder failures or recalls may be provided by them as well as the respiratory protection equipment manufacturer and NIOSH.

Filling Breathing-Air Cylinders
[NFPA 1500: 7.10.1, 7.13.5, 7.13.6]
[NFPA 1404: 9.2.1, 9.2.2, 9.2.3]
[NFPA 1852: 7.3.1, 7.3.2, 7.3.3, 7.3.4, 7.3.5]

Breathing-air cylinders that are less than 90 percent of their rated capacities must be removed from service and refilled. Cylinders may be filled from stationary or portable cascade systems or from stationary or portable breathing-air compressors. A cascade system consists of a series of large-capacity cylinders containing at least three 300 cubic-foot (eight 490 L) cylinders of breathing air connected by a manifold to a regulated fill station (**Figure 9.35**). The cascade system may be located in an apparatus room, maintenance facility, or on an apparatus or specially designed trailer. As cylinders are expended, they are replaced with fresh cylinders or the system is replenished from a breathing-air compressor.

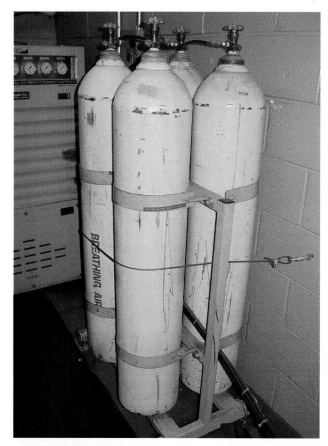

Figure 9.35 A breathing-air cascade system includes large-capacity compressed-air cylinders that are properly secured (such as these shown).

The breathing-air compressor is specifically designed to provide Type 1 Grade D breathing air (**Figure 9.36**). Note that only compressors certified for this purpose may be used to provide breathing air. These compressors may be installed in a facility or on board an apparatus. In either case, the ambient air must be free of pollutants to ensure that the filtration system can provide the best quality of raw air.

Breathing-air compressors must be equipped with in-line air-purifying sorbent beds or filters (**Figure 9.37**). The manufacturer's maintenance, replacement, or refurbishment schedule and recommendations must be followed. Breathing-air compressors that are not oil lubricated must maintain carbon monoxide (CO) levels of less than 10 parts per million (ppm). Oil-lubricated breathing-air compressors must be equipped with a high-temperature or CO alarm (or both) to monitor the CO level. If the compressor is equipped with only the high-temperature alarm, then the air supply must be monitored at sufficient intervals to

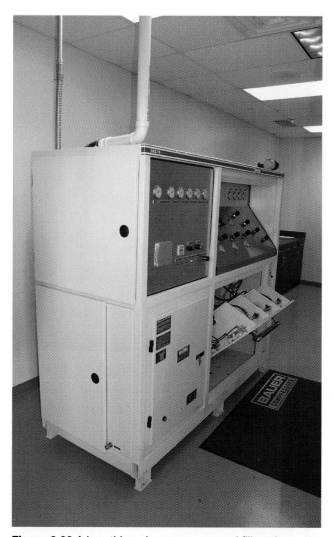

Figure 9.36 A breathing-air compressor and fill station must be located away from vehicle exhausts in a well-ventilated space.

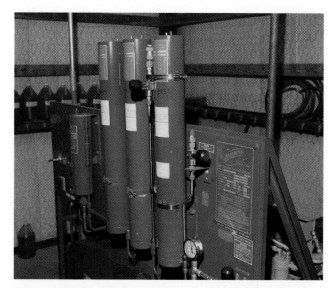

Figure 9.37 The filtration system for a breathing-air compressor requires periodic inspection and maintenance. Filter element replacement is usually determined by the hours of operation of the unit.

ensure that the CO does not exceed 10 ppm. See Air-Quality Testing section for further information.

Both the cascade system and the compressor system have fill stations connected to them. The fill station provides the fill hoses and connections, pressure-regulating valves and gauges, and the fragmentation shielding to protect personnel from a rupture (**Figure 9.38**). Filling procedures should be posted on the fill station and must follow the manufacturer's recommendations and regulations for ranges and rates to avoid excessive overheating in the cylinder. No matter how the cylinders are filled, the following safety precautions apply:

• Only trained personnel should operate the fill equipment.

• Cylinders must be inspected before filling.

• Hearing and eye protection must be worn during fill operations.

• Cylinders must be placed in the shielded fill station.

• Cylinders must be filled slowly to prevent overheating.

• Cylinders must be filled to their capacity.

• Cylinders must not be overfilled.

Maintenance of the cascade and compressor systems, including the replacement of the filter elements, must follow the manufacturer's specifications. This responsibility is usually assigned to the respiratory protection equipment technician. The technician should be trained and

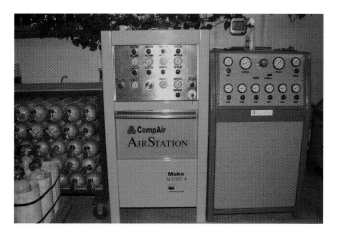

Figure 9.38 Breathing air-compressors and cascade systems include fill stations as part of the system. Fill stations (like the one shown) have enclosed and shielded areas for the cylinders to prevent injury in the event of a rupture during the filling process. *Courtesy of Bob Parker.*

certified by the system manufacturer for performing this maintenance.

Some SCBA manufacturers provide refill connections on the regulator that allow the filling of cylinders without removing them from the backpack assembly (**Figure 9.39**). This procedure has the advantage of decreasing the time for refilling or replacing the cylinder during an emergency operation. It also has the disadvantage of reducing the opportunity for evaluating the physical condition of the wearer. After the use of a cylinder of air, the wearer should be evaluated before returning to the hot zone.

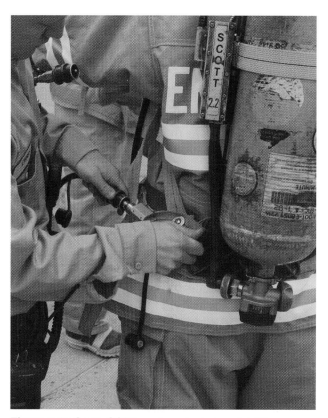

Figure 9.39 Some SCBA systems include quick-fill connections that permit the breathing air-cylinder to be filled without removing it from the wearer's backpack assembly.

Air-Quality Testing
[NFPA 1500: 7.10.2, 7.10.3, 7.10.4, 7.10.5]

[NFPA 1404: 9.1]

The air quality must be tested to ensure that the breathing air used in SCBA and SAR respiratory protection systems meets requirements and standards of OSHA, NFPA, CSA (such as CAN/CSAZ180.1-00, Compressed Breathing Air Systems), and others. The health and safety officer or other designated person is responsible for taking a sample from the discharge air of the breathing-air compressor or cascade system (**Figure 9.40**). The sample is then sent to a third-party testing laboratory that tests the air for purity and moisture content. The written results of the test are provided to the fire and emergency services organization and maintained on file as part of the respiratory protection records files. The breathing air must be tested quarterly and following any maintenance on the system. Breathing-air cylinders that are rented, leased, or purchased from an outside vendor must also be tested quarterly or the vendor must provide certification of the air quality. Breathing air must be Type 1 Grade D or better air quality based on American National Standards Institute (ANSI)/CGA Commodity Specification for Air (G-7.1-1989), OSHA, and NFPA requirements. Breathing air must meet the following minimum requirements:

- Oxygen content of 19.5 to 23.5 percent

- Hydrocarbon content of 5 milligrams per cubic meter of air or less

- Carbon monoxide content of 10 parts per million or less

- Carbon dioxide (CO_2) content of 1,000 parts per million or less

- Lack of any noticeable odor

Oxygen for Closed-Circuit SCBA

Most fire and emergency services organizations use compressed medical-grade oxygen for medical emergencies. Medical-grade oxygen is usually purchased from medical gas suppliers (**Figure 9.41**). It may be delivered to the fire and emergency services organization in large Type K cylinders for transfer to smaller cylinders or the small cylinders that are refilled by the supplier. Either way, the use and storage of oxygen and filling cylinders with oxygen must meet the requirements of CGA, DOT, OSHA, NFPA, and any other applicable regulations and standards. This same oxygen may be used for closed-circuit SCBA when it is contained in the proper cylinder for the SCBA system. When working with oxygen cylinders, specific requirements must be met, including the following:

- All personnel must be trained in the use of the oxygen cylinders.

- Smoking must be prohibited during filling operations and use.

- Oily rags and gloves must not be used or stored around oxygen cylinders.

- Cylinders that are empty should be marked or tagged *EMPTY* (**Figure 9.42**).

- Cylinder valve caps must be in place when hoses are not connected to cylinders and during transportation.

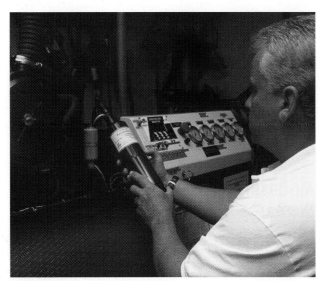

Figure 9.40 The health and safety officer or other designated member of the organization may be responsible for drawing a sample of the breathing air from the breathing-air compressor or cascade system. This sample is then tested for purity by a third-party laboratory.

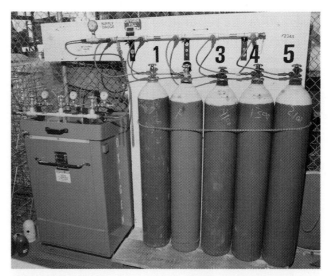

Figure 9.41 Oxygen used in closed-circuit systems and for medical emergencies may be purchased from a vendor in quantity and then transferred to the appropriate size cylinders for use. Organizations should consult the appropriate governmental agency concerning restrictions that are placed on oxygen handling and filling operations.

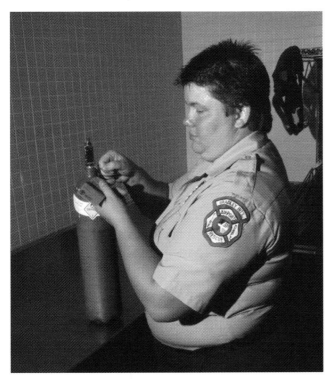

Figure 9.42 An oxygen cylinder that requires filling must be prominently marked with the word *EMPTY*.

Respiratory Protection Equipment Disposal and Retirement

The local authority having jurisdiction establishes the requirements for disposing of or retiring respiratory protection equipment and components. Depending on the value of the equipment, the process may be determined by the purchasing agent or the user department/organization. In some jurisdictions, the value and life expectancy of the equipment will place it into one of two categories: capital purchases or noncapital purchases.

Capital purchases have a value greater than a predetermined sum such as $1,000, have a life expectancy of greater than 1 year, are maintained on a fixed-assets inventory list, and are purchased with designated funds. Capital items are usually disposed of through a controlled auction or they are included as a trade-in for a new similar item or donated to another agency or authority. Complete SCBA and SAR systems fall into the capital-purchase category. Noncapital purchases have a value of less than the predetermined sum, have a life expectancy of less than 1 year, and are purchased with operation funds that do not specify the exact item to be purchased, only a general category. This category includes repair parts, filters, canisters, cartridges, and APR systems. These items are usually disposed of when they are expended, damaged, or obsolete. Descriptions of disposal/retirement procedures for the various items are given in the sections that follow.

Air-Purifying Respirator Devices

APR filter, canister, and cartridge disposal depends on the following factors:

● Type of contamination

● OSHA requirements

● Manufacturer's recommendations

The manufacturer's recommendations should be consulted first. Disposal recommendations are found in the written instructions with the filter, canister, or cartridge. Recommendations may be based on the type of contaminant and exposure time, odor break-through, resistance to breathing, and hours of operation or on the end-of-service-life indicator on the canister or cartridge. OSHA specifies that the canister or cartridge be replaced following each use and that high efficiency particulate air (HEPA) filters be replaced at least annually (**Figure 9.43**). Information available on each of the specific contaminates also provides an indication of when and how to dispose of the canister or cartridge. If there is any doubt, remove the filter, canister, or cartridge and replace it with a fresh element; dispose of the old one.

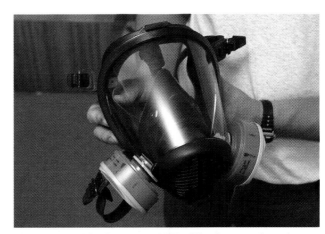

Figure 9.43 If full facepiece APRs (like the one shown) are stored with filter cartridges in place, they should be inspected periodically and the filter cartridge replaced if they are out of date.

How expended filters, canisters, and cartridges are disposed of depend on the type of contaminate that they are used to protect against. Filters used to protect against biological hazards should be disposed of with other medical/biological waste in accordance with local protocol. Biologically contaminated filters may go to a designated landfill for burial or an incinerator for burning. Canisters and cartridges that have been exposed to gases or vapors must be disposed of using the protocol for hazardous waste. Contaminated canisters and cartridges may be sealed in designated containers and stored or buried in a hazardous waste site or burned in a designated incinerator, depending on the hazardous waste protocol (**Figure 9.44**). Filters, canisters, and cartridges that have not been exposed to medical/biological or hazardous materials may be disposed of with other waste material to be buried in a landfill or burned in an incinerator.

Dispossession of the basic APR system, facepiece, harness, and canister holder, may be through auction, donation, or waste removal. The decision on which method is chosen depends on the local protocol, condition of the equipment, and potential liability that is associated with used equipment. The fire and emergency services organization should consult the legal department or the purchasing department for guidance.

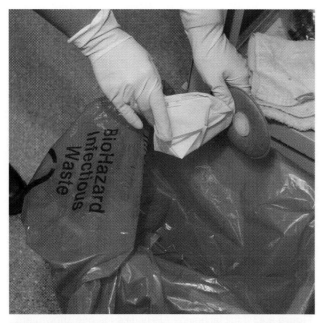

Figure 9.44 Used and contaminated APR filters should be disposed of with other medical waste. Personnel must wear personal protection such as medical gloves when handling contaminated filters, particulate masks, or cartridges.

Open-Circuit SCBA and Supplied-Air Respirator Devices

[NFPA 1852: 4.6.1, 4.6.2, 4.6.2.1, 4.6.2.2, 4.6.3, 4.6.4, 4.6.5, 4.6.6, 7.2.4.1, 7.2.4.2, 7.2.4.3, 7.2.4.4, 7.2.4.5]

SCBAs and SARs are usually disposed of when they are obsolete, they fail to meet minimum test standards, repairs are no longer cost-effective, or they are no longer needed. As mentioned earlier, these systems are usually considered capital purchases, exist on a fixed-assets inventory, and must be disposed of according to an established protocol. They may be traded in when new equipment is purchased, sold at auction, or donated to another agency. This type of retirement only applies to equipment that is known to operate correctly and has been tested and certified. Damaged and nonrepairable equipment should not be sold or donated; it should be destroyed to prevent injury to another user.

SCBA and SAR components may be disposed of as solid waste or scrap metal. The only restriction involves the disposal of breathing-air cylinders. Composite cylinders must be disposed of in accordance with DOT regulations on the 15th anniversary of the date of manufacture. Steel and aluminum cylinders may remain in service as long as they continue to pass hydrostatic tests. All breathing air cylinders that are to be disposed of must be destroyed and made inoperative by removing the cylinder valve and then cutting the cylinder in half, drilling holes in it, or crushing it (**Figure 9.45**). The remains are sent to metal salvage or disposed of in accordance with local protocols.

Closed-Circuit SCBA Devices

Closed-circuit SCBA systems may be considered capital purchases and are placed in the same category as the open-circuit SCBA systems. With the exception of the oxygen-generating canister, used parts and components are also treated in the same manner as the open-circuit SCBA systems. Therefore, dispossession requirements would follow similar guidelines.

As mentioned in the Air and Oxygen Cylinder Inspections and Maintenance section, the expended oxygen-generating canister is not only a hazardous material, it also presents a fire and

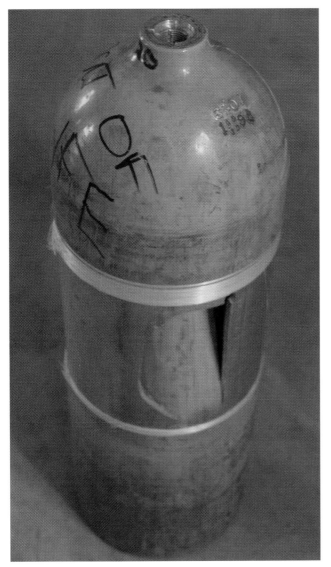

Figure 9.45 Damaged or out-of-date breathing-air cylinders must be cut in such a way as to prevent the chance of any further use. The cylinder in this photo has been cut open on the right side and the metal bent inward.

explosion hazard in both the fresh and expended form. Any petroleum product introduced into the open neck of the canister is extremely dangerous. The canister can also generate heat that requires the wearing of protective gloves when handling. The manufacturer's disposal requirements must be followed. The manufacturer suggests that holes be punched in the front, back, and bottom of these canisters. Then gently place the canister into a bucket of clean water that covers the unit by at least

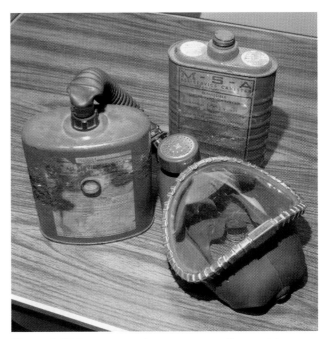

Figure 9.46 Because used oxygen-generating canisters (like the ones shown) may create a further hazard when they are disposed of, the local authority having jurisdiction must establish a disposal protocol for such items.

3 inches (76 mm). When the bubbling stops, the canister can be disposed of along with other hazardous waste. The water, which is caustic, must be disposed of according to local environmental codes. (**Figure 9.46**).

Summary

Personnel who are assigned the use of respiratory protection equipment must be thoroughly trained in all aspects of its care, cleaning, maintenance, testing, and disposal to ensure that the equipment is available for immediate use. Proper training at all levels provides not only a safe working environment but also a cost-efficient means of maintaining the respiratory protection equipment. Training and certification should be renewed on a periodic basis and also when the respiratory protection program is altered or an evaluation indicates a need for additional training. Increased familiarity with the equipment helps to ensure that it is properly used during emergency incidents.

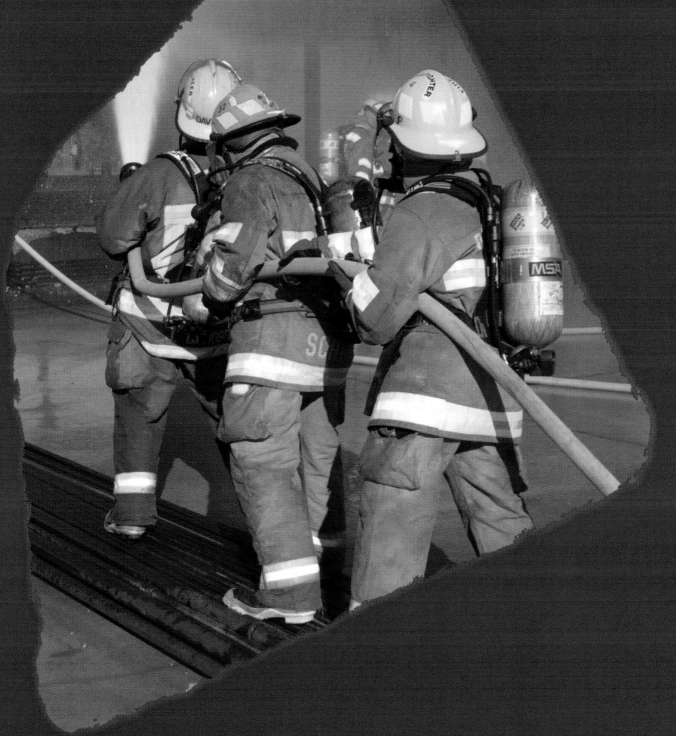

Chapter 10

Emergency Scene Use

This chapter provides information that will assist the reader in meeting the following job performance requirements from NFPA 1404, *Standard for Fire Service Respiratory Protection Training*, 2002 Edition, and NFPA 1500, *Standard on Fire Department Occupational Safety and Health Program*, 2002 Edition.

NFPA 1500

7.1.1 The fire department shall provide each member with the appropriate protective clothing and protective equipment to provide protection from the hazards to which the member is or is likely to be exposed. Such protective clothing and protective equipment shall be suitable for the tasks that the member is expected to perform.

7.1.2 Protective clothing and protective equipment shall be used whenever the member is exposed or potentially exposed to the hazards for which it is provided.

7.2.1 Members who engage in or are exposed to the hazards of structural fire fighting shall be provided with and shall use a protective ensemble that shall meet the applicable requirements of NFPA 1971, *Standard on Protective Ensemble for Structural Fire Fighting*.

7.3.1.1 The proximity protective coat and proximity protective trousers, or the proximity protective coverall, shall meet the applicable requirements of NFPA 1976, *Standard on Protective Ensemble for Proximity Fire Fighting*.

7.4.1 Members who perform emergency medical care or are otherwise likely to be exposed to blood or other body fluids shall be provided with emergency medical garments, emergency medical face protection devices, and emergency medical gloves that meet the applicable requirements of NFPA 1999, *Standard on Protective Clothing for Emergency Medical Operations*.

7.5.1.1 Members who engage in operations during hazardous materials emergencies that will expose them to known chemicals in vapor form or to unknown chemicals shall be provided with and shall use vapor-protective suits.

7.5.1.4 All members who engage in operations during hazardous materials emergencies that will expose them to known chemicals in vapor form or to unknown chemicals shall be provided with and shall use SCBA that meet the applicable requirements of Section 7.11 of this chapter.

7.5.1.4.1 Additional outside air supplies shall be permitted to be utilized in conjunction with SCBA, provided such systems are positive pressure and have been certified by NIOSH under 42 *CFR* 84.

7.5.2.4 All members who engage in operations during hazardous chemical emergencies that will expose them to known chemicals in liquid-splash form shall be provided with and shall use either SCBA that meet the applicable requirements of 7.11.1 or respiratory protective devices that are certified by NIOSH under 42 *CFR* 84 as suitable for the specific chemical environment.

7.5.2.4.1 Additional outside air supplies shall be permitted to be utilized in conjunction with SCBA, provided such systems are positive pressure and have been certified by NIOSH under 42 *CFR* 84.

7.5.2.5.1 Only vapor-protective suits specified in 7.5.1 of this chapter and SCBA specified in 7.11.1 of this chapter shall be considered for use.

7.8.2 Members who engage in or are exposed to the hazards of wildland fire-fighting operations shall be provided with and use protective garments that meet the requirements of NFPA 1977, *Standard on Protective Clothing and Equipment for Wildland Fire Fighting*.

7.9.5 An adequate reserve air supply shall be provided by use of reserve cylinders or by an on-scene refill capability, or both.

7.9.7 When engaged in any operation where they could encounter atmospheres that are immediately dangerous to life or health (IDLH) or potentially IDLH or where the atmosphere is unknown, the fire department shall provide and require all members to use SCBA that has been certified as being compliant with NFPA 1981, *Standard on Open-Circuit Self-Contained Breathing Apparatus for the Fire Service*.

7.9.8 Members using SCBA shall not compromise the protective integrity of the SCBA for any reason when operating in IDLH, potentially IDLH, or unknown atmospheres by removing the facepiece or disconnecting any portion of the SCBA that would allow the ambient atmosphere to be breathed.

7.13.5 During filling of SCBA cylinders, all personnel and operators shall be protected from catastrophic failure of the cylinder.

7.13.6 Due to the possibility of catastrophic failure of SCBA cylinders during filling, cylinders shall not be filled while being worn by the user.

7.13.7 In an emergency situation where an individual is trapped or injured and cannot be moved to a safe atmosphere and danger of additional serious injury or death is likely, a supplied-air source shall be the preferred method of providing a safe source of breathing air.

7.13.8 If a supplied source is not immediately available, transfilling of cylinders shall be done in accordance with the manufacturer's instructions.

7.14.2 Each member shall be provided with, use, and activate their PASS device in all of the following situations:

(1) Fire suppression

(2) Rescue

(3) Other hazardous duty

7.16.2 The full facepiece of SCBA shall constitute face and eye protection when worn.

7.16.2.1 SCBA that has a facepiece-mounted regulator that, when disconnected, provides a direct path for flying objects to strike the face or eyes, shall have the regulator attached in order to be considered face and eye protection.

8.4.4 Members operating in hazardous areas at emergency incidents shall operate in crews of two or more.

8.4.5 Crew members operating in hazardous areas shall be in communication with each other through visual, audible, or physical means or safety guide rope, in order to coordinate their activities.

8.4.6 Crew members shall be in proximity to each other to provide assistance in case of emergency.

8.4.7 In the initial stages of an incident where only one crew is operating in the hazardous area at a working structural fire, a minimum of four individuals shall be required, consisting of two individuals working as a crew in the hazard area and two individuals present outside this hazard area available for assistance or rescue at emergency operations where entry into the danger area is required.

8.4.8 The standby members shall be responsible for maintaining a constant awareness of the number and identity of members operating in the hazard area, their location and function, and time of entry.

8.4.9 The standby members shall remain in radio, visual, voice, or signal line communication with the crew.

8.4.13.1 The full protective clothing, protective equipment, and SCBA shall be immediately accessible for use by the outside crew if the need for rescue activities inside the hazard area is necessary.

8.4.14 The standby members shall don full protective clothing, protective equipment, and SCBA prior to entering the hazard area.

8.4.28 The incident commander shall ensure arson investigators or other members that enter an IDLH atmosphere or hazardous area use the appropriate personal protective equipment and/or SCBA.

8.5.2.1 Rapid intervention crews/company shall be fully equipped with the appropriate protective clothing, protective equipment, SCBA, and any specialized rescue equipment that could be needed given the specifics of the operation underway.

NFPA 1404
6.6.2 Fire department members shall be trained to handle problems related to the following situations that can be encountered during the use of respiratory protection equipment:

(1) Low temperatures

(2) High temperatures

(3) Rapid temperature changes

(4) Communications

(5) Confined spaces

(6) Vision

(7) Facepiece-to-face sealing problems

(8) Absorption through or irritation of the skin

(9) Effects of ionizing radiation on the skin and the entire body

(10) Punctured or ruptured eardrums

(11) Use near water

(12) Overhaul

6.7.2 Understanding the Safety Features and Limitations of SCBA. The training program of the authority having jurisdiction shall evaluate the ability of members to perform the following skills:

(1) Describe the operational principles of warning devices required on a SCBA

(2) Identify the limitations of the SCBA used by the authority having jurisdiction

(3) Describe the limitations of the SCBA's ability to protect the body from absorption of toxins through the skin

(4) Describe the procedures to be utilized if unintentionally submerged in water while wearing a SCBA

(5) Demonstrate the possible means of communications when wearing a SCBA

(6) Describe the emergency bypass operation

(7) Describe how to recognize medical signs and symptoms that could prevent the effective use of respirators

6.7.3 Donning and Doffing SCBA. The training program of the authority having jurisdiction shall evaluate the ability of members to demonstrate the following:

(1) Techniques for donning and doffing all types of SCBA used by the authority having jurisdiction while wearing the full protective clothing used by the authority having jurisdiction

(2) That a proper face-to-facepiece seal has been achieved by using the seal check

6.7.4 Practical Application in SCBA Training. The training program of the authority having jurisdiction shall evaluate the ability of members to demonstrate the following:

(1) Knowledge of the components of respiratory protection

(2) Use of all types of SCBA utilized by the authority having jurisdiction under conditions of obscured visibility

(3) Emergency operations that are required when a SCBA fails

(4) Emergency techniques using a SCBA to assist other members, conserve air, and show restrictions in use of bypass valves

(5) Use of a SCBA in limited or confined spaces

(6) Proper cleaning and sanitizing of the facepiece

6.8.1 Understanding the Components of a SAR. The training program of the authority having jurisdiction shall evaluate the ability of members to perform the following skills:

(1) Describe the air source, air hose limitations, and NIOSH approved inlet pressure gauge range

(2) Identify the components of facepieces, regulators, harnesses, manifold system, and cylinders or compressors used by the authority having jurisdiction

(3) Describe the operation of the SAR used by the authority having jurisdiction

(4) Describe the limitations of the escape cylinder

(5) Describe the potential incompatibility of different makes and models of SAR units

(6) Describe proper procedures for inspection, cleaning, and storage of SAR units

6.8.3 Donning and Doffing SAR. The training program of the authority having jurisdiction shall evaluate the ability of members to demonstrate the following:

(1) Proper techniques for donning and doffing all types of SAR used by the authority having jurisdiction while wearing the full protective clothing

(2) That a proper face-to-facepiece seal has been achieved by using the seal check

(3) Proper methods for tending SAR air hoses

6.8.4 Practical Application in SAR Training. The training program of the authority having jurisdiction shall evaluate the ability of members to perform the following skills:

(1) Demonstrate knowledge of the components of the SAR System

(2) Understand that the use of SAR is prohibited for fire fighting

(3) Demonstrate the use of SAR utilized by the authority having jurisdiction under conditions of obscured visibility

(4) Demonstrate the emergency operations that are required when the SAR fails

(5) Demonstrate the use of SAR when using hazardous materials personal protective equipment if utilized by the authority having jurisdiction

(6) Demonstrate the use of SAR in limited or confined spaces

(7) Demonstrate the proper cleaning and sanitizing of the facepiece

6.9.2 Understanding the Safety Features and Limitations of FFAPR. The training program of the authority having jurisdiction shall evaluate the ability of members to perform the following skills:

(1) Describe the operational principles of the FFAPR

(2) Identify the limitations of the FFAPR used by the authority having jurisdiction

(3) Describe the limitations of the FFAPR's ability to protect the body from absorption of toxins through the skin

(4) Describe the procedures for determining canister and cartridge selection by color-coded as well as NIOSH-approved labeling

(5) Understand labels are not to be removed from canisters or cartridges

(6) Understand that the use of FFAPR is prohibited for fire fighting

(7) Describe the limitations of FFAPR in fire ground activities

6.9.3 Donning and Doffing FFAPR. The training program of the authority having jurisdiction shall evaluate the ability of members to demonstrate the following:

(1) Proper techniques for donning and doffing all types of FFAPR used by the authority having jurisdiction while wearing the full protective clothing

(2) That a proper face-to-facepiece seal has been achieved

6.9.4 Practical Application in FFAPR Training. The training program of the authority having jurisdiction shall evaluate the ability of members to demonstrate the following:

(1) Knowledge of the components of respiratory protection

(2) Limits of communications when wearing an FFAPR

(3) Use of FFAPR utilized by the authority having jurisdiction under conditions of obscured visibility

(4) Correct selection and installation of canisters and cartridges for a given situation

(5) Proper method of donning and doffing the FFAPR

(6) The positive pressure and the negative pressure facepiece-to face leak test

(7) Use of FFAPR in limited or confined spaces

(8) Proper cleaning and sanitizing

The final element of an effective respiratory protection program is the proper use of respiratory protection equipment. Situations that may require the need for respiratory protection equipment include but are not limited to the following:

- *Fireground operations*
  - Fire suppression
  - Forcible entry
  - Search and rescue
  - Loss control
  - Ventilation
  - Investigation
- *Special operations*
  - Hazardous materials incidents
  - Technical rescues
    † Confined spaces
    † Trenches
    † Extrications
  - Emergency medical services (EMS)
- *Special situations*
  - Unique structures
    † High-rise buildings
    † Open-plan buildings
    † Subterranean structures
  - Temperature extremes

To be able to reduce the hazards posed by these situations, the fire and emergency responder must understand and know proper size-up techniques, respiratory equipment donning and doffing techniques, emergency incident field service, standard exit indications and techniques, and emergency escape indications and techniques. This chapter covers each of these emergency-scene categories and situations and the necessary skills to meet them.

Hazardous Situation Size-Up

[NFPA 1500: 7.9.7, 7.9.8]
[NFPA 1404: 1.3.2]

Proper size-up is the key to controlling any hazardous situation. The type of hazard, its scope, weather and environmental conditions, incident duration, resource requirements (which includes determining respiratory equipment requirements), resource availability, and the degree of risk posed by the hazard to life, property, and the environment are essential considerations when making an initial size-up. Size-up begins with the pre-incident planning of potential hazards that may produce conditions that could result in high life and financial loss, require maximum resources, involve hazardous materials, or create exposure hazards to the population or environment (**Figure 10.1**). Pre-

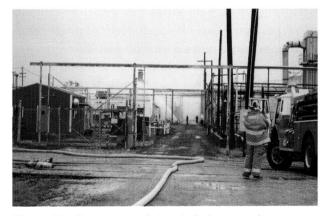

Figure 10.1 Petroleum and chemical plants require a thorough and detailed preplan inspection to provide responders with the information necessary when responding to an emergency at the site. *Courtesy of Chris Mickal.*

incident planning involves site inspections by code enforcement officers and emergency responders, analyses of hazards, development of attack plans, and training for all units and emergency personnel who may respond to the site. Detailed information on pre-incident planning may be found in the IFSTA **Fire Department Company Officer** manual.

However, developing a pre-incident plan for all emergency incidents may not be possible. Therefore, response personnel must be trained to make rapid evaluations of situations upon arrival at an emergency scene. These evaluations (or size-ups) are based on visual indicators, dispatch information, and information gained from witnesses in addition to any previous knowledge of the site, the situation, departmental/organizational policies, or standards/regulations.

As mentioned in earlier chapters, both NFPA standards and Occupational Safety and Health Administration (OSHA) regulations require the use of proper and adequate respiratory protection equipment. NFPA 1500, *Standard on Fire Department Occupational Safety and Health Program*, states that respiratory protection equipment shall be worn by all personnel when they are *"engaged in any operations where they might encounter atmospheres that are immediately dangerous to life or health (IDLH) or potentially IDLH or where the atmosphere is unknown."* NFPA 1404, *Standard for Fire Service Respiratory Protection Training*, further states that respiratory protection equipment is required for all members who might be exposed to respiratory hazards in the performance of their duties. Further, this standard requires the use of respiratory protection equipment in confined spaces and belowground levels or where the possibility of a contaminated or oxygen-deficient atmosphere exists. Fire and emergency services personnel must be aware that respiratory hazards may exist in all types of emergency situations, and they should be prepared for such hazards through the proper use of respiratory protection equipment. The respiratory protection decision tree shown may be used as a basic guide for all respiratory protection emergencies.

Respiratory Protection Decision Tree

Respiratory protection equipment must be worn in the following situations:

- An unknown atmosphere is suspected to be present.
- The atmosphere is known to be hazardous due to the presence of smoke, toxic vapors, dust, biological contaminants, or other particulates.
- The incident requires that emergency responders operate belowground level or in any confined space.

Fireground Operations

[NFPA 1500: 7.1.1, 7.1.2]

Respiratory hazards may be encountered on the fireground during fire suppression, forcible entry, search and rescue, loss control, ventilation, and investigation operations. The respiratory hazards may be generated by fires in structures, vehicles, large trash receptacles, vessels or boats, and aircraft or by other types of miscellaneous fire situations. Training in each type of fireground activity during the various types of emergencies must be accomplished while wearing respiratory protection equipment. Basic training for Firefighter I and II certifications are found in the **Essentials of Fire Fighting** manual, which includes training in the use of respiratory protection equipment (**Figure 10.2**).

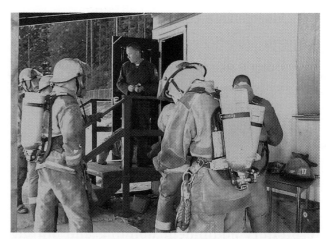

Figure 10.2 Thorough training in the use of respiratory protection equipment is necessary during entry-level training. This training is then followed by annual training and recertification of emergency responders. *Courtesy of Lloyd Lees.*

In all types of incidents, hazard assessments must be conducted to determine the levels of respiratory protection necessary. The respiratory protection decision tree can be used to aid in the assessment process.

Fire Suppression

[NFPA 1500: 7.2.1, 7.3.1.1, 7.8.2, 7.9.7, 7.9.8, 7.14.2, 7.16.2, 7.16.2.1, 8.4.4, 8.4.5, 8.4.6, 8.4.7, 8.4.8, 8.4.9, 8.4.13.1, 8.4.14]

Fire and emergency services personnel involved in fire-suppression operations must wear self-contained breathing apparatus (SCBA) during interior fire attacks in structures, on board ships, and in tunnels and other confined spaces and during other fire-suppression situations such as vehicle fires, large trash receptacle fires, aircraft fires, and other miscellaneous-type fires. Air-purifying respirators (APRs) designed for specific hazards may be used during situations that do not involve IDLH or oxygen-deficient conditions and when the type of respiratory hazard is known and has been quantified. Full protective ensembles may consist of structural fire fighting clothing and other high-temperature protective clothing such as proximity or fire-entry suits.

Structures

Structure fires generate toxic fire gases and high temperatures, and they create oxygen-deficient atmospheres both within the structure and adjacent to it. All personnel who are engaged in fire-suppression operations inside or outside structures must be equipped with SCBA. Personnel working inside structures must wear SCBA, activate personal alert safety system (PASS) devices, operate in teams, maintain contact (physical, visual, or verbal) with team members, and listen for end-of-service-time alarms. Personnel who are assigned to a rapid intervention crew (RIC) or to exterior operations within a hot zone must have SCBA donned but may not need to have facepieces in place until needed (**Figure 10.3**). PASS devices must be activated at all times when personnel are in hot zones. Personnel outside hot zones should have SCBA readily accessible.

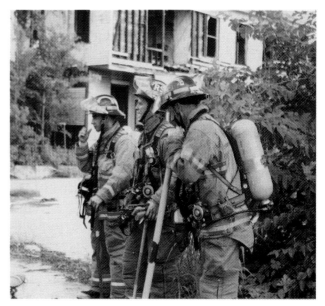

Figure 10.3 Members of the rapid intervention crew (RIC) are fully equipped and ready to respond when needed. *Courtesy of Chris Mickal.*

Vehicles

Vehicle fires may occur in open terrain, inside buildings, or in parking garages both above- and below-grade levels. If a burning vehicle is located within a structure, then the requirements for respiratory protection are the same as those for an interior fire-suppression operation. Vehicles that are located in open terrain should be approached as a potential respiratory hazard, and SCBA should be worn and activated during the suppression, rescue, loss control, and investigation phases of incidents (**Figure 10.4**). This protocol should be followed because the types of toxic fire gases and the nature of

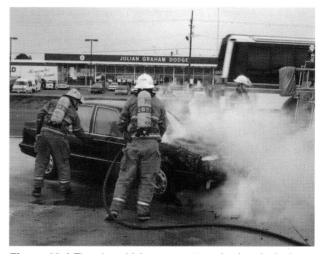

Figure 10.4 Fires in vehicles generate toxic chemicals that require the use of respiratory protection equipment. *Courtesy of Chris Mickal.*

burning material in vehicles may not be known. This protocol applies to passenger vehicles as well as transport trucks.

Large Trash Receptacles

Onc of thc more common fire locations is in large metal trash receptacles such as Dumpsters™ that are used for trash, rubbish, and waste materials. Dumpsters™ are found at multifamily dwellings, commercial facilities, industrial sites, and construction sites. The receptacle's contents are widely varied and usually unknown to emergency responders. Some may even contain materials that will react violently with water. Therefore, full personal protective equipment including respiratory protection should be used during fire-suppression operations (**Figure 10.5**).

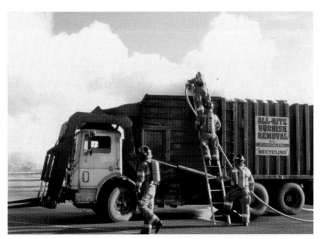

Figure 10.5 Fires in waste-removal vehicles such as this one can create a respiratory hazard for responders. The unknown types of materials that are involved and the reaction with other materials within the container mandate the use of respiratory protection equipment. *Courtesy of R. J. Bennett.*

Vessels

Fires on board vessels are similar to fires in high-rise and below-grade level structures. Vessels contain flammable materials in the form of interior finishing materials, furniture, fuel, and cargo. All of this material is confined in metal-enclosed spaces that usually do not have openings to the outside. Heat, smoke, and toxic fire gases are held within the spaces during fires while levels of oxygen are rapidly depleted. Backdrafts may occur due to the presence of Class B fuels that have high heat-release rates. Ventilation and fire-suppression activities

must be coordinated to prevent flashover when fresh air is admitted to these spaces. In addition to the hazards created by fires, the design and construction of vessels may create peculiar hazards. Access to fires may be difficult, and mazelike passageways, vertical and horizontal openings, and large open spaces filled with machinery or cargo may increase escape times. Interior shipboard fire fighting must only be attempted by personnel who are trained to perform it and properly equipped with personal protective equipment. SCBA equipped with high-pressure cylinders designed to provide extended use should be used (**Figure 10.6**). Information on shipboard fire fighting may be found in the IFSTA **Marine Fire Fighting** and **Marine Fire Fighting for Land-Based Firefighters** manuals.

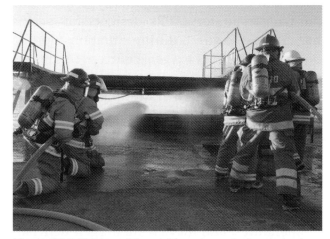

Figure 10.6 Shipboard fires (either above deck or below) require the use of complete personal protective equipment, including respiratory protection. This training evolution depicts a petroleum fire on a tanker.

Aircraft

Due to the potential respiratory hazards associated with aircraft fires and crashes, personnel responding to such incidents must wear the appropriate types of respiratory protection (see Protective Ensembles section). Fire and emergency services personnel operating in and around aircraft involved in fire face the same toxic hazards they would encounter in typical structural fires. Besides the smoke and toxic fire gases generated by fires, aircraft construction materials are composed of various composites that may generate harmful vapors. In addition, carbon and graphite fibers used in aircraft construction may be released into the atmosphere.

Other unknown materials are found in cargo compartments of aircraft and contribute to the toxic atmosphere. Finally, fuels, oils, lubricants, and hydraulic fluids used in aircraft may produce high heat and harmful vapors in either burned or unburned conditions. SCBA must be worn as part of the full personal protective ensemble (**Figure 10.7**). Aircraft incidents that occur on or near airports are usually the responsibility of fire and emergency responders who are equipped and trained specifically for aircraft incidents. Aircraft incidents that occur in rural or residential areas are the responsibility of fire and emergency responders who are trained and equipped for structural incidents. Once aircraft fires are extinguished and atmospheres have been monitored for air quality, air-purifying respirators or particulate respirators may be worn during the investigation and overhaul phases. Further information on aircraft fire fighting may be found in the IFSTA **Aircraft Rescue and Fire Fighting** manual.

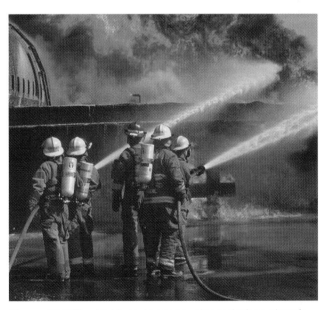

Figure 10.7 The highly toxic gases released when aircraft construction materials burn combined with the extremely high temperatures generated by aviation-grade fuels produce major challenges to fire and emergency responders. The responders shown in training here are equipped with standard structural fire fighting clothing. *Courtesy of Terry Chronkhite.*

Miscellaneous Fires

Miscellaneous fires include wildland fires, rubbish fires, landfill fires, outdoor equipment fires, power pole and electrical equipment fires, and other nonstructure, nonvehicle fires. Generally, oxygen deficiency is not a problem during these incidents. However, toxic fire gases and smoke create respiratory hazards. Therefore, the appropriate type of respiratory protection equipment based on the hazard must be worn (**Figure 10.8**). When in doubt, an SCBA should be used until the atmosphere can be monitored. Wildland, trash, and electrical fires may only require the use of APR units, while a fire in a landfill or tire-disposal site may require an SCBA. Wildland fires may also expose emergency responders to pesticides and herbicides that may cause respiratory injuries. Local protocols dictate the level of required protection for these various types of fires. Information on wildland fire fighting may be found in the IFSTA **Fundamentals of Wildland Fire Fighting** manual.

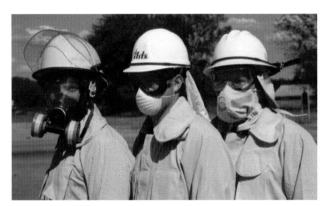

Figure 10.8 Respiratory protection may be required for personnel engaged in wildland fire fighting to protect them from airborne particulates.

Protective Ensembles

Depending on the responding organization, the full protective ensemble for fire suppression may consist of structural fire fighting clothing, proximity clothing, or entry clothing. High-temperature protective clothing such as proximity or fire-entry suits are designed for situations other than structural fire fighting (for example, aircraft crashes/fires). This clothing is designed to protect personnel from short-term exposures to high temperatures. The outer layers of materials may be aluminized to help reflect radiant heat. SCBA is worn inside each type of suit.

Structural fire fighting clothing. Structural fire fighting protective clothing consists of helmet, protective hood, turnout coat, turnout pants, boots, gloves, PASS device, and SCBA. The ensemble is designed, tested, and certified to NFPA 1971, *Standard on Protective Ensemble for Structural Fire Fighting*. The structural ensemble protects the wearer against limited direct flame contact, convected and radiant heat, physical hazards, water penetration, and airborne contamination. The fabrics used in the construction of the ensemble and SCBA harness assembly must meet a thermal-protective performance that ensures adequate protection in conditions normally encountered by fire and emergency services personnel during structural fires and other nonstructural incidents.

Proximity suits. These suits are designed for exposures of short duration and close proximity to flames and radiant heat, which can allow the rapid advancement of hoselines into an area. The outer shell is a highly reflective, aluminized fabric over an inner shell made of a flame-retardant fabric (**Figure 10.9**). This clothing is not designed to provide any substantial chemical or vapor protection. Proximity suits are often used in aircraft crash incidents.

Fire-entry suits. This clothing offers complete, effective protection for short-duration entry into a total flame environment. They are designed to withstand exposure to radiant heat levels up to 2,000°F (1 093°C). A fire-entry suit consists of a coat, pants, and a separate hood assembly. These suits are constructed of several layers of flame-retardant materials, with the outer layer often aluminized (**Figure 10.10**). Fire-entry suits are useful for accomplishing fireground operations such as valve shutdowns in flammable or liquid storage facilities. Disadvantages to the use of fire-entry suits are the lack of mobility and flexibility, limited potential use, and high cost of the units.

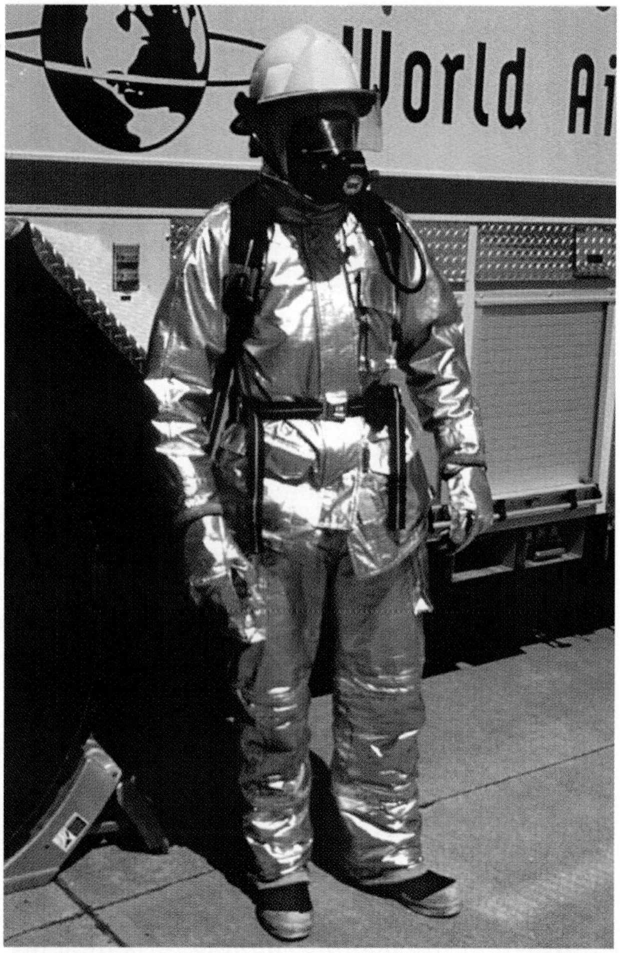

Figure 10.9 Personal protective proximity clothing is based on the design used for structural clothing and places the respiratory protection equipment on the outside of the garment.

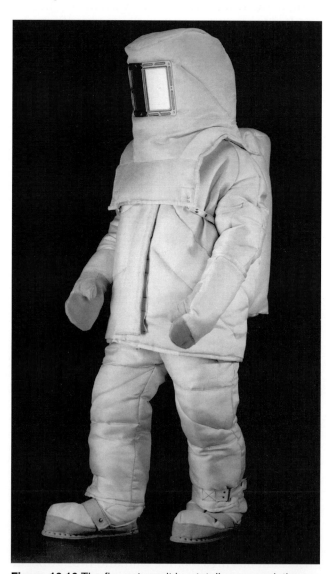

Figure 10.10 The fire-entry suit is a totally encapsulating design that protects the wearer from high temperatures for a short time. *Courtesy of Fyrepel Industries, Inc.*

Forcible Entry

In order to gain access to a fire or perform a rescue, fire and emergency services personnel may be required to force entry into a structure, vehicle, vessel, or aircraft. Forcible-entry techniques require specialized skills and equipment ranging from hand tools to power tools. Forcible-entry skills are usually provided in the entry-level training programs provided by the fire and emergency services organization. Because personnel are forcing entry into an unknown condition, full personal protective equipment including SCBA must be worn (**Figure 10.11**). The act of opening a closed area can contribute to hazards by adding fresh oxygen to a smoldering fire or by releasing pressure from a vapor spill or chemical. As long as the situation on the other side of the barrier is unknown, SCBA must be used during forcible entry.

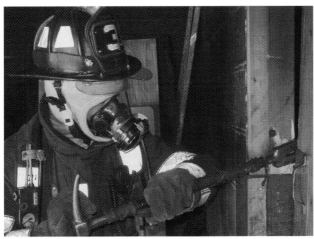

Figure 10.11 Full protective clothing and respiratory protection are required when making forcible entry into an area because often the conditions inside are unknown. *Courtesy of Kenneth Baum.*

Search and Rescue

Once access has been gained to the structure, aircraft, vessel, or vehicle, search and rescue and fire-suppression operations can begin. Due to the size and construction similarities of structures and vessels, search and rescue techniques usually take the same form. Search and rescue techniques at aircraft and vehicle incidents vary, depending on the size of the aircraft or vehicle and the fireground conditions at the time of the initial response. Response personnel who are assigned to make a search should make an initial exterior size-up to determine alternative paths of egress in the event that their main route becomes blocked. In addition, witnesses should be questioned to determine if anyone is known to be inside and to learn the most likely locations of victims.

Two objectives of a structure or vessel search are finding victims (searching for life) and obtaining information about the extent of the fire (searching for fire extension). In most structure and vessel fires, the search for life requires two types of searches: primary and secondary. The *primary search* is a rapid but thorough search that is performed either before or during fire-suppression operations. The *secondary search* is a thorough search conducted after the fire is under control and hazards are considerably reduced. In both cases, full personal protective clothing, respiratory protection equipment, communications systems, and forcible-entry tools are required for the search teams (**Figure 10.12**). A detailed description of search and rescue techniques may be found in the IFSTA **Essentials of Fire Fighting**, **Marine Fire Fighting,** and **Marine Fire Fighting for Land-Based Firefighters** manuals.

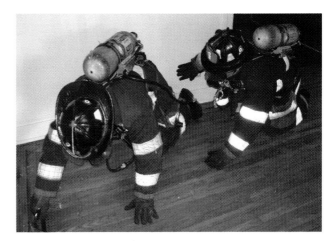

Figure 10.12 Search teams are trained to operate in pairs. Team members are fully equipped with personal protective equipment and remain in contact at all times. This team is practicing making a primary search for the victim of a structure fire.

Loss Control

The relatively new term *loss control* encompasses the older concepts of salvage and overhaul. Loss-control methods are intended to minimize damage to property and to provide good customer service to the incident victim.

Salvage operations consist of those methods and operating procedures associated with fire fighting that aid in reducing primary and secondary damage during fire fighting operations (**Figure 10.13**). The fire causes primary damage; secondary damage is the result of fire-suppression activities. Salvage operations begin when sufficient personnel have arrived at the incident. Property may be removed from the structure or stacked within the structure and covered by salvage covers to reduce smoke and water damage.

Overhaul operations consist of searching for and extinguishing hidden or remaining fires (**Figure 10.14**). Protecting the scene after a fire and preserving evidence of the fire's origin and cause are also components of overhaul. Overhaul operations are not normally started until a fire is under control. Overhaul activities include cutting into walls, removing window and door moldings, opening ceilings and floors, and removing built-in cabinets. Hidden fires are then extinguished, and the extent of fire travel in hidden spaces is determined.

Because fire and emergency services personnel are performing loss-control activities in an area that has been exposed to fire, SCBA must be worn until

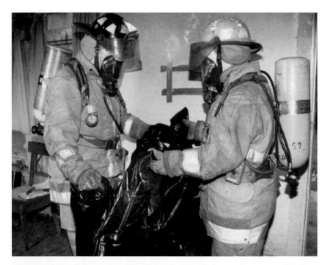

Figure 10.13 Emergency responders who enter a contaminated area to perform salvage operations (such as spreading salvage covers over property) must wear the appropriate level of respiratory protection.

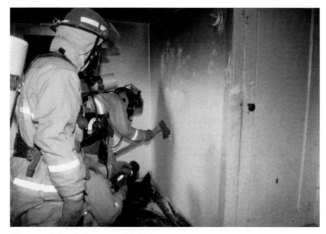

Figure 10.14 Overhaul operations may uncover smoldering or free-burning materials that produce smoke and other hazardous particles. Respiratory protection equipment must be worn during this phase of the operation.

the air can be monitored. If it is determined that the atmosphere is safe, APR or particulate respirators may be used during the remainder of the loss-control operations. These types of respirators protect against the large particulates that may be released during overhaul. However, constant monitoring of the air in the work area is necessary while the APRs are in use. The IFSTA **Fireground Support Operations** manual provides additional information regarding these activities.

Ventilation

Ventilation is both the systematic removal and replacement of heated air, smoke, and gases from a structure or vessel involved in fire with cooler air. Horizontal, vertical, and forced ventilation methods can be used. The cooler air improves atmospheric conditions, facilitates entry by fire and emergency services personnel, and contributes to increased life safety during rescue, loss-control, and fire-suppression operations. Ventilation improves visibility and reduces the chance of flashover or backdraft if it is performed properly. At the same time, ventilation can expose fire and emergency services personnel to the heated air, smoke, and gases that they are attempting to remove from the structure. Ventilation activities also include roof operations. Although fire and emergency response personnel may not initially encounter IDLH conditions on the roof, the very reason that roof operations are being conducted could possibly involve IDLH conditions. Potential IDLH conditions may evolve from either roof collapse or effective ventilation practices that release super heated and toxic fire gases. For these reasons, respiratory protection in the form of SCBA (with facepieces in place and regulators on) must be worn during all types of ventilation operations (**Figure 10.15**). Ventilation also provides breathable air during postsuppression activities. Although SCBA may not be required during these activities, APRs are still needed to protect fire and emergency responders from particulates in the atmosphere.

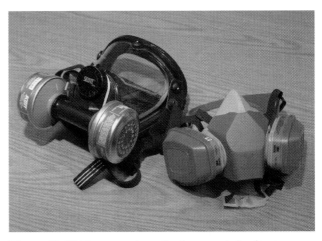

Figure 10.16 Fire-cause investigators must also be provided with respiratory protection. The level of protection may range from full SCBA to APRs like the full- and half-facepiece models shown.

Special Operations

Although fireground operations may constitute the majority of activities that require respiratory protection, they do not include all of the respiratory breathing hazards faced by fire and emergency services personnel. *Special operations* are those activities that require additional or specialized training and equipment in order to mitigate particular hazards, although the definition may vary from jurisdiction to jurisdiction. Special operations may include training in hazardous materials recognition and responses, technical rescues, and emergency medical responses.

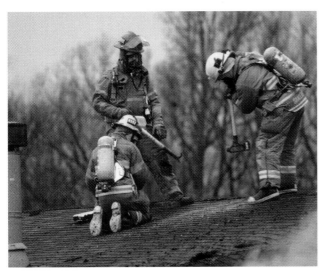

Figure 10.15 Roof ventilation operations require the use of respiratory protection equipment even though the work is being performed in the open atmosphere. Once the roof is opened, smoke and other unburned products of combustion are released into the immediate area of emergency responders. *Courtesy of Michael Watiker.*

Investigation

[NFPA 1500: 8.4.28]

Determining fire origin and cause usually occurs following the extinguishment of a fire and during overhaul activities. Until the atmosphere in a structure can be monitored and declared safe, SCBA must be worn. Once the levels of toxic fire gases are at an acceptable level and the oxygen content is between 19.5 and 23 percent, SCBA may be removed and APR units worn. Fire investigators must adhere to the same respiratory protection policy that fire-suppression personnel do. Therefore, they must be provided with full respiratory protection equipment, including both SCBA and APR units as well as personal protective equipment (**Figure 10.16**). Further guidelines for fire investigators may be found in the IFSTA **Introduction to Fire Origin and Cause** and **Fire Investigator** manuals.

> # WARNING!
> Special operations must only be attempted by personnel who are properly trained and equipped to accomplish the tasks.

Hazardous Materials Incidents

[NFPA 1500: 7.5.1.1, 7.5.1.4, 7.5.1.4.1, 7.5.2.4, 7.5.2.4.1, 7.5.2.5.1]

The United States Department of Transportation (DOT) defines a hazardous material as *"any substance or material in any form which may pose an unreasonable risk to health and safety or property when transported in commerce."* Because hazardous materials are routinely transported by rail, water, air, and road, every area of a jurisdiction contains potential sites for hazardous materials incidents. Such fixed locations as industrial sites, storage facilities, or retail outlets are also likely to present fire and emergency services personnel with a variety of hazardous materials situations.

Hazardous materials can range from chemicals in liquid or gas form to radioactive materials to etio-logic (disease-causing) agents. When these materials burn, they can pose an even greater danger. The release of hazardous materials may be the result of an equipment malfunction, human error, or an intentional act of terrorism. The use of respiratory protection is mandatory when dealing with hazardous materials incidents, both from a health and safety standpoint and because it is required by

Environmental Protection Agency Hazardous Materials Protection Levels

- Level A protection is worn when the highest level of respiratory, skin, eye, and mucous membrane protection is needed; it consists of positive-pressure self-contained breathing apparatus (SCBA) and a fully encapsulating chemical-resistant suit **(Figure 10.17)**.

- Level B protection is worn when the highest level of respiratory protection is needed with a lesser level of skin and eye protection; it consists of positive-pressure SCBA and a chemical-resistant coverall or splash suit. The Level B ensemble is the minimum level recommended for initial site entries until the health and safety officer or hazardous materials officer defines the hazards by

monitoring, sampling, and other reliable methods of analysis **(Figure 10.18)**.

- Level C protection is worn when the type of airborne substance is known, the concentration has been measured, criteria for air-purifying respirators (APRs) is met, and skin and eye exposure are unlikely; it consists of a full facepiece air-purifying respirator and chemical-resistant coverall or splash suit. Periodic air monitoring is required **(Figure 10.19)**.

- Level D protection is worn when respiratory or skin hazards do not exist. This level is primarily a work uniform. It should not be worn on any site where respiratory or skin hazards exist **(Figure 10.20)**.

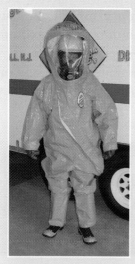
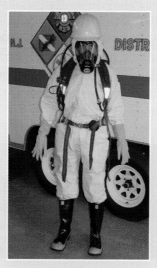
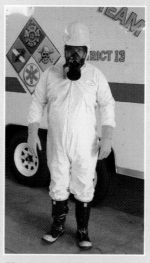
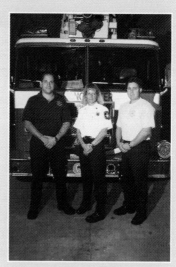

Figure 10.17 The EPA Level A protective ensemble includes a fully encapsulating suit worn over an SCBA as shown. *Courtesy of Kenneth Baum.*

Figure 10.18 The EPA Level B protective ensemble includes the chemical-resistant coverall or splash suit with the SCBA worn on the outside of the garment. *Courtesy of Kenneth Baum.*

Figure 10.19 The EPA Level C protective ensemble consists of a full-facepiece APR and chemical-resistant coverall. This ensemble is only used when the type and concentration of airborne substances are known and the air has been monitored. It is not used in oxygen-deficient atmospheres. *Courtesy of Kenneth Baum.*

Figure 10.20 The EPA Level D protective ensemble is worn when no respiratory or skin hazard exists and is usually the standard work uniform as defined by the local jurisdiction.

OSHA Title 29 (Labor) *CFR* 1910.120, Hazardous Waste Operations and Emergency Response Requirements.

Current hazardous materials regulations require extensive training and specialized equipment for anyone responding to a hazardous materials incident. Information on hazardous materials response protocol, clothing, and decontamination procedures are found in the IFSTA **Hazardous Materials for First Responders** and the FPP *Hazardous Materials: Managing the Incident* manuals.

Determining the type of respiratory protection required for the various types of hazardous materials incidents, carbon monoxide responses, and incidents involving weapons of mass destruction follows the decision tree presented in the Hazardous Situation Size-Up section. The respiratory protection system becomes part of the personal protection ensembles.

Respiratory Protection Ensembles

The level of protection required for the specific hazard determines the level of respiratory protection at a hazardous materials incident. The U.S. Environmental Protection Agency (EPA) has developed four levels of protection against hazardous chemical exposure: Level A, Level B, Level C, and Level D. The EPA defined these levels of protection for personnel assigned to hazardous waste sites where emergency conditions do not normally exist.

Personal protective clothing used with respiratory protection is available in a wide variety of types and designs. Structural fire fighting protective clothing, chemical protective clothing (including nonencapsulating chemical protective clothing and fully encapsulating personal protective clothing), and high-temperature clothing (including proximity and entry suits) provide varying levels of protection to the wearer during hazardous materials incidents. High-temperature clothing and structural fire fighting protective clothing as worn on the fireground was described in the Protective Ensembles section.

The structural fire fighting protective clothing ensemble should only be worn when the chance of physical contact from splashes is unlikely and the total atmospheric concentrations do not contain high levels of chemicals that are toxic to the skin

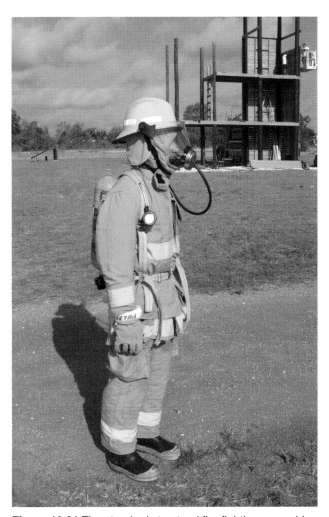

Figure 10.21 The standard structural fire fighting ensemble includes helmet, protective hood, turnout coat and pants, gloves, boots, PASS device, and SCBA. *Courtesy of Bob Parker.*

(**Figure 10.21**). Structural fire fighting protective clothing is commonly used at hazardous materials incidents when the following conditions are met:

- Contact with splashes of extremely hazardous materials is unlikely.

- Total atmospheric concentrations do not contain high levels of chemicals that are toxic to the skin. There are no adverse effects from chemical exposure to small areas of unprotected skin.

Encapsulating chemical protective clothing is manufactured in several configurations. They can be categorized by the manner in which respiratory protection is provided as follows:

- *Type 1 suit* — This suit allows for the SCBA to be worn underneath the suit. It is the most common design and provides total vapor protection (**Figure 10.22**).

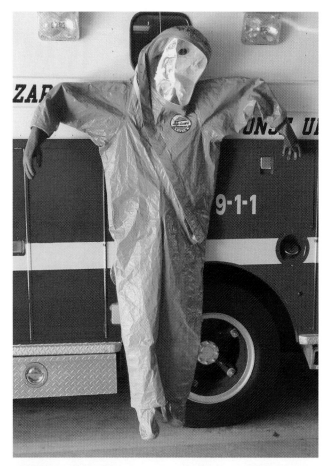

Figure 10.22 The Type 1 encapsulating chemical-protective suit shown is the most common design and provides total vapor protection. It is worn over the SCBA. *Courtesy of Kenneth Baum.*

- *Type 2 Suit* — The SCBA is worn over the suit, exposing the unit to potential contamination. The SCBA facepiece is either incorporated into the suit hood or worn over the hood (**Figure 10.23**).

- *Type 3 Suit* — This suit completely encapsulates the user but relies upon an airline hose respirator for respiratory protection. The airline is connected to a fitting in the shell of the garment and an emergency breathing support system (EBSS) is worn inside the unit.

Regardless of the type of chemical-protective clothing worn at an incident, it must be decontaminated before storage or disposal. Emergency response personnel who are engaged in the decontamination process (like those shown) must also be fully encapsulated and provided with respiratory protection during the process (**Figure 10.24**).

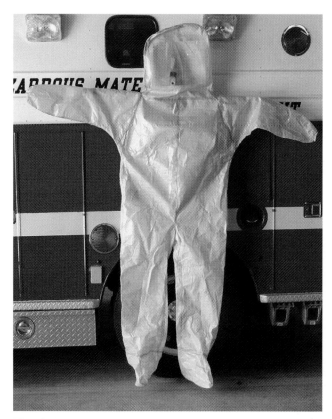

Figure 10.23 The Type 2 encapsulating chemical-protective suit shown here is worn with the SCBA on the outside. *Courtesy of Kenneth Baum.*

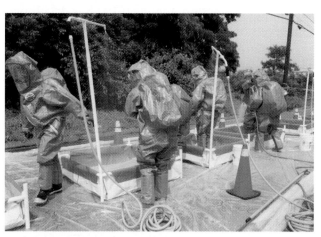

Figure 10.24 Personnel who are engaged in decontamination must also wear full personal protective clothing as shown in this photo. *Courtesy of Joseph J. Marino.*

Carbon Monoxide Responses
[NPFA 1500: 7.9.7, 7.9.8]

Concentrations of carbon monoxide (CO) may be the result of fire or incomplete combustion in heat-producing equipment such as furnace units. Changes in building codes in recent years have included the requirement for carbon monoxide detectors in many types of residential occupancies.

This, in turn, has increased the volume of CO alarms. Receipt of a CO alarm is an automatic indication for the need for respiratory protection (in the form of SCBA) by fire and emergency responders (**Figure 10.25**).

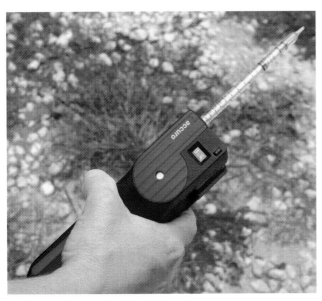

Figure 10.25 Because carbon monoxide (CO) is a colorless odorless gas, handheld monitoring devices (such as this one) must be used to determine when it is safe to enter an area without wearing SCBA.

Weapons of Mass Destruction

As mentioned in Chapter 1, Introduction to Respiratory Protection, terrorist attacks have increased during the last half of the twentieth century. Fire and emergency services personnel may respond to incidents involving the use of weapons of mass destruction that may involve the release of hazardous materials, radiation, or etiological and biological agents. Such incidents must be treated with the same caution and level of protection as nonterrorist hazardous materials incidents. Local fire and emergency services personnel are the initial responders and have to maintain the situation until the arrival of rapid reaction units. In the initial responses, all personnel must be equipped with full personal protective equipment including SCBA, supplied-air respirators (SARs), or APRs (if the incident does not require breathing air) (**Figure 10.26**).

Technical Rescues

While rescue incidents may occur in a variety of locations including highways, industrial sites, agricultural sites, and structural sites, technical res-

cue situations requiring the use of respiratory protection and special equipment can be reduced to three general areas: confined space, trench, and extrication. It is possible for any of these rescue situations to occur at any of the named locations.

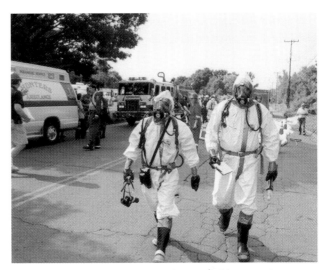

Figure 10.26 With the increased potential for terrorist attacks using chemical, biological, or nuclear weapons, local emergency response organizations must be equipped to handle the initial response. Hazardous materials teams, such as these responders dressed in Type 2 encapsulating suits, may have to control the situation until additional assistance arrives. *Courtesy of Joseph J. Marino.*

Confined Spaces

Rescue operations involving confined spaces can be especially difficult. Typical examples of confined spaces include empty storage tanks, silos, rail tank cars, utility manholes, wells, septic tanks, compost pits, mines, tunnels, and caves. In addition to the problems posed by small cramped spaces with limited access, the atmosphere in these spaces is often oxygen deficient and may contain toxic gases. Only personnel who are trained and equipped for confined-space rescue should perform it. All personnel entering a confined space must use SCBA and SAR equipped with EBSS (**Figure 10.27**). While the space may prevent the wearing of structural personal protective clothing, some protective clothing must be used. Hard hats, gloves, long-sleeved coveralls, and boots must be worn in addition to the respiratory protection equipment, PASS devices, and tag lines.

Structural collapse may also create a confined-space situation requiring specialized training and equipment. Structural collapse may occur as a result of fires, weather conditions, earthquakes, explosions, structural age, or terrorist activities. Pockets or voids are created within the debris as it collapses onto itself (**Figure 10.28**). The voids provide access routes to spaces where victims may be trapped. The potential for oxygen deficiency, toxic gases, natural gas leaks, or airborne particulates (including asbestos) makes the use of respiratory protection equipment by rescue workers mandatory.

Respiratory protection equipment used in confined-space incidents is primarily SCBA and SAR with EBSS. To protect against airborne particulates, APR units may be used once the oxygen content of the atmosphere is determined to be 19.5 percent or greater. Information on rescue operations is contained in the IFSTA **Essentials of Fire Fighting** and **Fire Service Rescue** manuals.

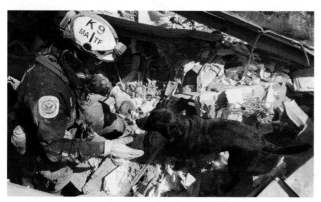

Figure 10.27 In situations involving confined-space or structural-collapse operations (such as this one), respiratory protection may take the form of SCBA, SARs, or APRs. *Courtesy of U.S. Federal Emergency Management Agency.*

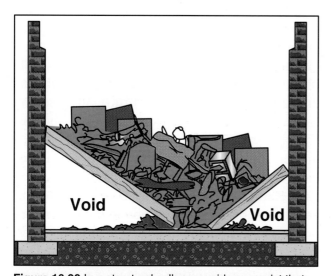

Figure 10.28 In a structural collapse, voids may exist that may contain survivors. Emergency responders equipped with respiratory protection equipment have to enter and search these areas.

Trenches

Trench construction occurs in virtually every jurisdiction in the United States and Canada on a daily basis. Cave-ins are likely to happen (and often do) with excavation activities. NIOSH estimates that an average of 60 people are killed annually in trench cave-ins. Of that number, 77 percent are construction workers and the other 23 percent are from other occupations, including fire and emergency services personnel. Many of those killed in trench incidents are would-be rescuers who fail to take proper safety precautions (including the use of respiratory protection) or do not stabilize the sides of the trench before entering it (**Figure 10.29**).

Excavation work done in the United States is covered by the OSHA regulations contained in Title 29 *CFR* 1926 (Safety and Health Regulations for Construction), Subpart P (Excavations), Sections 650–652. These regulations apply not only to the construction industry but also to the fire and emergency services personnel who respond to these sites. OSHA considers some excavation sites to be confined spaces, and most (if not all) of the hazards that are common to other confined spaces may also be found in trenches.

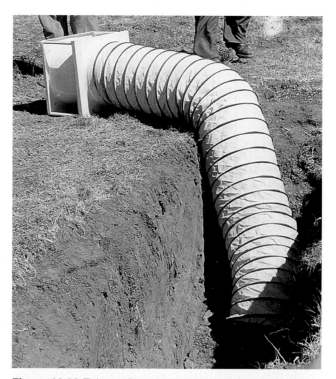

Figure 10.29 Exhaust fans are used to remove contaminants and draw fresh air into trenches during trench-rescue operations.

Respiratory hazards in trenches can be created in a number of different ways and may take different forms. However, the potential for their existence makes it critically important that the atmosphere within a trench be sampled with properly calibrated instruments before entry and continuously monitored throughout the rescue operation (**Figure 10.30**). Until the atmosphere in the trench has been monitored, personnel entering the trench must wear SCBA and SAR units. In addition, mechanical

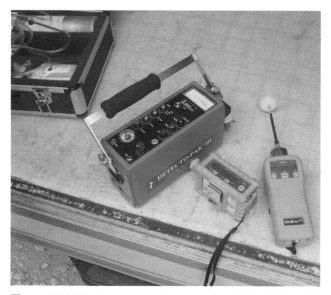

Figure 10.30 Various types of air-sampling instruments are available, depending on the type of information that is required during an incident.

ventilation should also be established to remove the potentially harmful gases and provide a breathable atmosphere for both the rescue workers and the victims. APRs may be used once the oxygen level is sufficient to support life. Respiratory hazards may include oxygen deficiency, flammable gases, and toxic gases and particulates.

Oxygen deficiency. The most common cause of oxygen deficiency in trenches is the displacing of the oxygen by heavier-than-air gases. With the exception of methane, all petroleum-based vapors and gases are heavier than air and tend to accumulate in low areas such as trenches. These vapors may originate from nearby machinery, broken gas lines, or high concentrations of traffic. Other gases (some highly toxic) are also heavier than air and may find their way into trenches (**Figure 10.31**).

Flammable gases. OSHA regulations also state that if the atmosphere within a trench contains a flammable gas, vapor, or mist in excess of 10 percent of its lower flammable limit (LFL), it is considered hazardous. This atmospheric concentration may result from a broken natural gas pipe in the trench or it may result from a volatile flammable liquid seeping in from a contaminated aquifer.

Toxic gases. Because the atmosphere within a trench tends to be relatively static, toxic gases and

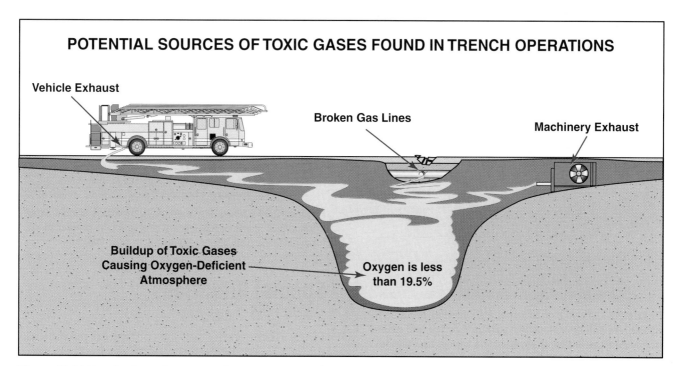

POTENTIAL SOURCES OF TOXIC GASES FOUND IN TRENCH OPERATIONS

Vehicle Exhaust

Broken Gas Lines

Machinery Exhaust

Buildup of Toxic Gases Causing Oxygen-Deficient Atmosphere

Oxygen is less than 19.5%

Figure 10.31 Heavier-than-air gases and vapors may seep into trenches, creating further hazards to victims and rescuers.

vapors that might otherwise be blown away by the wind can remain at harmful concentrations in the trench. Other sources may be biological activity such as the decomposition of waste materials or gases trapped in sewer lines or a liquid residue that is vaporizing.

Extrications

Extrication incidents involve the removal and treatment of victims who are trapped by some type of man-made machinery or equipment. Extrication may be required when victims are trapped in vehicles following collisions, under heavy equipment, in transportation crashes, or in structural collapses. Extrication activities use both hand-operated tools and power tools that are activated by air pressure, hydraulic power, electricity, or gasoline power. Personnel who are responsible for extrication activities must be trained in the use of such equipment (**Figure 10.32**).

Because a need for extrication usually results from incidents involving machinery, the potential for hazardous materials in the atmosphere exists. Petroleum vapors that are harmful to breathe also create an explosion hazard. Personnel involved in extrication must be fully equipped with personal protective clothing and have respiratory protection equipment available if warranted.

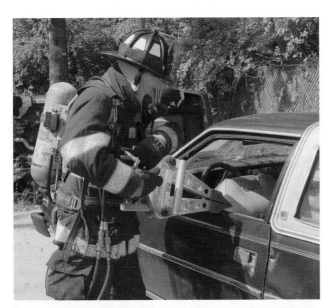

Figure 10.32 Even extrication operations may require the use of respiratory protection equipment by fire and emergency services responders. Gasoline vapors that are both toxic and explosive may be present following a vehicle collision. *Courtesy of Kenneth Baum.*

Emergency Medical Responses
[NFPA 1500: 7.4.1]

In some areas of North America, emergency medical services are provided by the local fire department. In other areas, the EMS organization is managed by a separate branch of government, nongovernmental agency, or civilian contractor. Regardless, all organizations that provide emergency medical services must provide their employees with respiratory protection. This protection usually takes the form of APRs and high efficiency particulate air (HEPA) filters to protect fire and emergency services personnel from airborne and bloodborne pathogens that may enter the respiratory system (**Figure 10.33**).

Just as the fire company officer must size up a fire incident, the EMS responder must size up the hazards present at a medical emergency. All victims must be considered to have communicable diseases, and the appropriate respiratory protection must be donned. This protection includes National Institute for Occupational Safety and Health (NIOSH)-approved eye, mouth, skin, and respiratory protection in the form of full facepiece or half facepiece APRs, eye shields or goggles, gloves, and long-sleeved disposable gowns. These items not only protect EMS workers but also victims.

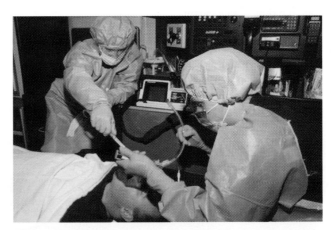

Figure 10.33 Emergency medical technicians should wear appropriate levels of respiratory protection to protect them from airborne pathogens. *Courtesy of Mike Nixon.*

Special Situations
[NFPA 1500: 7.9.7, 7.9.8]

Fire and emergency services personnel periodically have to deal with special situations that involve or require the use of respiratory protection. These situations may involve unique types of structures or environmental situations resulting from temperature extremes.

Unique Structures

Both fire and nonfire incidents can occur in high-rise buildings, large open-plan buildings, and subterranean structures. Response personnel working on elevating platforms may also be required to perform tasks while wearing respiratory protection equipment. The use of respiratory protection equipment, PASS devices, accountability systems, and RIC procedures are required for all these unique structural situations just as they are during standard fire-suppression operations.

High-Rise Buildings

Incidents involving fires, gas and vapor leaks, smoke odors, and carbon monoxide alarms in high-rise buildings pose challenges to fire and emergency services responders. High-rise structures are usually classified as those buildings of seven stories or higher above-grade level. Rescue, search, and fire-suppression operations become increasingly difficult because most floors are above the reach of aerial devices (**Figure 10.34**). Other factors that contribute to the difficulty are increased setbacks from the street, parking garages on the lower floors, and permanently sealed large-pane windows. Access to the involved floor must be made by interior stairways and controlled elevators operated to floors beneath the incident floor.

To provide support for personnel involved in rescue, search, and fire-suppression operations, a staging area is usually established in the lobby and on the second floor below the incident floor. These staging areas are used for gathering resources, initiating operations, rehabilitation of personnel, and exchanging SCBA cylinders. Having reserve air-cylinder supplies in the staging area allows responders to replenish air cylinders and return quickly to the involved floor without having to exit the structure. The shuttling of cylinders up stairways, however, requires additional response personnel. The use of a controlled elevator may be faster and require fewer personnel, but it is affected by the structure's power supply. Alternatives to SCBA cylinder exchange may include locating a portable fill station at the upper staging area, extending a ground-level large-capacity cascade system with hose and fill regulator up the stairway, or using static breathing-air supply piping and associated connections located in stairwells (**Figure 10.35**). If exterior access to upper floors is available,

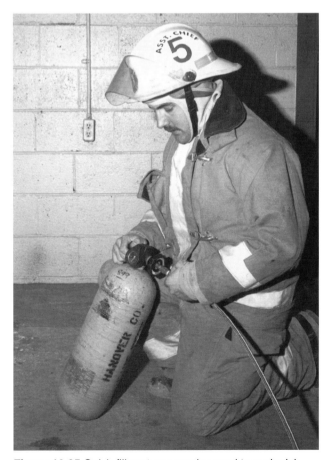

Figure 10.35 Quick-fill systems can be used to replenish breathing-air cylinders at upper-level command posts or staging areas.

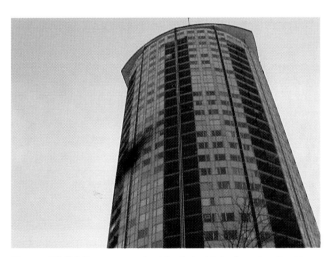

Figure 10.34 Emergency incidents in high-rise structures (such as this apartment fire) present many tactical and logistical challenges for emergency responders. *Courtesy of Tulsa (OK) Fire Department.*

replacement breathing air can be provided by the system installed on aerial apparatus platforms. Regardless of the method that is chosen for resupplying breathing air, preplanning in its operation is crucial.

NFPA 1901, *Standard for Automotive Fire Apparatus*, provides an option that aerial devices equipped with platforms may have a breathing-air system that is capable of supplying breathing air for at least two persons in the platform (**Figure 10.36**). Multiple connections are provided in the platform. These connections are supplied by a minimum of 400 cubic feet (11 363 liters) of breathing air carried on the apparatus (**Figure 10.37**). This amount of breathing air is intended to give the personnel in

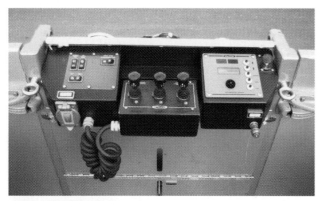

Figure 10.36 Aerial device platforms are equipped with SAR-type fittings to provide the personnel in the platform with a continuous supply of breathing air. EBSS or SCBA must also be provided in the event of system failures. *Courtesy of Bob Parker.*

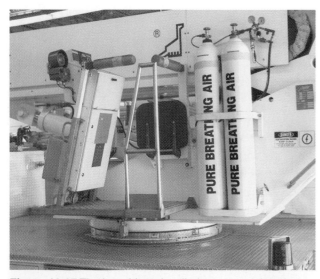

Figure 10.37 The breathing-air cylinders on aerial devices are usually located on the turntable (as shown) or on the side of the aerial ladder or boom. *Courtesy of Lloyd Lees.*

the platform extended operating time when using the breathing-air system. SCBA units may also be required for personnel in the platform as an additional escape system. Aerial devices without platforms may have a connection for one person and supply a minimum of 200 cubic feet (5 663 liters) of breathing air. As mentioned, the systems may also be used to resupply personnel wearing SCBA on upper levels of a structure. Personnel assigned to aerial platform apparatus must be thoroughly trained in the use of the breathing-air systems and the local policies that requires their use.

Open-Plan Buildings

Another type of structure that poses special problems is the large open-plan building. This type of building construction may be found in warehouses, manufacturing facilities, and retail sales outlets such as grocery stores, hardware and lumber supply houses, department stores, and electronic and computer stores (**Figure 10.38**). Factors that contribute to problems in open-plan buildings are as follows:

- Absence of standard floor plans or layouts
- Limited exits and ventilation points
- Varied populations
- Varied fuel loads based on material types
- Truss roofs
- High ceilings
- High-stack storage
- Long distances between walls

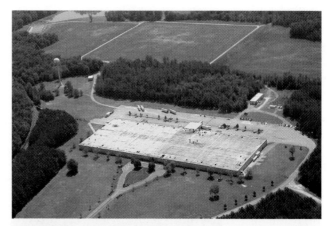

Figure 10.38 Large, open-plan structures like this manufacturing facility present special problems that impact the use of respiratory protection. Long travel distances and mazelike interior arrangements may rapidly deplete breathing-air supplies. *Courtesy of Captain Jack Photo Services, Inc.*

In buildings of this type, emergency responders run the risk of becoming disoriented and lost during search, rescue, and fire-suppression operations. Pre-incident planning, company inspection tours of facilities, and extensive training are essential to successful operations in these types of occupancies. In particular, personnel must be familiar with their individual air-consumption rates, able to calculate points of no return for their air-supply sources, and know emergency escape procedures. Command staff personnel must monitor the locations of interior teams by using accountability systems, calculating air supply times, and monitoring incident radio communications traffic (**Figure 10.39**).

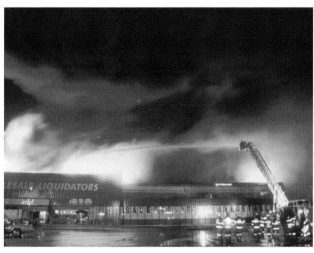

Figure 10.39 A fire in a large-area structure such as the one shown can accelerate out of control rapidly. It is essential that incident commanders monitor the locations of personnel working inside these types of structures at all times. *Courtesy of Bill Tompkins.*

Subterranean Structures

Subterranean or underground structures including subways, tunnels, basements, and parking garages present particular challenges for fire and emergency services personnel. In addition, windowless buildings (though not necessarily underground) share similar characteristics. Once again, these situations demand pre-incident planning, company inspections, training, SCBA or SAR respiratory protection equipment, PASS devices, and accountability systems (**Figure 10.40**). These types of structures (like high-rise and large open-plan structures) present special problems such as the following:

- Limited egress and exit access
- Limited ventilation

- Lack of exterior available lighting
- Long travel distances
- Absence of standard floor plans
- Various ceiling heights
- Special hazards such as boilers, furnaces, and electrified rails
- Potential concentrations of heavier-than-air gases

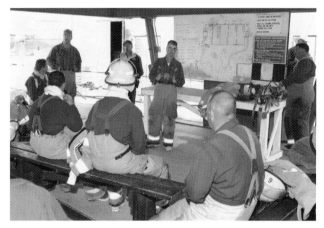

Figure 10.40 Training for special situations such as high-rise, large-area, and subterranean emergency operations is essential for successful resolutions.

Temperature Extremes

[NFPA 1404: 6.6.2]

Fire and emergency services personnel seldom encounter temperature extremes for very long, but they should know what can happen to their respiratory protection equipment in temperatures ranging from -40°F to 200°F (-40°C to 93°C). An SCBA works well in naturally hot temperatures. The biggest problem with its use in high temperatures is not with the functioning of the equipment but with the effects of heat on the user. Hot temperatures commonly cause fluid loss and fatigue. Low-temperature extremes, however, can adversely affect the performance of SCBA. Response personnel should exercise extreme caution while using open-circuit SCBA during freezing weather. The *NIOSH Emergency Information Bulletin on the Use of SCBA in Low Temperatures* contains the following important precautions:

- Be sure that moisture in the air cylinders is kept at an absolute minimum. Even small amounts of moisture in the air supply may freeze and result in failure of the breathing apparatus. Moisture

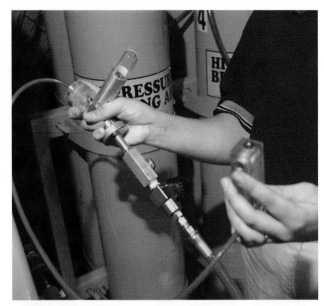

Figure 10.41 Periodic air-quality sampling of an organization's breathing-air supply will detect the presence of moisture that may cause regulators to freeze in subfreezing weather. Samples are drawn from the air cylinders with devices such as the one shown.

content is controlled by the filtration system on the compressor. Regular air testing will alert the department/organization if moisture content exceeds minimum requirements **(Figure 10.41)**.

- Always use a nose cup in the SCBA facepiece when temperatures are below freezing. Failure to use a nose cup under such circumstances can result in facepiece fogging and severely impaired vision. Chemical anti-fog agents do not perform adequately in low temperatures.

- Prepare for a cold weather response in advance by carefully reading the approval label on the respirator to determine whether it is necessary to install special accessories before use in subfreezing weather. Certain old models of SCBA approved by the U.S. Bureau of Mines before March 25, 1972, require such low-temperature accessories.

- Learn in advance the procedures for coping with exhalation valves that have frozen open or closed in low temperatures. Contact the manufacturer for specific instructions.

- Always place the respirator facepiece in the turn-out coat to keep it warm if it is to be quickly reused when leaving an extremely hot environment (such as a fire scene) and entering cold air (below or near freezing). Respirators can freeze

due to moisture buildup when they are not being actively breathed.

- Use special care to remove all moisture after washing respirator facepieces and breathing tubes. Water drainage can freeze in the regulator.

- Make visual checks of the remote air pressure gauge when SCBAs are used in freezing conditions; SCBA end-of-service-time indicators (ESTIs) can fail in low temperatures.

- Use extreme caution if SCBA are used in temperatures below -25°F (-32°C). SCBA are NIOSH-laboratory approved for use in temperatures as low as -25°F (-32°C), but at extremely low temperatures, metal can fatigue and crack. In addition, anything at -25°F (-32°C) causes the skin to freeze if it comes into contact with it.

- Observe the following general precautions:
  — Use Compressed Gas Association (CGA) 6-7.1, Type I Grade D air or an air of equivalent specifications.
  — Follow all information listed on the NIOSH/Mine Safety and Health Administration (MSHA)-approval label for the specific SCBA in use.
  — Follow the manufacturer's recommendations included in the instruction and maintenance manual accompanying the SCBA.
  — Follow all applicable federal, state, and local regulations regarding the use of SCBA.
  — Keep SCBA in a warm location between uses.

These precautions may also be applied to SAR units and full facepiece APRs as applicable. The manufacturer's recommendations for the use of APRs in temperature extremes must be followed.

Donning and Doffing Respiratory Protection Equipment

Although some emergency situations may not require the use of respiratory protection equipment, the majority of them do. Emergency responders must consider all situations as life threatening and be equipped with adequate respiratory protection and prepared to deal with the worst possible situation. This preparation means donning respiratory protection equipment while approaching the incident or before entering the hot zone (**Figure 10.42**). Therefore, emergency personnel must be trained in the proper donning and doffing procedures to rapidly provide and, when necessary, remove respiratory protection equipment as needed.

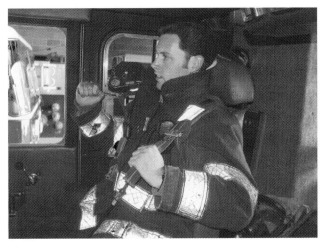

Figure 10.42 While traveling to the emergency incident scene, responders must be able to safely don respiratory protection equipment. Seat-mounted SCBA can be donned while the responder is safely buckled into the seat. *Courtesy of Kenneth Baum.*

Donning Procedures

Fire and emergency services personnel must be able to don respiratory protection equipment quickly and correctly. The manufacturers of SCBA, SAR, and APR provide specific donning instructions. However, general techniques may be applied to each type of respiratory protection device. In each case, the donning method depends on the storage method for the unit. Emergency personnel must be trained in the appropriate method for donning the equipment based on the type of equipment, manufacturer's recommendations, and the storage method. Appendix K, Donning and Doffing Procedures for SCBA Respirators, contains a step-by-step description of general SCBA donning and doffing procedures. The steps for donning and doffing SAR and APR are similar to those for SCBA. Also review the IFSTA **Essentials of Fire Fighting** manual for proper procedures.

Self-Contained Breathing Apparatus

[NFPA 1404: 6.7.3]

The procedures given in this section are general in nature; emergency responders should be aware that there are different steps for donning different SCBA makes and models. Therefore, the instructions given should be adapted to the specific type of SCBA used. Always follow the manufacturer's instructions when donning, doffing, and operating SCBA.

SCBA may be stored in a case, a seat back or side bracket in the crew compartment, or an apparatus storage compartment bracket. Several methods of donning the backpack can be used, depending upon how the SCBA is stored. These methods include the following:

- Over-the-head
- Cross-armed coat
- Regular coat
- Seat mount
- Side or rear mount
- Compartment or backup mount

Donning procedures that are the same for all of these methods are as follows:

- Check the cylinder gauge to make sure that the air cylinder is within 90 percent of its rated capacity (**Figure 10.43**). Open the cylinder valve

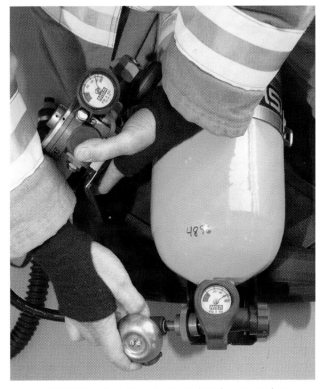

Figure 10.43 The first steps in most donning procedures are to make certain that the breathing-air cylinder is full and that the regulator and cylinder gauges read within 10 percent of each other.

slowly and listen for the audible alarm as the system pressurizes. Then, open the cylinder valve fully. If the audible alarm does not sound or if it sounds but does not stop, place the unit out of service by tagging it and notifying an officer. Use another unit.

- Check the regulator gauge. Both the cylinder and regulator gauges should register within 10 percent of each other — if increments are in pounds per square inch (psi) (kilopascals [kPa]) — when the cylinder is pressurized to its rated capacity. If increments are in other measurements, such as fractions or minutes, they should correspond. If the unit has a donning switch (for units with facepiece-mounted regulators), leave the cylinder valve open and the unit in the donning mode. If the unit is positive pressure only, refer to the manufacturer's instructions concerning the cylinder valve.

- Extend the harness straps to their fullest extents.

The steps for donning differ with each model of SCBA, but once the SCBA is on the body, the method of securing the unit is the same. The shoulder, chest, and waist straps are pulled snug to prevent the unit from shifting on the body (**Figure 10.44**).

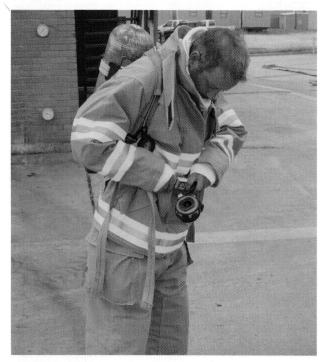

Figure 10.44 The waist strap (and chest strap when present) must be pulled snug to the body. The loose ends of the straps should be tucked into the waist strap to prevent them from snagging on objects.

Methods for donning the facepiece differ depending upon the manufacturer, the model, or whether the regulator is harness-mounted or facepiece-mounted. The facepiece should be stored in a ready-to-use condition, with the head straps extended fully. General procedures for donning any facepiece are as follows:

- Put on the protective hood and pull it over the head until the face opening is around the neck.

- Turn up the collar of the turnout coat.

- Grasp the harness of the facepiece by the straps and spread the straps apart.

- Push the top of the harness up the forehead to remove hair that may be present between the forehead and the sealing surface of the facepiece.

- Center the chin in the chin cup and position the harness so that it is centered at the rear of the head.

- Tighten the head straps by pulling them evenly and simultaneously to the rear. Start with the lower straps followed by the temple straps and finally the top strap.

- Check the facepiece seal by covering the end of the low-pressure hose or by attaching the regulator to the facepiece and using the DON position. The facepiece should draw up to the face when the user inhales, indicating a tight seal.

- Attach the low-pressure hose to the regulator and activate the flow of air.

- Pull the protective hood into place, making certain that all exposed skin is covered and that the hood does not obscure vision (**Figure 10.45**).

- Don the helmet with earflaps covering the sides and back of the head. Tighten the helmet chin strap.

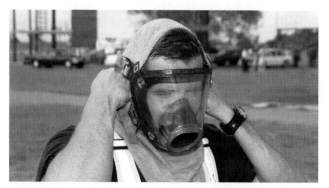

Figure 10.45 With the facepiece straps tightened, the protective hood is pulled over the head and facepiece material, covering all exposed skin. Ensure that the lens still provides adequate vision when the hood is in place. *Courtesy of Bob Parker.*

Supplied-Air Respirator

[NFPA 1404: 6.8.3]

Specific procedures for operating, donning, and doffing SAR systems are provided by the manufacturer, and training should be based on those procedures. In general, however, some of the donning procedures are the same as those listed for SCBA units:

- Remove the portable supplied-air respirator system from the apparatus and locate it near the entrance to the incident. If the air supply is permanently mounted on the apparatus, locate the vehicle so that the air-supply hoses are protected from traffic or other sources of damage (**Figure 10.46**).

- Check the air-supply source to ensure that it is operating properly and that the cylinders are full.

- Extend the air-supply hoses and attach them to the air-supply source.

- Don the harness, regulator, and EBSS and pull the harness straps snugly to prevent movement of the harness.

- Check the EBSS cylinder for proper operation and to ensure that the cylinder is full (**Figure 10.47**).

- Don the facepiece using the method described for the SCBA facepiece or the manufacturer's recommended method.

- Connect the facepiece to the air-supply hose or regulator.

- Don hard hat, helmet, or other protective equipment.

- Attach the tag line (**Figure 10.48**).

Emergency personnel who are assigned to monitor a SAR team should remain with the air-supply equipment and ensure that air-supply hoses do not become snared on obstacles. They must also maintain communications with the team either through radio or physical connection by way of the tag lines. These individuals may also perform the function of the rapid intervention crew. As such, they must be fully equipped with protective clothing, respiratory protection (SCBA), and forcible-entry tools.

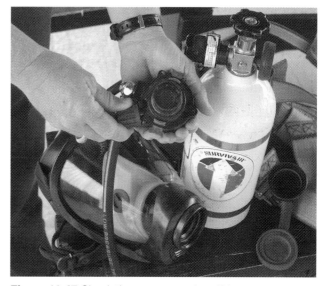

Figure 10.47 Check the emergency breathing support system (EBSS) to ensure proper operation.

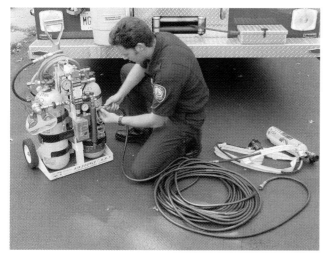

Figure 10.46 The supplied-air respirator unit is removed from the apparatus, assembled, and prepared for operation. This activity should be performed in a protected area and away from traffic. *Courtesy of Kenneth Baum.*

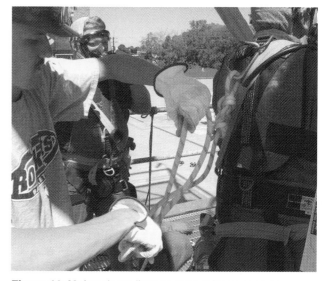

Figure 10.48 Attach tag lines to rescue harnesses on emergency responders who are using SAR in confined-space operations.

Air-Purifying Respirator

[NFPA 1404: 6.9.3, 6.9.4(6)]

The donning procedures for air-purifying respirators are not defined in the NFPA standards or OSHA regulations. The manufacturer of each brand and model specifies the proper procedures to use. Some basic guidelines that may apply to some if not all APRs are as follows:

- Inspect the APR to ensure that the cartridge, filter, or canister is unused, undamaged, and not out of date (**Figure 10.49**).

- Don the harness and pull the straps snug to the body if the canister or cartridge case is mounted on a harness.

- Don the facepiece following the steps given for the SCBA facepiece or use the manufacturer's recommended method.

- Check the seal to ensure that it is complete.

- Check the exhalation valve for proper operation.

- Don remaining protective clothing.

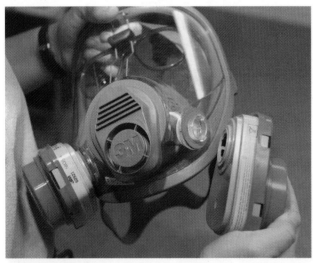

Figure 10.49 Check APR filters and canisters for proper operation and to ensure that they are approved for the type of hazard that has been encountered.

Doffing Procedures

Doffing or removing respiratory protection equipment should only occur when it is determined that the atmosphere is safe to breath. This situation occurs when the user leaves the hot zone and moves to a safe area or when the atmosphere in the hot zone is tested for contamination and oxygen content and found to be safe. Proper doffing procedures

(as defined by the manufacturer) ensure that the respiratory protection equipment will not be damaged or exposed to excessive wear and will be ready for use at the next emergency. General doffing procedures for SCBA, SAR, and APR are given in the sections that follow.

Self-Contained Breathing Apparatus

[NFPA 1404: 6.7.3]

General procedures to follow when doffing SCBA are as follows:

- Remove the helmet, and pull the protective hood down around the neck.

- Close the air-supply valve on the regulator, disconnect the low-pressure hose from the regulator, or place the facepiece-mounted regulator in the donning mode.

- Loosen the facepiece harness strap buckles and remove the facepiece.

- Extend the facepiece harness straps completely.

- Place the facepiece in the case, the carrying bag, or some other protected area while doffing the rest of the system. The facepiece is not stored until it has been inspected and cleaned.

- Unbuckle the waist strap and extend the straps fully.

- Disconnect the chest strap.

- Lean forward to support the weight of the unit on the back and release the shoulder straps and extend them fully.

- Grasp the shoulder straps, slip one arm free, and swing the unit off the remaining shoulder.

- Lower the unit to the ground while preventing the regulator or cylinder valve from striking the ground (**Figure 10.50**).

- Close the cylinder valve and bleed the remaining pressure from the rest of the system.

- Inspect and clean the unit and replace the cylinder as needed before returning the unit to service.

Supplied-Air Respirator

[NFPA 1404: 6.8.3]

When it is determined that it is safe to doff the SAR, follow the manufacturer's recommendations. In general, they include the following procedures:

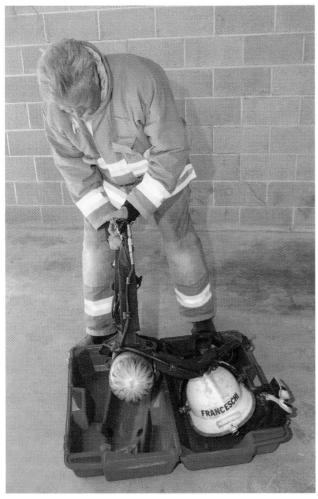

Figure 10.50 Gently lower the SCBA into its case or onto the ground when doffing it. The cylinder valve, cylinder, and regulator must be protected from damage during the doffing process.

- Remove the helmet, and pull the protective hood down around the neck.

- Close the air-supply valve on the regulator, disconnect the low-pressure hose from the regulator, or place the regulator in the donning mode.

- Loosen the facepiece harness strap buckles and remove the facepiece.

- Extend the facepiece harness straps completely.

- Place the facepiece in the case, the carrying bag, or some other protected area while doffing the rest of the system. The facepiece is not stored until it has been inspected and cleaned.

- Turn off the air supply at the source, bleed the air-supply line, and disconnect it from the regulator.

- Loosen the shoulder and waist harness, extend the straps completely, and remove the harness assembly, setting it on the ground (**Figure 10.51**).

- Inspect the system, replace the EBSS if used, replenish the air-supply cylinders, clean the system, and store it properly.

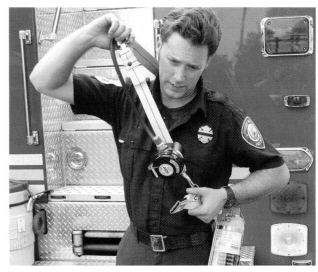

Figure 10.51 Loosen the shoulder strap of the SAR/EBSS system, and lift it over the head. *Courtesy of Kenneth Baum.*

Air-Purifying Respirator
[NFPA 1404: 6.9.3]

Doffing air-purifying respirators follows similar procedures as those used for doffing the SCBA or SAR facepiece. Once the facepiece has been removed, it should be inspected, cleaned, and stored. Nonreusable filters, canisters, or cartridges should be disposed of and replaced (**Figure 10.52**).

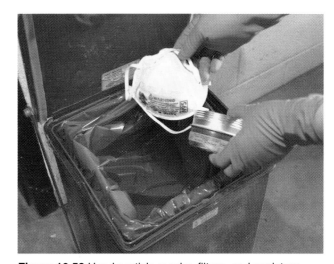

Figure 10.52 Used particle masks, filters, and canisters should be disposed of according to the established protocol for medical or hazardous waste.

Emergency Incident Field Service

Respiratory protection equipment may require replacement or replenishment while personnel are operating at an emergency incident. Personnel must be aware of warning alarms, end-of-service-time indicators, how alarms/indicators function, and how to replenish the air supply to return the equipment to service.

End-of-Service-Time Warnings

Both NFPA and NIOSH require that two end-of-service-time indicators be installed on SCBA and SARs but not on APRs. The function of the ESTI is to provide the user with a warning that the system is reaching its air-supply limit and it is time to leave the contaminated atmosphere. The warning is provided by an audible alarm, tactile alarm, visual alarm, or a combination of alarms. Fire and emergency services personnel must be thoroughly trained in the type of alarm that is provided for each type of respiratory protection equipment that they use.

Self-Contained Breathing Apparatus

NFPA 1981, *Standard on Open-Circuit Self-Contained Breathing Apparatus for the Fire Service*, certifies that SCBA must have two end-of-service-time indicators as part of the system. These alarms activate when the cylinder pressure reaches the manufacturer's preset level, usually between 20 and 25 percent of the cylinder's capacity. The indicators are both an audible alarm (like a bell, electronic beep, or high-pitched siren) and a flashing light or physical vibration (**Figure 10.53**). They cannot be turned off until the air-cylinder valve is closed and the system is bled of all remaining pressure. When the indicators activate, the user and other personnel who entered the area at the same time should retrace their steps and exit the contaminated area.

Supplied-Air Respirators

[NFPA 1404: 6.8.1 (4), 6.8.4 (4)]

End-of-service-time indicators or alarms on SARs are located at the air-supply source if the unit relies on air cylinders. This placement allows the personnel monitoring the air supply to replace a cylinder while the remaining cylinder continues to operate or notify the team working in the hazardous atmo-

sphere that it is time to withdraw. Currently, no ESTIs are located at the regulator end of SAR systems. Therefore, a wearer must depend on communications by the tag line or be aware of the symptoms of a system failure.

If the primary air supply is lost due to damage to the air-supply line or failure of part of the system, the user must be able to activate the emergency breathing support system. The specific steps to activate it depend on the manufacturer's recommended procedures. When the EBSS is activated, the user must leave the contaminated atmosphere immediately. Depending on the design, the EBSS may provide from 5 to 15 minutes of breathing air (**Figure 10.54**).

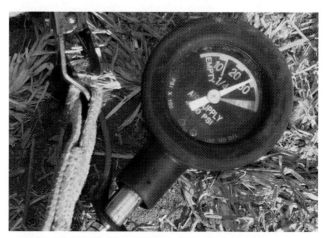

Figure 10.53 The breathing-air supply gauge on the regulator of an SCBA is the visual component of the end-of-service-time indicator for the system.

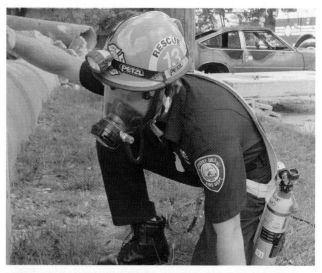

Figure 10.54 All SAR systems must be equipped with EBSSs to provide additional safety factors. The length of escape time must be calculated and the appropriate-sized EBSS cylinder selected. *Courtesy of Kenneth Baum.*

Air-Purifying Respirators

[NFPA 1404: 6.9.2]

NIOSH-certified respirators do not have end-of-service-time indicators like the ones found on SCBA. Instead, the canisters and cartridges have visual end-of-service-life indicators (ESLIs) (**Figure 10.55**). These indicators show when the air cleanser has become totally saturated and is no longer providing breathable air. These indicators should be checked visually before entering contaminated atmospheres and periodically during the work period. If it appears that the canister or cartridge is reaching its saturation level, the user should exit the area and replace the canister or cartridge.

Other clues or symptoms that the canister, cartridge, or filter is losing its ability to protect the user are time, taste, smell, and resistance-to-breathing indicators (**Figure 10.56**). The user should estimate

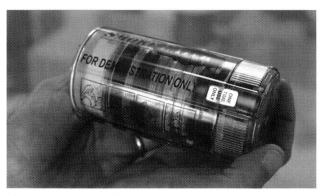

Figure 10.55 This APR demonstration cartridge illustrates the internal filter arrangement of the cartridge. The end-of-service-life indicator (not shown) lets the user know when the filters have reached full saturation.

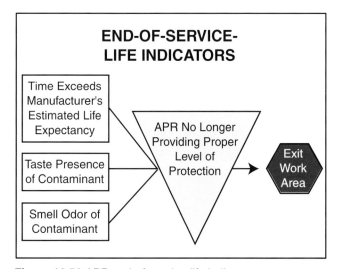

Figure 10.56 APR end-of-service-life indicators are depicted in this illustration.

the amount of time that the work in the contaminated area will take and compare it to the manufacturer's estimated life expectancy for the canister, cartridge, or filter. When the estimated time approaches, the user should exit the area. If the user can taste the contaminant (similar to the taste fit test experience), the unit is no longer providing the proper level of protection. If the user can smell the contaminant, the unit is no longer working, and it is time to exit the area. Finally, filters that have reached their saturation level cause resistance in the breathing process. The wearer experiences a sensation of labored breathing. APRs are not certified for use in IDLH atmospheres. Therefore, the atmospheres that they are certified for provide a measure of safety once the user is aware that the unit is no longer working.

Air-Replenishment Methods

[NFPA 1500: 7.9.5, 7.13.5, 7.13.6, 7.13.7, 7.13.8]

Replenishing expended breathing-air supplies is required when the incident is major in duration or size or when the incident is finished and units must return to service. Currently, most fire apparatus carry one spare SCBA cylinder for each complete unit assigned to the vehicle. These spare cylinders allow fire companies to return to service more quickly or to operate for a longer period of time while additional air supplies are dispatched. Dedicated rescue units may carry a greater quantity of spare cylinders. In addition, spare cylinders are usually maintained at the fire station or centrally located facilities. As mentioned in Chapter 9, Inspection, Care, and Maintenance, breathing-air cylinders can be filled at a permanent facility, from a portable cascade system, or from a vehicle-mounted breathing-air compressor.

The quickest method of replenishing air for SCBA at the emergency incident is to replace the cylinder with a full one. The user may do this by removing the SCBA harness assembly, closing the cylinder valve, disconnecting the cylinder from the air-supply hose, opening the cylinder clamp, and removing the cylinder from the backpack. A new cylinder is then placed into the backpack, secured, and attached to the air-supply hose. If a second person is available to assist, the cylinder can be removed and exchanged without taking off the backpack assembly (**Figure 10.57**). The IFSTA **Essentials of Fire Fighting** manual contains the specific steps for both of these evolutions. Empty cylinders are appropriately marked and placed in a controlled area to prevent their reuse before refilling.

Most manufacturers provide a quick-fill connection that allows an SCBA cylinder to be filled from a portable cascade system or apparatus-mounted breathing-air compressor. The filling takes longer than replacing the cylinder but allows the complete unit to return to service and gives the user a brief rest (**Figure 10.58**). NFPA 1500 prohibits the filling of cylinders while emergency responders wear them. This prohibition is based on the potential for catastrophic failure of the cylinder during the filling process. The authority having jurisdiction should determine whether this fill procedure should be used or not based on a review of local standards and the manufacturer's instructions.

Mobile or portable fill stations may consist of either large-capacity cascade systems or breathing-air compressors. SCBA and SAR cylinders are filled directly from these sources. The SCBA cylinder may be filled while still being worn by the user (if permitted by the local authority) or in a portable fill station. The fill station is similar to the permanently mounted unit and includes fragmentation sleeves to protect personnel from a cylinder rupture. SAR cylinders that are too large to fit into the fill station may be filled while in their carrying carts. Regardless of the filling source or system, the same care must be taken during emergency-scene cylinder filling that is taken during routine cylinder filling.

APR canisters, cartridges, and filters are replaced according to the manufacturer's recommendations. Used materials are disposed of in the manner prescribed in Chapter 9, Inspection, Care, and Maintenance.

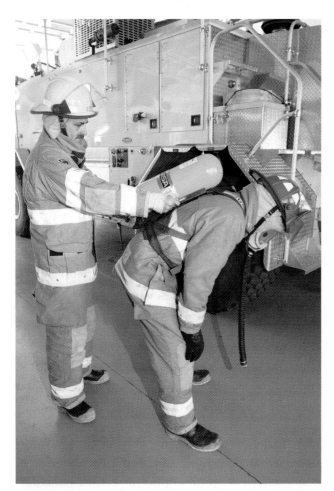

Figure 10.57 A second person can assist in the replacement of an expended breathing-air cylinder without removing the harness, regulator, or facepiece.

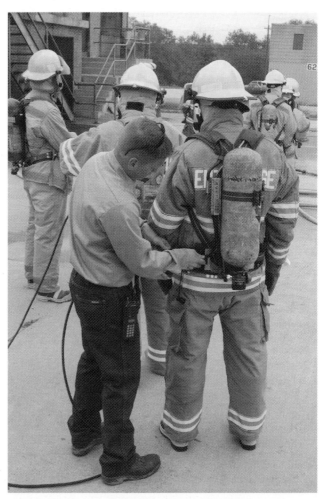

Figure 10.58 The quick-fill connection provided on some SCBA permits a rapid replenishment of breathing air at emergency incidents or during training as shown.

Exit Indications and Techniques

Initially, all emergency situations may be considered "out of control." Therefore, emergency responders should be prepared to make a rapid withdrawal or exit if the situation warrants. The most common exit procedures are those used at the majority of incidents and are referred to as *standard exit procedures*. Less common, but far more important, are *emergency exit procedures* that are used in life-threatening situations such as regulator failures and catastrophic changes in the incident.

Under both standard and emergency conditions, proper exit techniques must be practiced during training and followed during emergency incidents. Both standard and emergency exit techniques are applied with all types of respiratory protection equipment.

Standard Exit Indications

Fire and emergency services personnel exit or leave contaminated or hazardous areas under various conditions. Standard situations that may require following exit procedures include the following:

- *End-of-service-time indications*
  - Low-pressure alarms
  - Respirator breakthrough symptoms (odor, taste, sound, or breathing resistance)
  - Respirator end-of-service-life indicators
- *Operations mode changes*
  - Increase or decrease in concentration of respiratory hazards
  - Permissible exposure limits (PELs) attained or exceeded
  - Environmental condition changes
  - Changes in types of hazards
    † Oxygen-level changes
    † Temperature changes
    † Indications of new hazards

End-of-Service-Time Indications

SCBA units are equipped with end-of-service-time indicators that sound when cylinder pressures reach 20 to 25 percent of the rated cylinder capacity (**Figure 10.59**). When the ESTI of a respiratory protection unit sounds, the user must exit the hot zone immediately. Since this alarm is an indication of the consumption rate of an individual, it is also an indication that other members of a work team may be reaching their limits also. SCBA air-capacity gauges should be checked and any members of a team who have low air supplies should begin the process of exiting the area. Replacement teams should be requested via radio to the command post. In no case should fewer than two members be left in the work area.

Supplied-air respirators are not required to have ESTI alarms on the portable cascade systems. Some manufacturers provide them with the units however (**Figure 10.60**). Constant monitoring of the cylinder pressure gauge is necessary while personnel are operating in the hot zone of an incident.

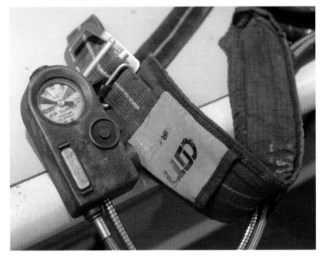

Figure 10.59 When the breathing-air supply of a cylinder reaches a predetermined quantity, an audible low-pressure alarm activates. A visual inspection of the gauge confirms that it is time to leave the area and replenish the air supply.

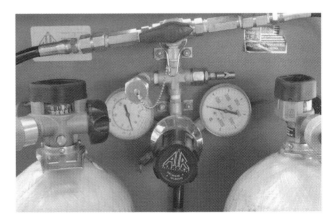

Figure 10.60 Portable cascade systems have pressure gauges that must be monitored during SAR operations. Some units are equipped with low-pressure alarms as options.

Air-purifying respirators may experience a breech or breakthrough that requires the wearer to exit the area. APR breakthroughs are indicated by odor, taste, sound, or breathing resistance. If the wearer senses a change in odor or taste within the APR, it is an indication that the filter or canister is no longer effective. An improper seal at the face or around the canister seal creates a sucking sound as air enters the facepiece. If the canister, filter, or cartridge has reached its capacity, resistance is created that causes difficulty in inhalation. APRs that are equipped with end-of-service-life indicators provide a visual means of determining when it is time to exit the area. Either the wearer or another team member should periodically check the ESLI reading (**Figure 10.61**).

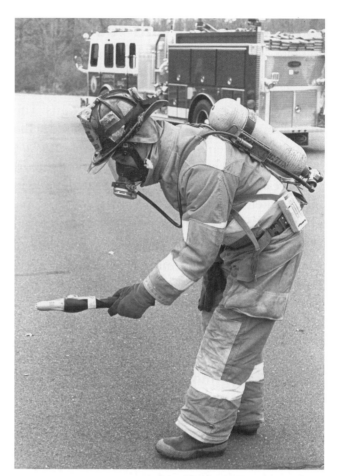

Figure 10.62 Constant monitoring of the atmosphere during hazardous materials operations gives the incident commander rapid information concerning the changes in respiratory hazards. Personnel who are engaged in monitoring the atmosphere must be fully protected from respiratory hazards. *Courtesy of Joe Marino.*

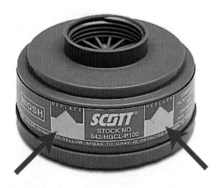

Figure 10.61 End-of-service-life indicators may be found on APR filters or cartridges. The form of the indicators varies among manufacturers. A use-by date, indicated with arrows, is also provided. *Courtesy of Scott Aviation.*

Operations Mode Changes

Changes in the operations mode of an incident may result from changes in respiratory hazards, permissible exposure limits, environmental conditions, or hazard types. An increase or decrease in the concentration of vapors or gases in the atmosphere may cause a change in the respiratory hazards. Emergency personnel operating in a hazardous environment while wearing an APR must exit the area when the permissible exposure limit for the material is exceeded. Constant monitoring of the environment provides personnel with an indication of changes in the PEL (**Figure 10.62**). When there is an increase in the concentration, personnel must exit the area and don the appropriate level of protection. SCBA or SARs provide the greatest level of protection in these circumstances. A decrease in the

level of concentration is an indication that respiratory protection is no longer required and respirators may be removed. This indication may only be determined by the use of accurate monitoring of the environment.

Oxygen-level changes may also create a need to exit the work area. Oxygen deficiency may cause APR wearers to experience light-headed sensations, disorientation, coordination losses, increased respiratory rates, and rapid fatigue. APRs equipped with canisters or cartridges exposed to increased levels of oxygen in excess of 23 percent may have unknown reactions. In either case, personnel must exit the site and don SCBA or SAR or use EBSS protection.

Environmental changes that may prompt a withdrawal from the scene include changes in wind direction and speed, increases or decreases in temperature, and increases in water level or speed within or near the incident site. The incident commander has the responsibility of monitoring the environment and making changes in the operation mode when it is warranted.

Developing situations may result in the creation of new hazards. When new hazards are identified, personnel may have to withdraw from the hot zone and don the appropriate level of personal protective equipment and respiratory protection (**Figure 10.63**). Emergency personnel should be ready to respond to withdrawal orders from the command post.

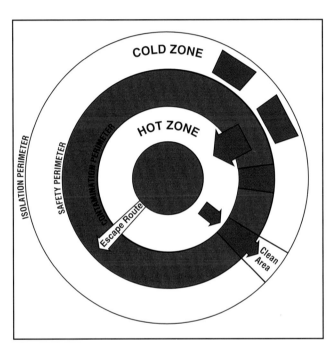

Figure 10.63 The Incident Management System has established the types of control zones around an incident. They include restricted access (hot zone) where full protective clothing and respiratory protection must be worn, limited access (warm zone) where protective equipment is worn but not activated, and support (cold zone) where protection is not required.

Standard Exit Techniques

Standard exit techniques may be required when end-of-service time indicators are present or changes in operational modes are necessary. Standard exit protocols should be developed to address each of these contingencies based on the Incident Management System (IMS) and accountability requirements of NFPA 1500. Train all personnel in standard exit techniques: buddy-system use, controlled breathing, entry/egress paths, and accountability systems.

Buddy System

In all hazardous atmospheres or situations, emergency responders should adhere to the buddy system: working in teams of at least two members (**Figure 10.64**). Each team member is responsible for the safety of the other member. When the need to exit the area becomes apparent (by alarm, change of conditions, or orders), then members of the team leave as a group or in pairs. Individual members must never be left alone in the hot zone. The only time when one member may be required to enter and work in an area alone is in a confined space where two members may not fit. In this instance, the second team member shall remain outside the area monitoring the tag line and ready to enter the space if the need for rescue arises.

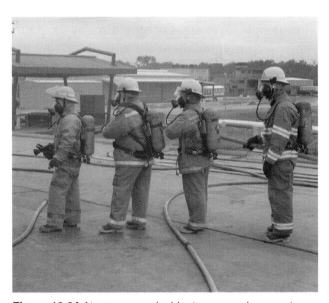

Figure 10.64 At emergency incidents, responders must work in teams of at least two members (buddy system). The four team members shown are preparing to enter a structure with an attack hoseline during a live-fire training exercise.

Controlled Breathing

Controlled breathing is a technique used to provide the most efficient use of air while working. It is a conscious effort to reduce air consumption by forcing exhalation from the mouth and allowing natural inhalation through the nose. Controlled breathing is primarily used when a person wears SCBA or SAR equipped with EBSS. Techniques can be applied to APR usage as a means of extending the life of the filter or canister and reducing the intake of toxins that might be present in a breakthrough. Fire and emergency services personnel should practice and perfect controlled breathing methods in training sessions until they become second nature. Training personnel to be conscious of breathing usually causes an immediate drop in breathing rates. Controlled breathing is important as an exit technique because it helps to decrease the amount of air consumed during the exit period.

Skip breathing is another breathing technique used to extend the use of the remaining air supply. To use this technique, the emergency responder inhales, exhales, inhales, inhales again, and then exhales. The responder should take normal breaths and exhale slowly to keep the carbon dioxide in the lungs in proper balance (**Figure 10.65**).

Entry/Egress Paths

Most people leave areas or structures by the paths they used to enter them because the paths are familiar, have familiar landmarks, and may be the most direct routes from the points of entrance. Emergency personnel should also use the same

BREATHING TECHNIQUES	
SKIP	**CONTROLLED**
Inhale Exhale Inhale Inhale Exhale + Normal Breaths Used to Extend the Use of Remaining Air While Keeping CO_2 in Lungs in Proper Balance	Normal Inhalation Through the Nose Forced Exhales Though Mouth + Decreases the Amount of Air Consumed

Figure 10.65 This illustration depicts the differences between skip and controlled breathing techniques.

paths to exit that they use to enter hot zones. This method is extremely important if emergency personnel are unfamiliar with the physical layout of an incident site such as a ship or large, open-plan structure (**Figure 10.66**). The method also

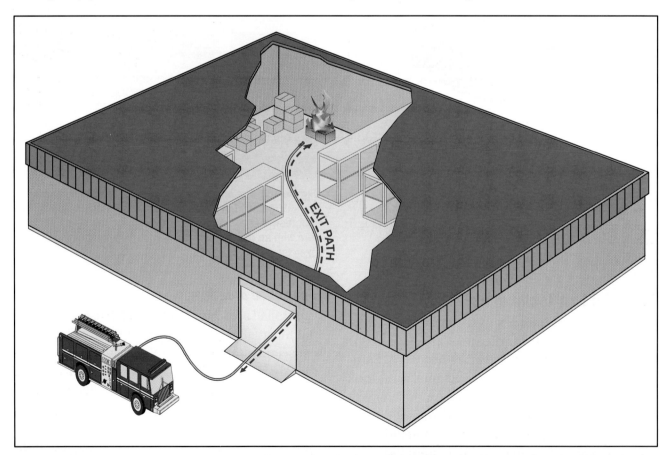

Figure 10.66 Because it is very easy to become disoriented and lost in a large-area structure, responders should be trained to follow proper exit techniques. The policy of exiting on the same path of entry and following the hoseline or tag line helps to ensure a safe withdrawal.

reduces the possibility of becoming lost and disoriented and allows personnel to calculate the time it will take to exit the area. In the case of fires, attack teams can follow hoselines or tag lines out of areas. Training should be used to reinforce this trait and make it a learned skill.

Accountability Systems

Finally, accountability plays a big part in normal exit procedures. No one who has not signed in with the accountability officer should be allowed into the hot zone. All emergency personnel and their locations and functions should be noted on a tracking board (**Figure 10.67**). When it is time to exit the scene, all personnel must check out with the accountability officer to ensure that no one is missing.

Emergency Exit Indications

Not all exits from the hot zone are made under normal conditions. Some occur during emergency situations. Fire and emergency services personnel must be trained to recognize these situations and to implement emergency escape procedures when necessary (**Figure 10.68**). In all cases, it is important to try and remain as calm as possible to reduce the consumption of air. Changes in conditions that may warrant following emergency exit procedures include the following:

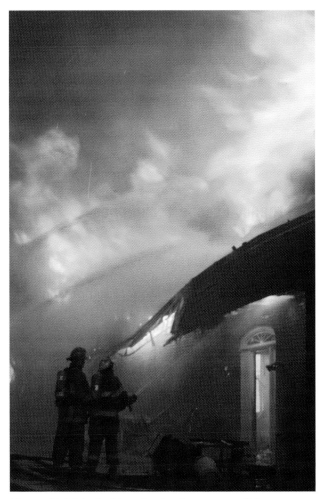

Figure 10.68 An incident that begins as a small fire can rapidly evolve into a fully involved structure fire. Emergency responders must be trained to recognize the indicators of situational changes and know the appropriate exit techniques to use when necessary. *Courtesy of Chris Mickal.*

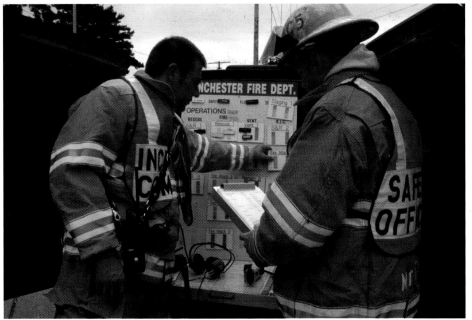

Figure 10.67 The incident command staff uses an accountability board to track the locations and activities of all personnel at an incident, which helps to ensure their safety.

- Equipment failures
  — Catastrophic failure of respiratory and/or personal protective equipment
  — Changes in priorities in response due to PASS-device malfunctions and activations
- Loss of cylinder air supplies
- Catastrophic mode changes
- Unintentional water submersions

Emergency Escape Techniques

[NFPA 1404: 6.7.4]

Emergency escape may become necessary during any type of hazardous situation. Emergency personnel must be trained in the proper escape techniques regardless of the type of respiratory protection equipment they are using. When SCBA or SARs malfunction in a contaminated atmosphere, emergency teams should immediately leave the structure or area. There may be times, though, when withdrawal may not be possible or when personnel may not have enough air to reach an exit. In these instances, emergency escape techniques may have to be used. Emergency escapes may require using emergency breathing system devices, cylinder transfilling systems, buddy-breather valves, and rapid intervention crews. Accidental water submersion requires knowledge of emergency escape techniques also.

> **WARNING!**
>
> **Various nonapproved respiratory breathing techniques exist and are practiced by some organizations. Any organization that uses nonapproved techniques must recognize the potential for personnel injury or death through their use. It is the responsibility of the organization to establish emergency escape procedures and train its members in their use. It is the responsibility of the individual members to understand the procedures and know when to apply them.**

SCBA Regulator Failures

[NFPA 1404: 6.7.2 (6)]

Although an SCBA's regulator usually works as designed, it can malfunction. The primary method of using SCBA when the regulator becomes damaged or malfunctions is to open the bypass valve or cycle the cylinder valve open and closed as warranted. Regulator failures are classified as either *failed closed* or *failed open*. When the failed-closed situation occurs, the regulator valve has sealed in the closed position preventing the flow of air into the facepiece. The bypass valve is opened in an intermittent fashion to introduce air into the facepiece and to conserve air in the cylinder. The bypass valve should be closed after the user takes a breath and then opened each time the next breath is needed. The failed-open situation occurs when the regulator freezes in the open position permitting continuous airflow that rapidly depletes the cylinder supply. Regulate the air supply by closing and opening the cylinder valve intermittently to provide sufficient air to allow the responder to exit the site (**Figure 10.69**).

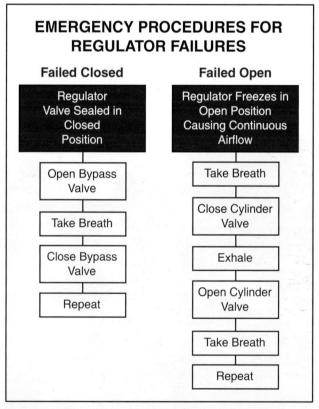

Figure 10.69 This illustration depicts the differences between failed-open and failed-closed failures on a breathing-air regulator.

Emergency Breathing Support System

When working in environments containing hazardous materials, emergency responders may be required to use an SAR supplied by an airline. Airlines are also used when personnel need a greater-than-normal supply of air. The airline is connected to a source of breathing air located away from the hazardous atmosphere or the working area and provides the user with a constant flow of breathing air. Emergency procedures for those using airlines should be included in the organization's respiratory protection program policies.

An EBSS can be used when the air supply through the airline is interrupted. A typical EBSS used with airline equipment consists of an auxiliary cylinder filled with a limited supply of air that is connected to the airline unit (**Figure 10.70**). When needed, the user can open the valve on the auxiliary cylinder. The user can then use this air supply while exiting the area. Normally, these devices are not associated with fire fighting but with other operations involving airlines such as hazardous materials and confined-space incidents. In the case of an EBSS regulator failure, open the cylinder valve and use the techniques listed under SCBA Regulator Failures section.

Another type of limited-duration escape device not approved for fire fighting use includes a small air cylinder and a hood or facepiece. Individuals in industrial situations who are not wearing SCBA

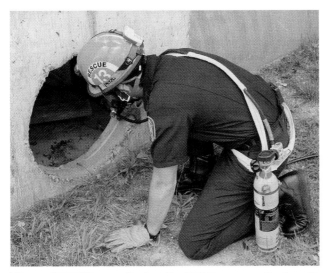

Figure 10.70 When activated, the EBSS can provide from 5 to 15 minutes of breathing air for the wearer, which should provide sufficient time to exit a confined space. *Courtesy of Kenneth Baum.*

more commonly use this escape device. Similar to this device is a filtration canister that can be attached to the facepiece of an SCBA for escape purposes only. The disadvantage of filters of this type is that the user is exposed to the toxic atmosphere while removing the regulator and inserting the canister (**Figure 10.71**).

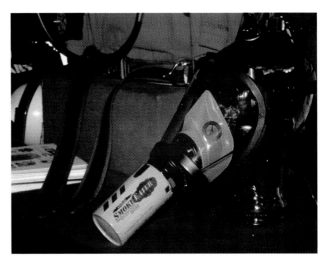

Figure 10.71 A recent option offered by some respiratory protection manufacturers is the filter canister that attaches to the facepiece in place of the regulator. It does not help, however, in oxygen-deficient atmospheres.

Cylinder Transfilling System

Some of the newer SCBA equipment designs include additional valves or valve adapters for transfilling capabilities. With this type of system, an empty or nearly empty cylinder of one SCBA can be filled with air from another SCBA air cylinder. This filling is done by connecting a hose with special connections on each end to special valve connections or valve adapters on two different SCBAs of the same make (**Figure 10.72**). The air pressure of the two air cylinders can then equalize. When transfilling, air from one cylinder flows to another and does not flow through the regulator of either SCBA. This system should not be confused with using an airline unit.

A major advantage of using a transfilling system is that the facepiece seal is not violated. Another advantage is that responders outfitted with encapsulated suits can refill their air supplies without exposing themselves to hazardous materials or without leaving the contaminated area. Additionally, a transfilling system can be used as an emergency breathing support system.

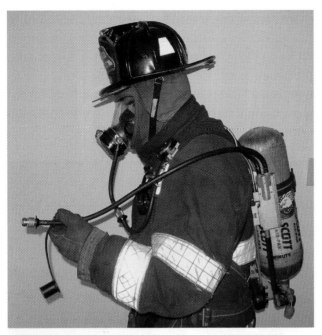
Figure 10.72 The transfill fittings on the cylinder first-stage regulator allow the sharing of breathing air in an emergency. *Courtesy of Kenneth Baum.*

There are, however, some disadvantages to using a transfilling system. The air supply of the donor (person supplying the air) is greatly reduced, shortening the length of time for escape. In addition, it may not be practical in some instances to use a transfilling system as an EBSS. For example, if the end-of-service-time indicator of the donor has sounded or begins to sound, transfilling should not be performed; both responders should exit immediately. By attempting to transfill in such a situation, neither responder may have an adequate air supply for escape. Emergency personnel should keep in mind also that transfilling should be done only in emergency situations in which one responder has an adequate air supply. Both responders should immediately exit after transfilling.

Fire and emergency services organizations having SCBA with transfilling capabilities should address their use in the organization's standard operating procedures (SOPs). The policies should include procedures for transfilling cylinders in emergency situations, situations in which transfilling should and should not be attempted, and any other guidelines or factors to be considered depending upon the organization's particular type of SCBA.

Buddy-Breather Valves

Similar to the transfilling systems are the new so-called buddy-breather adapters/valves. These adapters/valves allow units with facepiece-mounted regulators to share the air from one cylinder. The responder without air connects the air hose into the buddy-breather valve of the donor unit. However, air does not flow from the full cylinder into the empty cylinder; these systems do not have transfilling capabilities. Air from the full SCBA cylinder of one responder travels through the regulator or a pressure-reducing assembly through a connecting hose to the SCBA and facepiece of the other responder (**Figure 10.73**). The hose must remain connected to both SCBAs while the responders escape. NFPA does not recognize buddy-breather valves, and NIOSH has not certified any of the current buddy-breather valves for use.

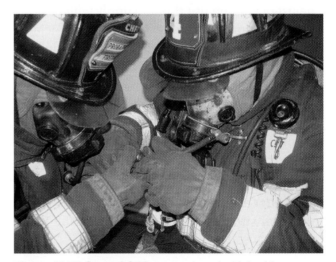
Figure 10.73 Some SCBA are equipped with buddy-breather valves that permit the sharing of air from one cylinder to another. *Courtesy of Kenneth Baum.*

Rapid Intervention Crews
[NFPA 1500: 8.5.2.1]

Sudden and catastrophic changes in the incident may prevent the use of standard exit procedures. Responders who find they are trapped due to collapse, fire extension, or other barriers to escape should remain calm, move to the safest accessible point, and report their situation and location to the incident commander or telecommunications center. Normal operations are halted, and a rapid intervention crew is directed to the location of the trapped crew.

Rapid intervention crews or teams are established before sending emergency personnel into hazardous situations. Tools and equipment carried by the RIC vary with the type of incident. Equipment is divided into two categories: personal equipment and team equipment. Personal equipment includes basic personal protective equipment, respiratory protection, personal survival gear (such as door chocks), medical trauma shears, rescue rope, and a life-safety belt or harness. Individuals should also be equipped with handheld radios, portable lights, forcible-entry tools, and spare respiratory protection units, although not every crew member needs each of these items (**Figure 10.74**). Team equipment depends on the type of incident. It may include hand-operated, forcible-entry tools, power extrication tools, search and rescue ropes, and other specialized rescue tools. The team equipment should be concentrated in the RIC staging area, preferably on an appropriately marked tarp.

Some emergency organizations have created RIC bags that contain tools and equipment specifically intended for use by the RIC. These bags may include basic rescue rope, trauma shears, hand light, blanket or small tarp, EBSS, or power tools. The contents vary depending on the training, funding, and intended duties of the crew (**Figure 10.75**). For a detailed description of the RIC concept, see the FPP publication, *Rapid Intervention Teams*.

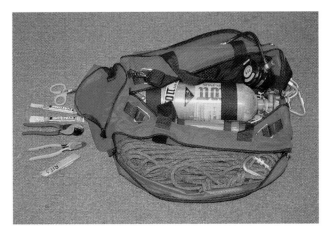

Figure 10.75 A RIC bag may contain an SCBA or EBSS, small hand tools, and medical instruments needed to aid in rescue or extrication. *Courtesy of Kenneth Baum.*

Accidental Water Submersion

[NFPA 1404: 6.7.2 (4)]

NFPA 1404 requires that emergency personnel wearing SCBA know what to do if they become unintentionally submerged in a body of water. SCBA is not self-contained underwater breathing apparatus (SCUBA) and is not intended for underwater use. Some emergency responders may routinely work near large bodies of water. Many others may work near swimming pools, ponds, rivers, or lakes or encounter flooded basements at incidents (**Figure 10.76**). Therefore, accidental submersion is possible, and emergency personnel must know how to react in such situations. Every fire and emergency services organization should include procedures for

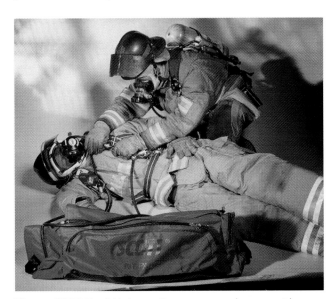

Figure 10.74 Rapid intervention crew members must be able to stabilize and remove a victim from a hazardous area. If the victim needs breathing air, a source may be a transfill fitting or an EBSS carried in a rapid intervention crew bag. *Courtesy of Scott Aviation.*

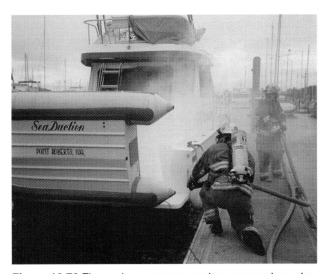

Figure 10.76 Fire and emergency services responders who respond to incidents (such as this small boat fire) around bodies of water must be trained in emergency procedures in the event they fall into the water while wearing respiratory protection equipment. *Courtesy of Captain John F. Lewis.*

dealing with accidental submersion in its SCBA training program. These procedures should follow the SCBA manufacturer's recommendations.

SCBA Operation

Whether or not SCBA offers any floatation assistance depends upon the particular type of SCBA being worn. Whether or not a person will be able to use the SCBA air supply also depends upon the type of SCBA worn. In a study conducted by Louisiana State University Firemen Training Program, various models of SCBA were tested to determine how each of the models was affected when submerged.

The test results revealed that SCBA might experience a complete loss of airflow, a free-flow condition, or no change in operation. Most of the regulators became free flowing. Only one unit experienced complete loss of air, but it worked with the bypass valve. Conversely, another model experienced no change in airflow. Only one of the models tested would not provide the user with air. All others continued in some manner to provide air. Those with free-flowing regulators continued to provide air to the user until the cylinder was empty.

Whether the individual sank (became negatively buoyant) or floated (became positively buoyant) depended upon the buoyancy the person maintained in the protective clothing, along with the buoyancy of the SCBA cylinder worn. Air trapped in the protective clothing provided some degree of buoyancy. Steel cylinders were negatively buoyant; aluminum cylinders were slightly negatively buoyant. Composite cylinders, conversely, were positively buoyant. Therefore, an individual having positive buoyancy (due to air trapped in clothing) and equipped with a steel cylinder will have slightly positive buoyancy and should be able to float. An individual equipped with an aluminum cylinder will most likely have positive buoyancy. An individual with a composite cylinder will have positive buoyancy; however, the more buoyant composite cylinder tends to move upward, positioning the individual face down in the water.

Another factor that helps determine an individual's buoyancy is the movement of the person while in the water. When submerged, a person must remain calm and control body movement. Exaggerated movements used to try and get out of the water can cause the individual to lose buoyancy and sink.

The emergency responder wearing SCBA should observe several guidelines when immersed in water. Most importantly, the responder should remain calm both mentally and physically. By staying calm, the responder is more likely to be able to maintain buoyancy and exit the water. More guidelines from the findings of tests conducted by the Louisiana State University Firemen Training Program for accidental submersion are as follows:

- Keep the facepiece in place to avoid breathing water.

- Remain calm; do not try to quickly swim or walk out of the water. Draw knees up to chest to trap air in boots. Air trapped in clothing provides buoyancy, and excessive movement can cause this air to escape.

- Use an explosive breathing technique: Hold the breath until ready for another one. Then rapidly exhale and rapidly inhale, and hold the breath again.

- Attempt to float in a horizontal position with face up. Then, keeping arms below the water surface, use a gentle backstroke to move to the water's edge. Remaining in a vertical position may force air from the clothing and cause the person to lose buoyancy (**Figure 10.77**).

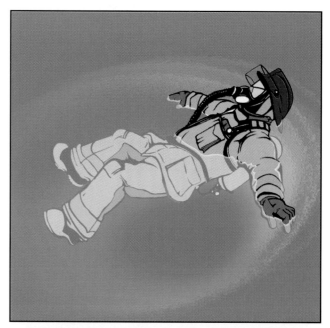

Figure 10.77 Fully equipped emergency responders can use the buoyancy provided by air trapped in their clothing to remain afloat during an accidental water submersion.

- Attempt to float in a horizontal position with face up and feet pointed in the direction of the current after a fall into a river or when overcome in a flash-flooded area. By doing so, obstacles can be seen and the feet are less likely to catch in down-stream obstructions. Do not attempt to stand. Remain in this position until reaching a point in the river where the current is not so swift such as at an inside bend in the river or at an area where the river is wider. Then gently swim to the inside river bend or river edge, locate shallow water, and walk out.

- Use proper techniques to control airflow if the regulator free flows upon submersion.

- Remove respirators that have been immersed in water from service. Tag them out of service, and send them for cleaning, repair, and inspection.

Summary

Fire and emergency services personnel are called upon to respond to a wide variety of situations that place them in hazardous environments. Training in the proper use of personal protective equipment, respiratory protection equipment, hazard size-up, response techniques, and special operations and situations will prepare them for such emergencies. However, no hazardous situation must ever be considered as "normal" or "taken for granted." Rapid changes in situations can result in the need to understand and be proficient at emergency exit techniques. Also, there may be times when fire and emergency responders experience situations in which respiratory protection equipment components do not function properly or where they no longer have adequate supplies of air. In such situations, an emergency responder should follow procedures for individual or team emergency escape techniques as outlined in the organization's policy. Any time emergency responders resort to using emergency breathing or escape techniques, they have overextended the use of the respiratory protection equipment. Supervisors should investigate and document each such occurrence to determine whether it was caused by equipment malfunction or improper respiratory protection equipment use.

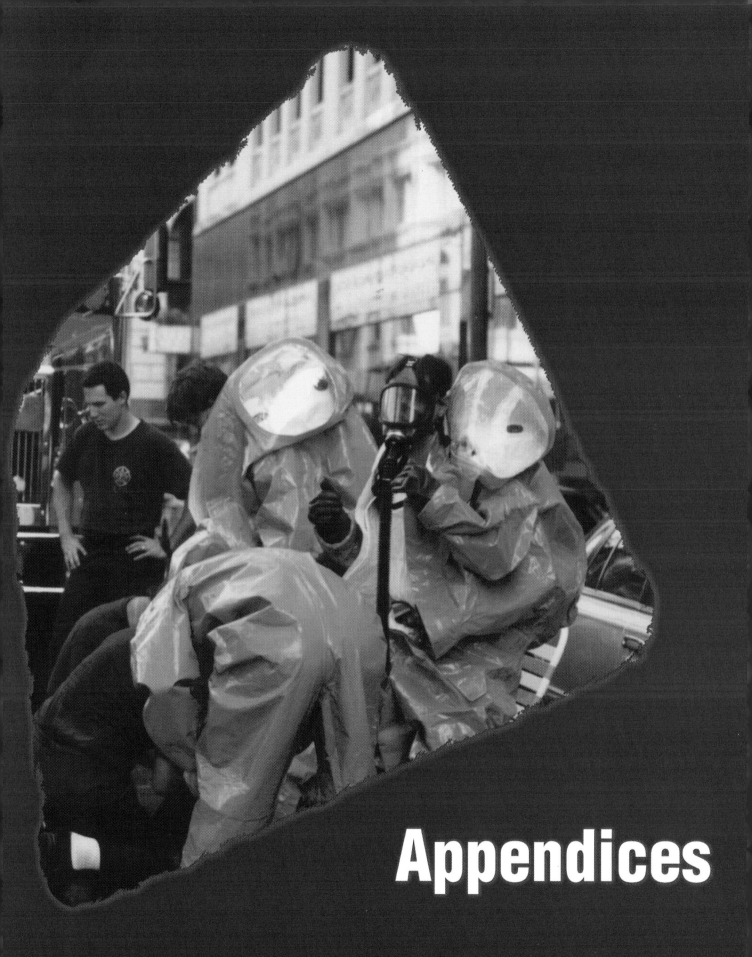

Appendices

Appendix A
Federal OSHA Office Directory
Directory of States with Approved Occupational Safety and Health Plans
[Last Updated: 16 July 2001]

Alaska Department of Labor and Workforce Development
P.O. Box 21149
1111 W. 8th Street, Room 306
Juneau, Alaska 99802-1149
Ed Flanagan, Commissioner (907) 465-2700
Fax: (907) 465-2784
Richard Mastriano, Program Director
(907) 269-4904 Fax: (907) 269-4915

Industrial Commission of Arizona
800 W. Washington
Phoenix, Arizona 85007-2922
Larry Etchechury, Director, ICA (602) 542-4411
Fax: (602) 542-1614
Darin Perkins, Program Director (602) 542-5795
Fax: (602) 542-1614

California Department of Industrial Relations
455 Golden Gate Avenue, 10th Floor
San Francisco, California 94102
Steve Smith, Director (415) 703-5050
Fax:(415) 703-5114
Dr. John Howard, Chief (415) 703-5100
Fax: (415) 703-5114
Vernita Davidson, Manager, Cal/OSHA Program
Office (415) 703-5177 Fax: (415) 703-5114

Connecticut Department of Labor
200 Folly Brook Boulevard
Wethersfield, Connecticut 06109
Shaun Cashman, Commissioner (860) 566-5123
Fax: (860) 566-1520
Conn-OSHA
38 Wolcott Hill Road
Wethersfield, Connecticut 06109
Donald Heckler, Director (860) 566-4550
Fax: (860) 566-6916

Hawaii Department of Labor and Industrial Relations
830 Punchbowl Street
Honolulu, Hawaii 96813
Leonard Agor, Director (808) 586-8844
Fax: (808) 586-9099
Jennifer Shishido, Administrator (808) 586-9116
Fax: (808) 586-9104

Indiana Department of Labor
State Office Building
402 West Washington Street, Room W195
Indianapolis, Indiana 46204-2751
John Griffin, Commissioner (317) 232-2378
Fax: (317) 233-3790
John Jones, Deputy Commissioner (317) 232-3325
Fax: (317) 233-3790

Iowa Division of Labor
1000 E. Grand Avenue
Des Moines, Iowa 50319-0209
Byron K. Orton, Commissioner (515) 281-6432
Fax: (515) 281-4698
Mary L. Bryant, Administrator (515) 242-5870
Fax: (515) 281-7995

Kentucky Labor Cabinet
1047 U.S. Highway 127 South, Suite 4
Frankfort, Kentucky 40601
Joe Norsworthy, Secretary (502) 564-3070
Fax: (502) 564-5387
William Ralston, Federal\State Coordinator
(502) 564-3070 ext. 240 Fax: (502) 564-1682

Maryland Division of Labor and Industry
Department of Labor, Licensing and Regulation
1100 North Eutaw Street, Room 613
Baltimore, Maryland 21201-2206
Kenneth P. Reichard, Commissioner (410) 767-2241
Fax: (410) 767-2986
Keith Goddard, Deputy Commissioner
(410) 767-2992 Fax: 767-2986
Cheryl Kammerman, Assistant Commissioner,
MOSH (410) 767-2215 Fax: 333-7747

Michigan Department of Consumer and Industry Services
Kathleen M. Wilbur, Director
Bureau of Safety and Regulation
P.O. Box 30643
Lansing, MI 48909-8143
Douglas R. Earle, Director
(517) 322-1814 Fax: (517) 322-1775

Minnesota Department of Labor and Industry
443 Lafayette Road
St. Paul, Minnesota 55155
Gretchen B. Maglich, Commissioner (651) 296-2342
Fax: (651) 282-5405
Rosyln Wade, Assistant Commissioner
(651) 296-6529 Fax: (651) 282-5293
Patricia Todd, Administrative Director, OSHA Management Team
(651) 282-5772 Fax: (651) 297-2527

Nevada Division of Industrial Relations
400 West King Street, Suite 400
Carson City, Nevada 89703
Roger Bremmer, Administrator (775) 687-3032
Fax: (775) 687-6305
Occupational Safety and Health Enforcement Section (OSHES)
1301 N. Green Valley Parkway
Henderson, Nevada 89014
Tom Czehowski, Chief Administrative Officer
(702) 486-9168 Fax:(702) 990-0358
[Las Vegas (702) 687-5240]

New Jersey Department of Labor
John Fitch Plaza - Labor Building
Market and Warren Streets
P.O. Box 110
Trenton, New Jersey 08625-0110
Mark B. Boyd, Commssioner (609) 292-2975
Fax: (609) 633-9271
Leonard Katz, Assistant Commissioner
(609) 292-2313 Fax: (609) 292-1314
Louis J. Lento, Program Director, PEOSH
(609) 292-3923 Fax: (609) 292-4409

New Mexico Environment Department
1190 St. Francis Drive
P.O. Box 26110
Santa Fe, New Mexico 87502
Peter Maggiore, Secretary (505) 827-2850
Fax: (505) 827-2836
Sam A. Rogers, Chief (505) 827-4230
Fax: (505) 827-4422

New York Department of Labor
W. Averell Harriman State Office Building 12, Room 500
Albany, NY 12240
Linda Angello, Commissioner (518) 457-2746
Fax: (518) 457-6908
Richard Cucolo, Director, Division of Safety and Health
(518) 457-3518 Fax: (518) 457-1519

North Carolina Department of Labor
4 West Edenton Street
Raleigh, North Carolina 27601-1092
Cherie Berry, Commissioner (919) 807-2900
Fax: (919) 807-2855
John Johnson, Deputy Commissioner, OSH Director (919) 807-2861 Fax: (919) 807-2855
Kevin Beauregard, OSH Assistant Director
(919) 807-2863 Fax:(919) 807-2856

Oregon Occupational Safety and Health Division
Department of Consumer & Business Services
350 Winter Street, NE, Room 430
Salem, Oregon 97310-0220
Peter DeLuca, Administrator (503) 378-3272
Fax: (503) 947-7461
David Sparks, Deputy Administrator for Policy
(503) 378-3272 Fax: (503) 947-7461
Michele Patterson, Deputy Administrator for Operations (503) 378-3272 Fax: (503) 947-7461

Puerto Rico Department of Labor and Human Resources
Prudencio Rivera Martínez Building
505 Muñoz Rivera Avenue
Hato Rey, Puerto Rico 00918
Víctor Rivera Hernández, Secretary
(787) 754-2119 Fax: (787) 753-9550
Brenda Sepúlveda, Assistant Secretary for Occupational Safety and Health
(787) 756-1100, 1106 / 754-2171 Fax: (787) 767-6051
José Droz, Deputy Director for Occupational Safety and Health
(787) 756-1100, 1106 / 754-2188 Fax: (787) 767-6051

South Carolina Department of Labor, Licensing, and Regulation
Koger Office Park, Kingstree Building
110 Centerview Drive
P.O. Box 11329
Columbia, South Carolina 29211
Rita McKinney, Director (803) 896-4300
Fax: (803) 896-4393
William Lybrand, Program Director (803) 734-9644
Fax: (803) 734-9772

Tennessee Department of Labor
710 James Robertson Parkway
Nashville, Tennessee 37243-0659
Michael E. Magill, Commissioner (615) 741-2582
Fax: (615) 741-5078
John Winkler, Acting Program Director
(615) 741-2793 Fax: (615) 741-3325

Utah Labor Commission
160 East 300 South, 3rd Floor
P.O. Box 146650
Salt Lake City, Utah 84114-6650
R. Lee Ellertson, Commissioner (801) 530-6901
Fax: (801) 530-7906
Jay W. Bagley, Administrator (801) 530-6898
Fax: (801) 530-6390

Vermont Department of Labor and Industry
National Life Building - Drawer 20
Montpelier, Vermont 05620-3401
Tasha Wallis, Commissioner (802) 828-2288
Fax: (802) 828-2748
Robert McLeod, Project Manager (802) 828-2765
Fax: (802) 828-2195

Virgin Islands Department of Labor
2203 Church Street
Christiansted, St. Croix, Virgin Islands 00820-4660
Cecil R. Benjamin, Acting Commissioner
(340) 773-1990 Fax: (340) 773-1858
Marcelle Heywood, Program Director
(340) 772-1315 Fax: (340) 772-4323

Virginia Department of Labor and Industry
Powers-Taylor Building
13 South 13th Street
Richmond, Virginia 23219
Jeffrey Brown, Commissioner (804) 786-2377
Fax: (804) 371-6524
Jay Withrow, Director, Office of Legal Support
(804) 786-9873 Fax: (804) 786-8418

Washington Department of Labor and Industries
General Administration Building
P.O. Box 44001
Olympia, Washington 98504-4001
Gary Moore, Director (360) 902-4200
Fax: (360) 902-4202
Michael Silverstein, Assistant Director [P.O. Box 44600] (360) 902-5495 Fax: (360) 902-5529
Steve Cant, Program Manager, Federal-State Operations [P.O. Box 44600] (360) 902-5430
Fax: (360) 902-5529

Wyoming Department of Employment
Workers' Safety and Compensation Division
Herschler Building, 2nd Floor East
122 West 25th Street
Cheyenne, Wyoming 82002
Stephan R. Foster, Safety Administrator
(307) 777-7786 Fax: (307) 777-3646

Appendix B
Respiratory Protection Program Sample

*[**NOTE:** This sample program is based on the program developed by the Centers for Disease Control and is intended to meet federal OSHA requirements.]*

1.0 INTRODUCTION

It is the policy of the _____ to provide employees with a safe and healthful working environment. This is accomplished by utilizing facilities and equipment that have all feasible safeguards incorporated into their design. When effective engineering controls are not feasible, or when they are being initiated, protection shall be used to ensure personnel protection.

This program does not apply to contractors as they are responsible for providing their own respiratory protection programs and respiratory protective equipment.

2.0 RESPONSIBILITIES

2.1 Office of Health and Safety

The Office of Health and Safety (OHS) is responsible for establishing and maintaining a respiratory protection program consistent with the goal of protecting _____ personnel. OHS will implement a Respiratory Protection Program which is designed and organized to ensure respirators are properly selected, used, and maintained by _____ personnel, and to meet federal regulatory standards (29 CFR 1910.134) and industry accepted standards (ANSI & NFPA).

OHS is also responsible for evaluating those tasks for which respiratory protection is thought to be necessary, determine the degree of hazard posed by the potential exposure, determine whether engineering or administrative controls are feasible, and will specify which respiratory protection device is to be used at each task. In addition, OHS will train personnel in the selection and use of respiratory protective devices, conduct qualitative and quantitative fit testing, and issue necessary protective devices.

2.2 Occupational Health Clinic, OHS

The Occupational Health Clinic is charged with establishing medical evaluation and surveillance procedures and reviewing the health status of all personnel who may be required to wear respiratory protective equipment in the completion of their assigned tasks.

2.3 Supervisor

Supervisors will ensure each employee under his or her supervision using a respirator has received appropriate training in its use and an annual medical evaluation. Supervisors will ensure the availability of appropriate respirators and accessories, provide adequate storage facilities, and encourage proper respirator equipment maintenance. Supervisors must be aware of tasks requiring the use of respiratory protection, and ensure all employees engaged in such work use the appropriate respirators at all times.

2.4 Respirator Wearers

It is the responsibility of each respirator wearer to wear his/her respirator when and where required and in the manner in which they were trained. Respirator wearers must report any malfunctions of the respirator to his/her supervisor immediately. The respirator wearer must also guard against mechanical damage to the respirator, clean the respirator as instructed, and store the respirator in a clean, sanitary location.

2.5 Others

Personnel, such as employees, inspectors, and visitors, who must enter an area where the use of respiratory protective equipment is required, even when their stay time in the area may be 15 minutes or less, shall be provided with and use appropriate equipment, including instructions regarding use and limitations. Personnel shall be fit tested and medically qualified to wear the respirator being issued prior to entry to the site.

Contractors are required to develop and implement a respiratory protection program for their employees who must enter into or work in areas where exposure to hazardous materials cannot be controlled or avoided. This program must meet OSHA regulations and include issuance of respirators, medical evaluations, fit testing and training.

3.0 MEDICAL EVALUATION

The Occupational Physician, Occupational Health Clinic, initially, and periodically thereafter, makes a determination as to whether or not an employee can wear the required respirator without physical or psychological risk. Based on the overall health of the individual and special medical tests (pulmonary function studies, EKG, etc.) as appropriate, the examining physician determines whether or not the individual will be restricted from wearing respiratory protective equipment. If a medical restriction is applied, the employee, his/her supervisor, and the Office of Health and Safety are formally notified of the restriction.

Specific medical tests and procedures will be determined by the Occupational Health Physician and will be in accordance with OSHA medical surveillance requirements and/or NIOSH recommendations.

4.0 SELECTION AND USE OF RESPIRATORY PROTECTIVE DEVICES

4.1 Respirator Use

Respiratory protection is authorized and issued for the following personnel:

A.   Workers in areas known to have contaminant levels requiring the use of respiratory protection or in which contaminant levels requiring the use of respiratory protection may be created without warning (e.g., emergency purposes such as hazardous material spill responses).

B.   Workers performing operations documented to be health hazardous and those unavoidably required to be in the immediate vicinity where similar levels of contaminants are generated.

C.   Workers in suspect areas or performing operations suspected of being health hazardous but for which adequate sampling data has not been obtained.

4.2 Respirator Use for Biohazards

Respirators for use in areas where biohazards are used or stored must be selected based on a review of the laboratory procedures, protocols, biohazardous agents proposed for use, etc. The Biosafety Branch, OHS, will conduct a risk assessment and determine the appropriate Biosafety Level for the laboratory and the corresponding level of personal protective equipment required.

4.3 Respirator Selection

Selection of the proper respirator(s) to be used in any work area or operation at _____ is made only after a determination has been made as to the real and/or potential exposure of employees to harmful concentrations of contaminants in the workplace atmosphere. This evaluation will be performed prior to the start of any routine or non-routine tasks requiring respirators. Respiratory protective devices will be selected by the Office of Health and Safety, using ANSI Z88.2, NIOSH Certified Equipment List, and/or the NIOSH Respirator Selection Decision Logic as a guide. The following items will be considered in the selection of respirators:

- Effectiveness of the device against the substance of concern;
- Estimated maximum concentration of the substance in the work area;
- General environment (open shop or confined space, etc.);

- Known limitations of the respiratory protective device;
- Comfort, fit, and worker acceptance; and
- Other contaminants in the environment or potential for oxygen deficiency.

Supervisors shall contact OHS prior to non-routine work that may expose workers to hazardous substances or oxygen deficient atmospheres. Examples of work that may require the use of respirators includes, but are not limited to:

- Asbestos contaminated areas
- Interior fire fighting and associated activities
- Medical responses
- Hazardous materials responses
- Cutting or melting metal surfaces
- Welding or burning
- Painting, especially with epoxy or organic solvent coatings
- Using solvents, thinners, or degreasers
- Any work which generates large amounts of dust
- Working in a confined space

A review of the real and/or potential exposures is made at least annually to determine if respiratory protection continues to be required, and if so, do the previously chosen respirators still provide adequate protection.

4.4 Types of Respirators

A. Air-Purifying Respirator

These respirators remove air contaminants by filtering, absorbing, adsorbing, or chemical reaction with the contaminants as they pass through the respirator canister or cartridge. This respirator is to be used only where adequate oxygen (19.5 to 23.5 percent by volume) is available. Air-purifying respirators can be classified as follows:

1. Particulate removing respirators, which filter out dusts, fibers, fumes and mists. These respirators may be single-use disposable respirators or respirators with replaceable filters.

NOTE: Surgical masks do not provide protection against air contaminants. They are never to be used in place of an air-purifying respirator. They are for medical use only.

2. Gas- and vapor-removing respirators, which remove specific individual contaminants or a combination of contaminants by absorption, adsorption or by chemical reaction. Gas masks and chemical-cartridge respirators are examples of gas- and vapor-removing respirators.

3. Combination particulate/gas- and vapor-removing respirators, which combine the respirator characteristics of both kinds of air-purifying respirators.

A. Supplied-Air Respirators

These respirators provide breathing air independent of the environment. Such respirators are to be used when the contaminant has insufficient odor, taste or irritating warning properties, or when the contaminant is of such high concentration or toxicity that an air-purifying respirator is inadequate. Supplied-air respirators, also called airline respirators, are classified as follows:

1. Demand

This respirator supplies air to the user on demand (inhalation) that creates a negative pressure within the facepiece. Leakage into the facepiece may occur if there is a poor seal between the respirator and the user's face.

2. Pressure-Demand

This respirator maintains a continuous positive pressure within the face piece, thus preventing leakage into the facepiece.

3. Continuous Flow

This respirator maintains a continuous flow of air through the facepiece and prevents leakage into the facepiece.

A. Self-Contained Breathing Apparatus (SCBA)

This type of respirator allows the user complete independence from a fixed source of air and offers the greatest degree of protection but is also the most complex. Training and practice in its use and maintenance is essential. This type of device will be used in emergency situations only.

4.5 Identification of Respirator Cartridges and Canisters

Respirator cartridges and canisters are designed to protect against individual or a combination of potentially hazardous atmospheric contaminants, and are specifically labeled and color-coded to indicate the type and nature of protection they provide.

The NIOSH approval label on the respirator will also specify the maximum concentration of contaminant(s) for which the cartridge or canister is approved. For example, a label may read:

"DO NOT WEAR IN ATMOSPHERES IMMEDIATELY DANGEROUS TO LIFE. MUST BE USED IN AREAS CONTAINING AT LEAST 20 PERCENT OXYGEN. DO NOT WEAR IN ATMOSPHERES CONTAINING MORE THAN ONE-TENTH PERCENT ORGANIC VAPORS BY VOLUME. REFER TO COMPLETE LABEL ON RESPIRATOR OR CARTRIDGE CONTAINER FOR ASSEMBLY, MAINTENANCE, AND USE."

4.6 Warning Signs of Respirator Failure

A. Particulate Air-Purifying

When breathing difficulty is encountered with a filter respirator (due to partial clogging with increased resistance), the filter(s) must be replaced. Disposable filter respirators must be discarded.

B. Gas or Vapor Air-Purifying

If, when using a gas or vapor respirator (chemical cartridge or canister), any of the warning properties (e.g., odor, taste, eye irritation, or respiratory irritation) occur, promptly leave the area and check the following:

- Proper face seal
- Damaged or missing respirator parts
- Saturated or inappropriate cartridge or canister

If no discrepancies are observed, replace the cartridge or canister. If any of the warning properties appear again, the concentration of the contaminants may have exceeded the cartridge or canister design specification. When this occurs an airline respirator or SCBA is required.

A. Service Life of Air-Purifying Respirator Canisters and Cartridges

The canisters or cartridges of air-purifying respirators are intended to be used until filter resistance precludes further use, or the chemical sorbent is expended as signified by a specific warning property, e.g., odor, taste, etc. New canisters, cartridges or filters shall always be provided when a respirator is reissued. When in doubt about the previous use of the respirator, obtain a replacement canister or cartridge.

B. Supplied-Air Respirator

When using an airline respirator, leave the area immediately when the compressor failure alarm is activated or if an air pressure drop is sensed. When using an SCBA leave the area as soon as the air pressure alarm is activated.

5.0 RESPIRATOR TRAINING

Respirator users and their supervisors will receive training on the contents of the _____ Respiratory Protection Program and their responsibilities under it. They will be trained on the proper selection and use, as well as the limitations of the respirator. Training also covers how to ensure a proper fit before use and how to determine when a respirator is no longer providing the protection intended.

OHS provides training of respirator wearers in the use, maintenance, capabilities, and limitations of respirators. Retraining is given annually thereafter and only upon successful completion of the medical evaluation.

The training program will include the following:

1. Nature and degree of respiratory hazard
2. Respirator selection, based on the hazard and respirator capabilities and limitations
3. Donning procedures and fit tests including hands-on practice
4. Care of the respirator, e.g., need for cleaning, maintenance, storage, and/or replacement
5. Use and limitations of respirator

Respirator training will be properly documented and will include the type and model of respirator for which the individual has been trained and fit-tested.

6.0 RESPIRATOR FIT TESTING

A fit test shall be used to determine the ability of each individual respirator wearer to obtain a satisfactory fit with any air-purifying respirator. Both quantitative and qualitative fit tests will be performed. Personnel must successfully pass the fit test before being issued an air-purifying respirator.

No employee is permitted to wear a negative-pressure respirator in a work situation until he or she has demonstrated that an acceptable fit can be obtained. Respirator fitting is conducted initially upon assignment to a task requiring use of a respirator. Refitting is conducted annually thereafter upon successful completion of the respirator training.

Fit testing will be conducted by the Office of Health and Safety and the test results will be the determining factor in selecting the type, model, and size of negative-pressure respirator for use by each individual respirator wearer.

6.1 Fit Checking

Each time a respirator is donned, the user will perform positive and negative pressure fit checks. These checks are not a substitute for fit testing. Respirator users must be properly trained in the performance of these checks and understand their limitations.

A. Negative Pressure Check

Applicability/Limitations: This test cannot be carried out on all respirators; however, it can be used on facepieces of air-purifying respirators equipped with tight-fitting respirator inlet covers and on atmosphere supplying respirators equipped with breathing tubes which can be squeezed or blocked at the inlet to prevent the passage of air.

Procedure: Close off the inlet opening of the respirator's canister(s), cartridge(s), or filter(s) with the palm of the hand, or squeeze the breathing air tube or block its inlet so that it will not allow the passage of air. Inhale gently and hold for at least 10 seconds. If the facepiece collapses slightly and no inward leakage of air into the facepiece is detected, it can be reasonably assumed that the respirator has been properly positioned and the exhalation valve and facepiece are not leaking.

B. Positive Pressure Check

Applicability/Limitations: This test cannot be carried out on all respirators; however, respirators equipped with exhalation valves can be tested.

Procedure: Close off the exhalation valve or the breathing tube with the palm of the hand. Exhale gently. If the respirator has been properly positioned, a slight positive pressure will build up inside the facepiece without detection of any outward air leak between the sealing surface of the facepiece and the face.

6.2 Qualitative Fit Testing

Federal regulations (29 CFR 1910.1001) require qualitative fit tests of respirators and describe step-by-step procedures. This test checks the subject's response to a chemical introduced outside the respirator facepiece. This response is either voluntary or involuntary depending on the chemical used. Several methods may be used. The two most common are the irritant smoke test, and the odorous vapor test.

A. Irritant Smoke

The irritant smoke test is an involuntary response test. Air-purifying respirators must be equipped with a high efficiency particulate air (HEPA) filter for this test. An irritant smoke, usually either stannic chloride or titanium tetrachloride, is directed from a smoke tube toward the respirator. If the test subject does not respond to the irritant smoke, a satisfactory fit is assumed to be achieved. Any response to the smoke indicates an unsatisfactory fit.

The irritant smoke is an irritant to the eyes, skin, and mucous membranes. It should not be introduced directly onto the skin. The test subject must keep his or her eyes closed during the testing if a full facepiece mask is not used.

B. Odorous Vapor

The odorous vapor test is a voluntary response test. It relies on the subject's ability to detect an odorous chemical while wearing the respirator. Air-purifying respirators must be equipped with an organic cartridge or canister for this test. Isoamyl acetate (banana oil) is the usual test. An isoamyl acetate-saturated gauze pad is placed near the facepiece-to-face seal of the respirator of the test subject's skin. If the test subject is unable to smell the chemical, than a satisfactory fit is assumed to be achieved. If the subject smells the chemical, the fit is unsatisfactory.

If the subject cannot smell the chemical, the respirator will be momentarily pulled away from the subject's face. If the subject is then able to smell the chemical, a satisfactory fit is assumed. If the subject cannot smell the chemical with the respirator pulled away from the face, this test is inappropriate for this subject, and a different test will be used.

This test is limited by the wide variation of odor thresholds among individuals and the possibility of olfactory fatigue. Since it is a voluntary response test it depends upon an honest response.

6.3 Quantitative Fit Testing

Quantitative fit testing, using the Portacount Plus fit test system, is generally performed on both full-face and half-face negative pressure respirators. Fit factors are determined by comparing the particle concentration outside the respirator with the concentration inside the respirator facepiece. An acceptable fit is achieved when the respirator wearer successfully completes a series of six programmed exercises (normal breathing, deep breathing, moving head up and down, moving head side to side, reading, and normal breathing) with a fit factor of 100 or more.

6.4 Special Problems

A. Facial Hair

No attempt is made to fit a respirator on an employee who has facial hair which comes between the sealing periphery of the facepiece and the face, or if facial hair interferes with normal functioning of the exhalation valve of the respirator.

B. Glasses and Eye/Face Protective Devices

Proper fitting of a respiratory protective device facepiece for individuals wearing corrective eyeglasses or goggles, may not be established if temple bars or straps extend through the sealing edge of the facepiece. If eyeglasses, goggles, face shield or welding helmet must be worn with a respirator, they must be worn so as not to adversely affect the seal of the facepiece. If a full-facepiece respirator is used, special prescription glasses inserts are available if needed.

6.5 Respirator User Cards

Respirator User Cards will be issued by OHS to workers who have been trained, fitted, and medically evaluated to use respirators. A Respirator User Card will include:

1. Name and identification number of the worker.

2. The statement: "(name) has been trained, fitted and medically evaluated to use the respirator(s) indicated."

3. The type(s), model(s), and size(s) of respirator(s) that the cardholder was issued.

4. Expiration date of card.

6.6 Record keeping

Respirator fit-testing shall be documented and shall include the type of respirator, brand name and model, method of test and test results, test date and the name of the instructor/tester.

7.0 MAINTENANCE AND ISSUANCE OF RESPIRATORS

7.1 Maintenance

The maintenance of respiratory protective devices involves a thorough visual inspection for cleanliness and defects (i.e., cracking rubber, deterioration of straps, defective exhalation and inhalation valves, broken or cracked lenses, etc.). Worn or deteriorated parts will be replaced prior to reissue. No respirator with a known defect is reissued for use. No attempt is made to replace components, make adjustments or make repairs on any respirator beyond those recommended by the manufacturer. Under no circumstances will parts be substituted as such substitutions will invalidate the approval of the respirator. Any repair to reducing or admission valves, regulators, or alarms will be conducted by either the manufacturer or a qualified trained technician.

7.2 Cleaning of Respirators

All respirators in routine use shall be cleaned and sanitized on a periodic basis. Respirators used non-routinely shall be cleaned and sanitized after each use and filters and cartridges replaced. Routinely used respirators are maintained individually by the respirator wearer. Replacement cartridges and filters are obtained by contacting OHS.

Cleaning and disinfecting respirators must be done frequently to ensure that skin-penetrating and dermatitis-causing contaminants are removed from the respirator surface. Respirators maintained for emergency use or those used by more than one person must be cleaned after each use by the user.

The following procedure is recommended for cleaning and disinfecting respirators:

1. Remove and discard all used filters, cartridges, or canisters.

2. Wash facepiece and breathing tube in a cleaner-disinfectant solution. A hand brush may be used to remove dirt. Solvents which can affect rubber and other parts shall not be used.

3. Rinse completely in clean, warm water.

4. Air dry in a clean area in such a way as to prevent distortion.

5. Clean other respirator parts as recommended by the manufacturer.

6. Inspect valves, headstraps, and other parts to ensure proper working condition.

7. Reassemble respirator and replace any defective parts.

8. Place in a clean, dry plastic bag or other suitable container for storage after each cleaning and disinfection.

7.3 Issuance of Respirators

Respiratory protective equipment shall not be ordered, purchased, or issued to personnel unless the respirator wearer has received respirator training and a fit test. New employees who require respiratory protective equipment, must be placed into the respirator program before being issued equipment.

OHS provides at least three types of devices: APR half-mask; APR, SAR, SCBA full-face; and powered air-purifying respirators (PAPR). These facepieces have a variety of canisters that may be worn with them; hence, the canisters and facepieces are packaged separately. At the time of issue the appropriate canister is determined, based on the user's needs, and is issued with the appropriate facepiece. In addition, disposable respirators with filter ratings N-95 and N-100 ratings are available for use under appropriate conditions.

7.4 Storage

After inspection, cleaning, and any necessary minor repairs, store respirators to protect against sunlight, heat, extreme cold, excessive moisture, damaging chemicals or other contaminants. Respirators placed at stations and work areas for emergency use shall be stored in compartments built for that purpose, shall be quickly accessible at all times and will be clearly marked. Routinely used respirators, such as half-mask or full-face air-purifying respirators, shall be placed in sealable plastic bags. Respirators may be stored in such places as lockers or toolboxes only if they are first placed in carrying cases or cartons. Respirators shall be packed or stored so that the facepiece and exhalation valves will rest in a normal position and not be crushed. Emergency use respirators shall be stored in a sturdy compartment that is quickly accessible and clearly marked.

8.0 PROGRAM SURVEILLANCE

The ANSI Z88.2-1980 document entitled "Practices for Respiratory Protection" specifies:

"Section 3.5.15 Respirator Program Evaluation. An appraisal of the effectiveness of the respirator program shall be carried out at least annually. Action shall be taken to correct defects found in the program."

The evaluation of the Respirator Program will include investigating wearer acceptance of respirators, inspecting respirator program operation, and appraising protection provided by the respirator. Evidence of excessive exposure of respirator wearers to respiratory hazards will be followed up by investigation to determine why inadequate respiratory protection was provided. The findings of the respirator program evaluation will be documented, and this documentation will list plans to correct faults in the program and set target dates for the implementation of the plans. These evaluations will be conducted at least annually.

9.0 RECORDKEEPING

The following records shall be developed and maintained for the Respirator Program:

Record	Location
Medical Evaluations	Office of Health and Safety
Training Records	Office of Health and Safety Training Center
Respirator Program Manual, IHP, and SOPs	Office of Health and Safety
Hazard Evaluations (Air sampling results, surveys, respirator selection records)	Office of Health and Safety

Record	Location
Biohazard Risk Assessments	Office of Health and Safety Medical Branch
Fit Test Records	Office of Health and Safety
Program Evaluations	Office of Health and Safety

Respirator Training Certification

I hereby certify that I have been trained in the proper use and limitations of the respirator issued to me. The training included the following:

1. Instruction on putting on, fitting, testing and wearing the respirator.

2. Instruction on inspection, cleaning, and maintaining the respirator.

3. Explanation of dangers related to misuse.

4. Instructions on emergency situations.

I further certify that I understand the use, care, and inspection of the respirator and have tested and worn the unit.

Date: _____

Signed:_____ SSN: _____

Respirator Type Issued: _____

Training Coordinator: _____

Fit Test Work Sheets
Qualitative Respirator Fit Test

Name: _____ SSN: _____

Clean Shaven? __Yes __No

Spectacle Kit? ___Yes ___No

Manufacturer/Model _____ Size: ___S ___M ___L

Irritant Smoke ___Pass ___Fail

Isoamyl Acetate ___Pass ___Fail

Manufacturer/Model_____ Size: ___S ___M ___L

Irritant Smoke ___Pass ___Fail

Isoamyl Acetate ___Pass ___Fail

Examiner _____ Date_____

Employee _____ Date _____

Quantitative Respirator Fit Test Report

Last Name _____

First Name_____

ID Number_____

Next Test Due_____

Operator Name_____

Respirator Model_____

- Size_____
- Manufacturer_____
- Approval number_____

Notes_____

Test Date_____

Test Time_____

Test Data

Fit Factor Pass Level: 100

Ex. (Part/cc)	Ambient (Part/cc)	Mask	Fit Factor	Pass/Fail
NB DB SS UD R NB				

Overall Fit Factor = _____

Operator _____ Date _____

Subject_____ Date _____

Appendix C
NIOSH Decision Logic Flow Chart

References found in flow chart refer to the original text published in the *NIOSH Respirator Decision Logic*, U. S. Department of Health & Human Services, Centers for Disease Control, May, 1987.

The Respirator Decision Logic Sequence is presented below in the form of a flow chart. This flow chart can be used to identify suitable classes of respirators for adequate protection against specific environmental conditions.

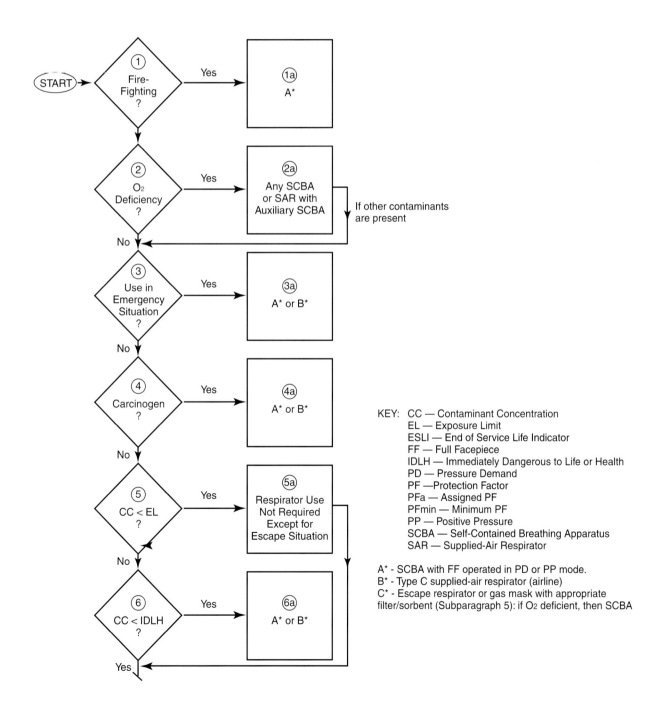

KEY: CC — Contaminant Concentration
EL — Exposure Limit
ESLI — End of Service Life Indicator
FF — Full Facepiece
IDLH — Immediately Dangerous to Life or Health
PD — Pressure Demand
PF —Protection Factor
PFa — Assigned PF
PFmin — Minimum PF
PP — Positive Pressure
SCBA — Self-Contained Breathing Apparatus
SAR — Supplied-Air Respirator

A* - SCBA with FF operated in PD or PP mode.
B* - Type C supplied-air respirator (airline)
C* - Escape respirator or gas mask with appropriate filter/sorbent (Subparagraph 5): if O$_2$ deficient, then SCBA

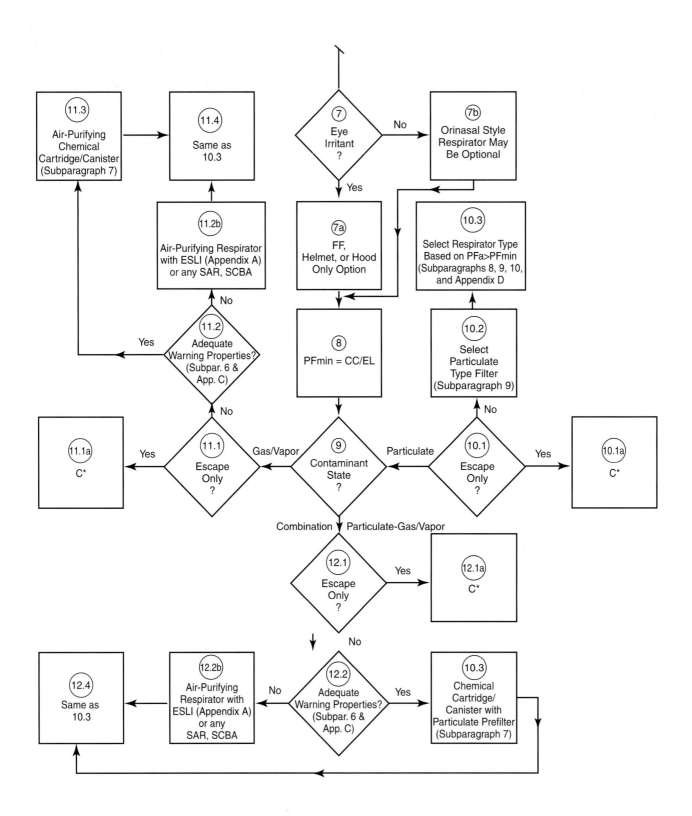

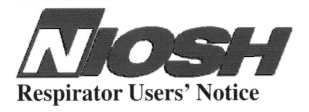

Respirator Users' Notice

June 12, 1998

The National Institute for Occupational Safety and Health (NIOSH) wishes to inform users of the Belt-Mounted Regulator (BMR) model self-contained breathing-apparatus (SCBA), manufactured by Mine Safety Appliances Company (MSA) that certain breathing tubes used on BMR SCBA may tear or separate unexpectedly. The Institute has recently received a number of reports indicating that breathing tubes can tear or completely separate, resulting in a loss of respiratory protection to the user. These breathing tubes are used on belt-mounted regulator type SCBA. The corrugated rubber tube connects the belt-mounted regulator to the facepiece and can be identified by the part numbers 801165, 803506, or 470734 stamped in yellow ink on one of the clamps at either end of the breathing tube.

Mine Safety Appliances Company is actively working to determine the cause of these breathing tube failures, along with the extent of the problem. Preliminary indications are that some breathing tubes may have recently been placed in service that are susceptible to premature failure. This could result in a complete loss of respiratory protection, in the event of breathing tube failure.

On May 29, 1998, MSA released a Safety Notice that reinforced the need to properly inspect breathing tubes for cracks, tears, cuts, perforations, and any deterioration or other signs of wear. The MSA Safety Notice is clear and should be followed when inspecting the breathing tube. However, Both NIOSH and MSA are concerned that this inspection procedure, by itself, may not be adequate to identify breathing tubes that are susceptible to tearing.

Therefore NIOSH is recommending that users immediately take the following actions to ensure that breathing tubes in their possession are safe for their intended use:

1. Perform the simple pull test developed by MSA that is described on the following pages.

2. Re-inspect the breathing tube following MSA's recommended procedure, paying particular attention to signs of cracking, ripping, or tearing, and to make certain the coupling/tube connection remains tight.

If the breathing tube passes both of these steps, the breathing tube can be returned to service. Any tube that shows signs of cracking, ripping, or tearing, however small, or the clamp has loosened, must be removed from service.

Mine Safety Appliances Company is actively working to determine the cause and extent of the breathing tube failures. Until a final resolution is reached, all breathing tubes in your possession should be inspected following the procedure outlined above.

Additional information on this subject may be obtained by contacting NIOSH at 1-800-35-NIOSH.

Appendix E
Sample Manufacturer's Warning

Current Events

July 17, 2000

Luxfer Announces New Inspection and Replacement Policy for Scuba Cylinders Manufactured in Australia and U.S.

RIVERSIDE, Calif.--Luxfer Gas Cylinders has announced a new inspection and replacement policy for scuba cylinders manufactured at its facilities in the United States. The primary purpose for the new policy is to clarify inspection and testing procedures for the two different aluminium alloys from which Luxfer scuba cylinders have been manufactured. The text of the policy is as follows:

Luxfer Scuba Cylinder Inspection and Replacement Policy

Section I: Inspection and Testing of Luxfer Scuba Cylinders Manufactured from 6351 Aluminium Alloy

Luxfer scuba cylinders were manufactured from 6351 aluminium alloy during the following periods:

- United States: 1972 through mid-1988
- England: 1967 through 1995
- Australia: 1975 through 1990

Luxfer requires that every Luxfer 6351-alloy all-aluminium scuba cylinder be visually inspected at least every 2.5 years by a properly trained inspector. As part of this inspection, Luxfer further requires that the cylinder neck be tested with an eddy-current device such as Visual Plus, Visual Eddy or equivalent non-destructive testing equipment. When properly used, eddy-current devices contribute significantly to early detection of difficult-to-observe sustained-load cracks in the necks of 6351-alloy cylinders. If the cylinder passes the inspection, the inspector will document that fact. If the cylinder fails the inspection, it must be removed from service immediately. *Do not use Luxfer 6351-alloy scuba cylinders that have not been both visually inspected and eddy-current tested and then properly documented.*

This Luxfer-required visual and eddy-current inspection is in addition to periodic requalifications (including retesting and inspections) required or recommended by various regulatory agencies around the world. The intervals between retests and inspections vary from country to country.

In addition to the required inspection and testing described above and in keeping with Australian and New Zealand scuba industry standards, Luxfer recommends that all Luxfer 6351-alloy scuba cylinders be visually inspected at least once each year by a properly trained inspector. For cylinders in heavy use (for example, those filled five or more times a week), Luxfer recommends visual inspection every four months. For more information, refer to Luxfer's *Scuba Cylinder Inspection Guide*, which is available by calling Luxfer at 800-764-0366 or by visiting the Luxfer web site at www.luxfercylinders.com.

Section II: Inspection and Testing of Luxfer Scuba Cylinders Manufactured from 6061 Aluminium Alloy

Luxfer began manufacturing scuba cylinders from a proprietary 6061 aluminium alloy in mid-1988 in the United States, and in 1995 in England and in 1990 in Australia. The majority of Luxfer scuba cylinders currently in service are made from this proprietary 6061 alloy, which Luxfer is still using.

Cylinders made from Luxfer's proprietary 6061 alloy are not susceptible to sustained-load cracks. Therefore, Luxfer does not deem it necessary to test these cylinders with eddy-current devices such as Visual Plus and Visual Eddy. In fact, field experience has shown that using such eddy-current devices with Luxfer 6061-alloy cylinders can result in misleading "false-positive" readings.

In keeping with U.S. scuba industry standards, Luxfer recommends annual visual inspection of Luxfer 6061-alloy cylinders by a properly trained inspector. For cylinders in heavy use (for example, those filled five or more times a week), Luxfer recommends visual inspection every four months. These recommended inspections are in addition to periodic requalifications (including retesting and inspections) required or recommended by various regulatory agencies around the world. The intervals between retests and inspections vary from country to country.

For more information, refer to Luxfer's *Scuba Cylinder Inspection Guide*, which is available by calling Luxfer at 880-764-0366 or visiting the Luxfer web site at www.luxfercylinders.com.

Section III: Luxfer Scuba Cylinder Replacement Policy

This replacement policy applies only to the original owner of a Luxfer scuba cylinder. If a properly inspected Luxfer scuba cylinder is found to have either sustained-load cracking (in the case of 6351-alloy cylinders) or a manufacturing defect (i.e., any imperfection that fails to meet product specifications at the time of manufacture), Luxfer will honor the following replacement policy:

- If the cylinder is 10 years old or less (based on the original hydrotest date), Luxfer will replace the cylinder at no charge with a new 6061-alloy cylinder. However, Luxfer will not replace cylinders that have been damaged, abused or mistreated.
- If the cylinder is more than 10 years old, the original owner may purchase an equivalent replacement cylinder for $50 (U.S.) for cylinders manufactured in the Unite States. For cylinders manufactured elsewhere, the purchase price of the replacement cylinder will be determined in the country of origin based on local currency rates.

For more information about this policy or Luxfer scuba cylinders, contact Luxfer Gas Cylinders, 3016 Kansas Avenue, Riverside, California 92507 U.S.A.; telephone toll-free 800-764-0366; fax 909-781-6598; on the web at www.luxfercylinders.com.

Appendix F
Risk Management Formulas

The following formulas may be used to calculate the frequency or incident rate and the severity of incidents. OSHA calculates the frequency (incident rate) as follows:

$$N/EH \times 200,000 = IR$$

N = number of injuries and/or illnesses
EH = total hours worked by all employees during the calendar year
$200,000$ = base for 100 full-time equivalent employees (provides standardization between agencies and companies)
IR = incident rate

OSHA calculates the severity as follows:

$$LWD/EH \times 200,000 = S$$

LWD = loss work days
EH = total hours worked by all employees during the calendar year
$200,000$ = base for 100 full-time equivalent employees
S = severity rate

Another method is to assign values to the frequency and severity in the following formula:

$$R = S \times IR$$

R = risk
S = severity
IR = incident rate

Assessment of Severity

8. Extreme	Multiple deaths or widespread destruction may result from hazard.
7. Very High	Potential death or injury or severe financial loss may result.
6. High	Permanent disabling injury may result.
5. Serious	Loss time injury greater than 28 days or considerable financial loss.
4. Moderate	Loss time injury of 4 to 28 days or moderate financial loss.
3. Minor	Loss time injury up to 3 days.
2. Slight	Minor injury resulting in no loss of time or slight financial loss.
1. Minimal	No loss of time injury or financial loss to organization.

Assessment of Incident Rate

7. Frequent	Occurs weekly.
6. Very Likely	Occurs once every few months.
5. Likely	Occurs about once a year.
4. Occasional	Occurs annually in the United States.
3. Rare	Occurs every 10 to 30 years.
2. Exceptional	Occurs every 10 to 30 years in the United States.
1. Unlikely	May occur once in 10,000 years within the global fire service.

Appendix G
Scott Aviation Flow Chart

The Scott Aviation Flow Chart is intended to provide a simplified process for determining the type of respiratory protection required, evaluating the various types of equipment available, specifying, purchasing, and accepting the systems. Most manufacturers can provide similar flow charts or process diagrams for fire and emergency service organizations to follow

SCBA Fire Service Purchase

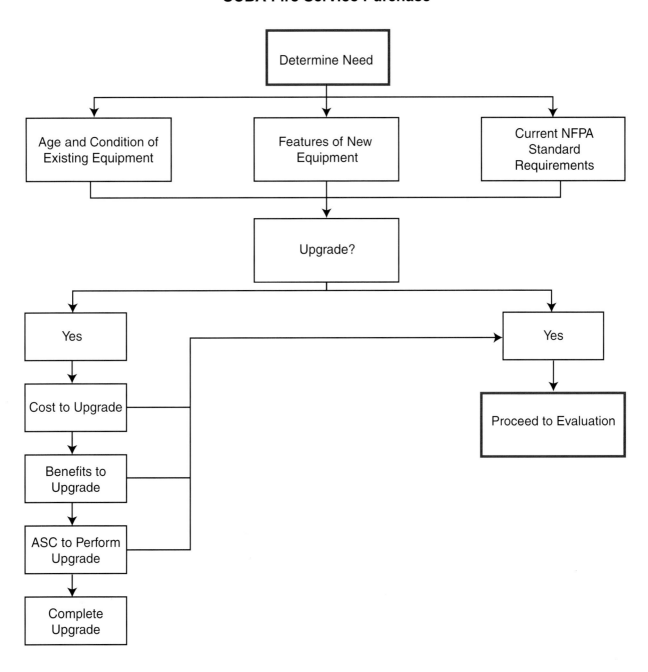

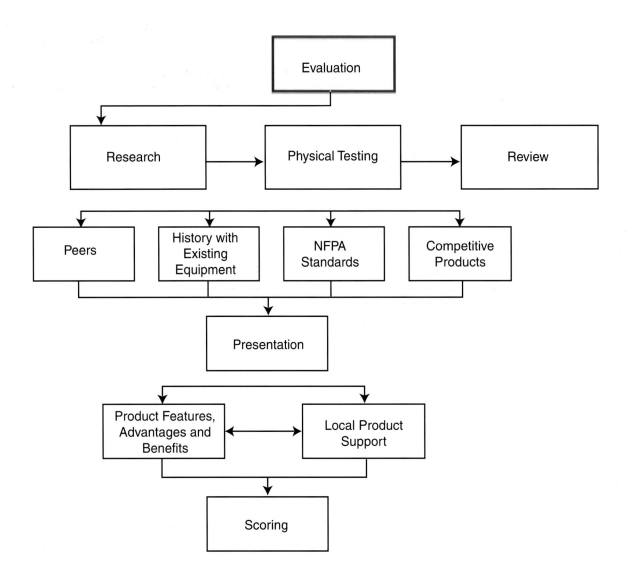

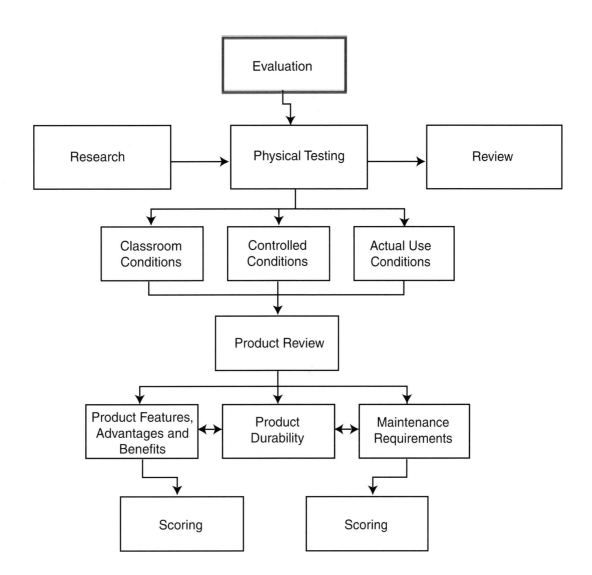

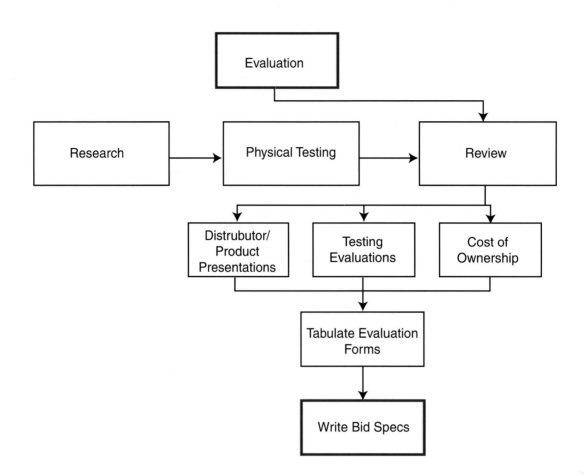

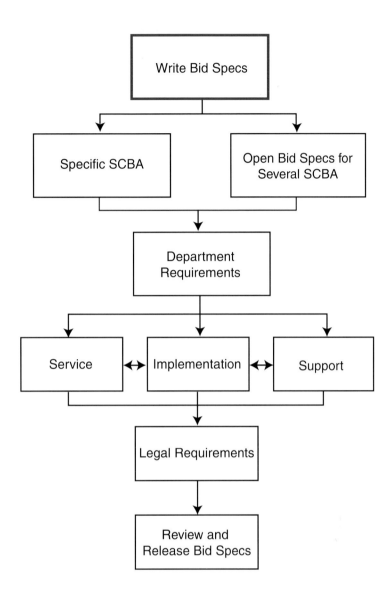

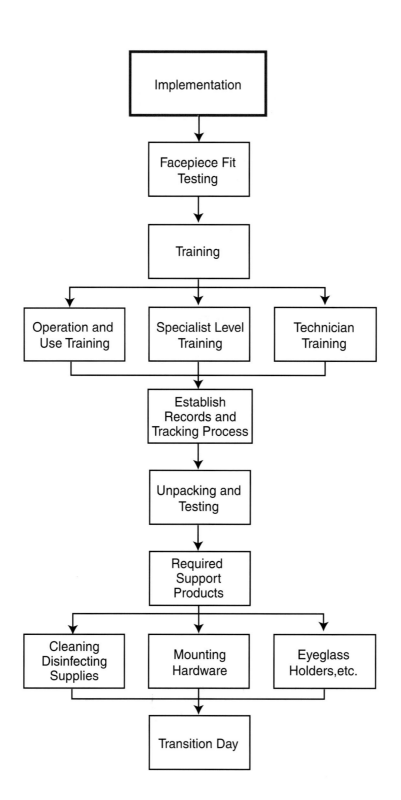

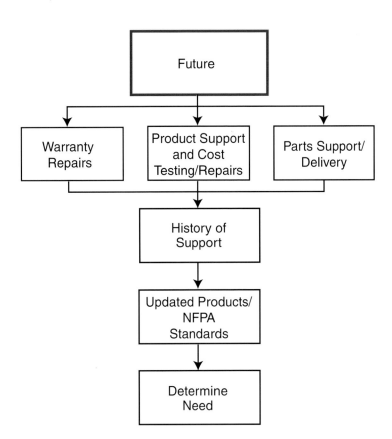

Appendix H
SCBA Survey Form

1. Primary Use Applications:

Fire fighting operations	Yes	No
Rescue operations	Yes	No
HAZ MAT operations	Yes	No
Other:	Yes	No

2. What features are most important for new SCBA?

NFPA compliance	Yes	No
Capable of future NFPA upgrade	Yes	No
Comfort	Yes	No
Communications	Yes	No
Individual facepiece and sizes	Yes	No
Electronic features	Yes	No
Low lifecycle cost	Yes	No
Ease of use while wearing protective clothing	Yes	No
Ease of cleaning/disinfecting	Yes	No
Proven performance	Yes	No
Distributor service and support	Yes	No
SCBA warranty	Yes	No
SCBA maintenance requirements	Yes	No

3. SCBA working pressure:

4 500 psig cylinders: • Lighter weight • Low profile • Choice of duration (30-45-60 minutes) 2 216 psig cylinders: • Lightweight (Composite cylinders) • Refill capability – cascade vs. compressor	4 500 psig	2 216 psig
Fill station capability	4 500 psig	2 216 psig

4. What accessory options are important?

Integrated PASS alarms	Yes	No
Buddy-breathing capabilities	Yes	No
Airline capabilities for extended duration – HAZ MAT/Confined space	Yes	No
Rapid cylinder refill option	Yes	No
Communications	Yes	No
• Amplification	Yes	No
• Radio interface	Yes	No

5. How many SCBA are required?

Total number of SCBA required	
Total number of spare cylinders required	
Rated duration: 30 Minute	
45 Minute (4 500 psig)	
60 Minute (4 500 psig)	

6. How will the department pay for this purchase?

Cash purchase	Yes	No
Lease-purchase options	Yes	No
• City/county/township finance	Yes	No
• Vendor finance programs	Yes	No
Other:	Yes	No

7. How many different SCBA will be considered?

Scott Air-Pak 2.2	Yes	No
Scott Air-Pak 3.0	Yes	No
Scott Air-Pak 4.5	Yes	No
MSA MMR	Yes	No
Survivair Panther	Yes	No
Draeger	Yes	No
ISI Viking	Yes	No
Interspiro	Yes	No

8. Which SCBA distributors will be considered?

Distributor	Contact Person and Phone	SCBA Supplied

9. Who will provide SCBA training after purchase?

SCBA distributor	Yes	No
Department training officer	Yes	No

10. Who will provide service and testing of SCBA after purchase?

SCBA distributor	Yes	No
Department personnel	Yes	No

11. Who will initiate SCBA?

Record format	Department	Distributor
SCBA identification	Department	Distributor
Facepiece fit testing and records	Department	Distributor

12. Will current SCBA be:

Kept for backup/training?	Yes	No
Traded in to offset purchase price?	Yes	No
Disposed of by SCBA distributor?	Yes	No
Sold by department?	Yes	No
Donated by department?	Yes	No

Appendix I
Sample Request for Proposal

Introduction

The _____Department is pursuing the evaluation and subsequent purchase of SCBA. To accomplish this, the department is requesting SCBA meeting the specifications shown in this request for proposal.

Through each of the major steps of the evaluation process, the SCBA evaluated will be assigned points based on a point system in the categories as follows:

SCBA Provider Support	30 points
Actual and/or Simulated Use Conditions	35 points
Classroom/Maintenance	35 points

Throughout the evaluation process each evaluation team member will review the features of the SCBA submitted and complete an evaluation form. The forms will be tabulated and totaled in each category.

The evaluation process will begin with distributor presentations and training of firefighters who are assigned to evaluate the SCBA. At the time of the presentation, the supplier must submit _____ SCBA meeting the specifications shown in this request for proposal and at least one spare cylinder for each SCBA to be used by the department for the evaluation period.

Each supplier is requested to complete the attached questionnaire and return it to:

_____

(Department Contact Person and Address)

The completed questionnaire should be returned no later than_____.

Pre-Qualification Questionnaire

All questions will be answered in detail on a separate sheet.

1. Location of Corporate/Business Headquarters:

    Company Name:
    Street:
    City, State, Zip:
    Phone:
    FAX:
    SCBA Supplied:

2. Location of the nearest office or distribution center with repair capabilities. Prompt facilitation of repairs will be a critical factor in pre-qualification. Describe in this section your ability to effectively perform maintenance service and repair functions.

    Company Name:
    Name of Person in Charge:
    Street:
    City, State, Zip:
    Phone:
    FAX:

3. Provide contact individuals, titles, and phone numbers of persons within your organization who will be responsible for supporting the department through the evaluation process as well as subsequent use and maintenance of SCBA.

4. How long has your firm been in the business of supplying SCBA and service?

5. What major fire department or industrial SCBA owner does your firm currently support? How many SCBA does this department/company own? How long has your firm supported this customer?

6. Indicate the approximate number of self-contained breathing apparatus sold during each of the past two years.

7. Indicate the approximate number of self-contained breathing apparatus overhauled/serviced during each of the past two years.

8. Will you furnish a finance program for this purchase? If so, include details of program.

9. Indicate if you will provide facepiece fit testing, equipment identification, and record format. Please provide details of how each process is conducted.

10. Will you furnish a written guarantee that sufficient replacement apparatus and/or replacement parts and components will be available at your facility if requested within a minimum 24-hour period?

11. Will your firm provide support including training and technical information for the evaluation units and subsequent purchased SCBA?

12. Will you provide a written copy of the manufacturer's warranty on the entire SCBA unit? State length of standard warranty and portions of unit covered as well as all requirements for the department to remain within warranty compliance.

13. Provider must state estimated ability to meet current and future NFPA standards.

14. Include any information that may be of interest to the _____ Department in this process.

15. Prospective provider must submit "Current Customer Profile" to allow the _____ Department full range of communication with current distributor customers.

Appendix J
Equipment Evaluation Form

Rank_____Name_____

Date_____Location_____

        (1) Strongly Disagree
        (2) Disagree
        (3) No Opinion or Not Applicable
        (4) Agree
        (5) Strongly Agree

1. The SCBA was easy to don.   1   2   3   4   5

_____

2. After donning, the SCBA fit comfortably.   1   2   3   4   5

_____

3. The facepiece is easy to don.   1   2   3   4   5

_____

4. The facepiece and head harness do not interfere
    with head protection.   1   2   3   4   5

_____

5. It is easy to breathe with the regulator undocked
    from the facepiece.   1   2   3   4   5

_____

6. The regulator is easy to dock/undock and
    remains secure.   1   2   3   4   5

_____

7. It is easy to breathe with air flowing.   1   2   3   4   5

_____

8. The purge/bypass is easy to operate.   1   2   3   4   5

_____

9. It is easy to determine when *my* PASS device activates.   1   2   3   4   5

_____

10. The PASS device is easy to reset.   1   2   3   4   5

_____

11. I felt balanced wearing the SCBA while:
     A. Walking   1   2   3   4   5
     B. Climbing ladder   1   2   3   4   5
     C. Crawling   1   2   3   4   5
     D. While raising arms and pulling   1   2   3   4   5

_____

12. The air-pressure gauge is easy to read.   1   2   3   4   5

_____

13. The low-air alarm is easy to hear and identify.   1   2   3   4   5

_____

14. The cylinder valve is easy to turn off.   1   2   3   4   5

_____

15. The cylinder is easy to change.   1   2   3   4   5

_____

16. Communication is clear with the facepiece on.   1   2   3   4   5

_____

17. The communication system is clear.   1   2   3   4   5

_____

Total Points _____/ 100 possible

Appendix K
Donning and Doffing Procedures for SCBA Respirators

Fire and emergency services personnel must be able to don and doff self-contained breathing apparatus quickly and correctly. Several general methods of donning the backpack can be used, depending upon how the SCBA is stored. These methods include the following

- Over-the-head
- Regular or cross-armed coat
- Donning from a seat
- Side or rear mount
- Compartment or backup mount

The steps for donning differ with each method, but once the SCBA is on the body, the method of securing the unit is the same. Methods for donning the facepiece differ, depending upon the manufacturer and whether the regulator is harness-mounted or facepiece-mounted.

The procedures in this appendix are intended to be general in nature. Fire and emergency services personnel should be aware that there are different steps for donning different makes and models. Therefore, the instructions given in this appendix should be adapted to the specific type of SCBA used. Always follow the manufacturer's instructions when donning, doffing, and operating SCBA.

Donning the Open-Circuit SCBA

Because many fire and emergency services personnel prefer to don the SCBA backpack first and then the facepiece, procedures for donning the backpack are covered in this section. Methods for donning different types of facepieces are covered in the section that follows.

Donning the Backpack

The donning methods for the over-the-head, cross-armed coat, regular coat, seat mount, side or rear mount, and compartment or backup mount are described in the sections that follow.

Over-the-Head Method

SCBA stored in carrying cases must be stored ready to don. The backpack straps should be arranged so that they do not interfere with grasping the cylinder. The emergency responder should put on the protective hood, pull it back, button the turnout coat, and turn the collar up so that the shoulder straps do not hold the collar down. The procedures for donning a backpack using the over-the-head method are as follows:

Step 1: Check the unit.

a. Crouch or kneel at the end opposite the cylinder valve, regardless of whether the unit is in its case or on the ground.

b. Check the cylinder gauge to make sure that the air cylinder is full. Open the cylinder valve slowly and listen for the audible alarm as the system pressurizes. Then, open the cylinder valve fully. If the audible alarm does not sound, or if it sounds but does not stop, place the unit out of service by tagging it and notifying an officer or supervisor; use another unit.

c. Check the regulator gauge. Both the cylinder and regulator gauges should register within 10 percent of each other when the cylinder is pressurized to its rated capacity (**Figure K.1**). If increments are in other measurements, such as fractions or minutes, they should correspond. If the unit has a donning switch (for units with facepiece-mounted regulators), leave the cylinder valve open and the unit in the donning mode. If the unit is positive pressure only, refer to the manufacturer's instructions concerning the cylinder valve.

Step 2: Spread the harness straps out to their respective sides.

Step 3: Grasp the backplate or cylinder with both hands, one at each side (**Figure K.2**). Make sure that the cylinder valve is pointed away from you. There should be no straps between the hands.

Step 4: Lift the cylinder, and let the regulator and harness hang freely (**Figure K.3**).

Step 5: Stand and raise the cylinder overhead; let the elbows find their respective loosened harness shoulder strap loops (**Figure K.4**). Keeping elbows close to the body, tuck the chin and grasp the shoulder straps as the SCBA begins to slide down the back. Let the straps slide through the hands as the backpack lowers into place.

Step 6: Lean forward to balance the cylinder on the back and partially tighten the shoulder straps by pulling them outward and downward (**Figure K.5**).

NOTE: It is sometimes necessary to lean forward with a quick jumping motion to properly position the SCBA on the back while tightening the straps.

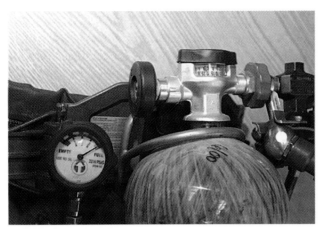

Figure K.1 Pressure gauges on the regulator and cylinder should register within 10 percent of each other when the cylinder is fully pressurized.

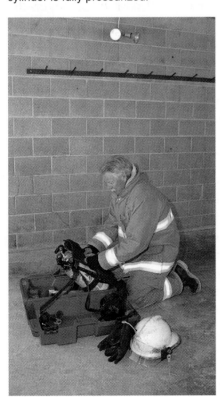

Figure K.2 With straps spread, grasp the cylinder through the shoulder straps, and lift it from the case.

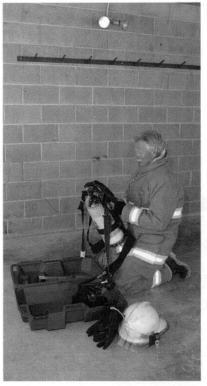

Figure K.3 Lift the cylinder, allowing the regulator and harness to hang freely.

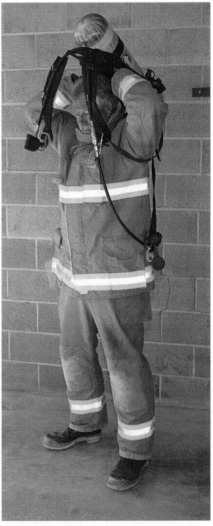

Figure K.4 Stand and raise the cylinder overhead, allowing the shoulder straps to fall outside the arms.

Step 7: Continue leaning forward on units equipped with chest straps, and then fasten the chest buckle if the unit has a chest strap.

NOTE: Depending upon the emergency responder's physique, it may be more comfortable to fasten the chest buckle before tightening the shoulder straps.

Step 8: Fasten and adjust the waist strap until the unit fits snugly (**Figure K.6**).

Step 9: Don the facepiece.

NOTE: This procedure is covered in the Donning the Facepiece section.

WARNING!

Some emergency services organizations have removed waist straps from SCBA. Without a waist strap fastened, the SCBA wearer suffers undue stress from side-to-side shifting of the unit and improper weight distribution of the unit. Even more important, removing waist straps permits the SCBA to be used in a nonapproved manner, which may violate NIOSH certification of the equipment and void the manufacturer's warranty.

Cross-Armed Coat Method

Self-contained breathing apparatus can be donned like a coat. The equipment should be arranged so that both shoulder straps can be grasped for lifting. Use the following steps:

Step 1: Check the unit.

　a. Crouch or kneel at the cylinder valve end of the unit, regardless of whether the unit is in its case or on the ground.

　b. Check the cylinder gauge to make sure that the air cylinder is full (**Figure K.7**). Open the cylinder valve slowly and listen for the audible alarm as the system pressurizes. Then, open the cylinder valve fully. If the audible alarm does

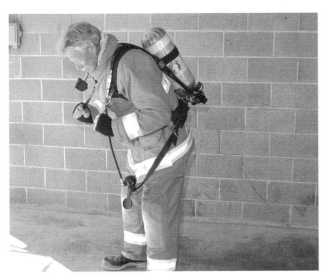

Figure K.5 Lean forward for balance and partially tighten the shoulder straps by pulling outward and downward.

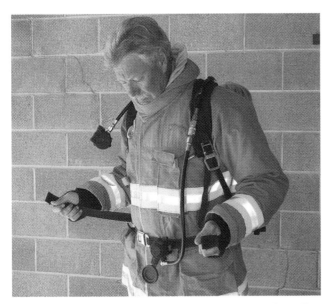

Figure K.6 Fasten and adjust the waist strap. Readjust all other straps until the unit fits snugly.

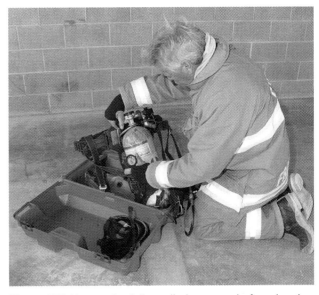

Figure K.7 Always check the cylinder gauge before donning the SCBA. Open the valve fully before donning the unit.

not sound, or if it sounds but does not stop, place the unit out of service by tagging it and notifying an officer or supervisor; use another unit.

c. Check the regulator gauge. Both the cylinder and regulator gauges should register within 10 percent of each other when the cylinder is pressurized to its rated capacity. If increments are in other measurements, such as fractions or minutes, they should correspond. If the unit has a donning switch, leave the cylinder valve open and the unit in the donning mode. If the unit is positive pressure only, refer to the manufacturer's instructions concerning the cylinder valve.

Step 2: Spread the harness straps out to their respective sides. Cross the arms, left over right. Grasp the shoulder straps at the top of the harness, left hand holding the left strap and right hand holding the right strap (**Figure K.8**).

Step 3: Stand and lift the SCBA. Using both arms, swing the unit around the right shoulder, and raising the left arm, continue bringing the unit behind the head and onto the back. Both hands should still be grasping the shoulder straps high on the harness (**Figures K.9, K.10,** and **K.11**).

Step 4: Slide the hands down the straps to the shoulder strap buckles, maintaining a firm grip on the straps. The elbows should be between the straps and the backpack.

Step 5: Lean slightly forward to balance the cylinder on the back; tighten the shoulder straps by pulling them outward and downward.

NOTE: It is sometimes necessary to lean forward with a quick jumping motion to properly position the SCBA on the back while tightening the straps.

Step 6: Continue leaning forward, and fasten the chest buckle if the unit has a chest strap.

NOTE: It may be necessary to fasten the chest strap before completely tightening the shoulder straps.

Step 7: Fasten and adjust the waist strap until the unit fits snugly (**Figure K.12**).

Step 8: Recheck all straps to see that they are correctly adjusted.

Step 9: Don the facepiece.

NOTE: This procedure is covered in the Donning the Facepiece section.

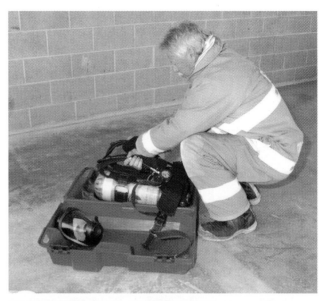

Figure K.8 Kneel and grasp the shoulder straps with arms crossed, left over right.

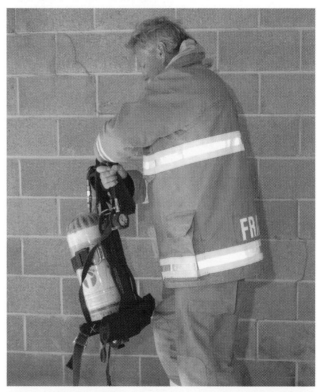

Figure K.9 While rising to a standing position, lift the SCBA, keeping wrists together.

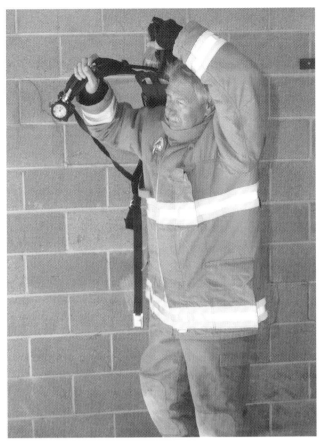

Figure K.10 Swing unit around the right shoulder, allowing wrists to separate.

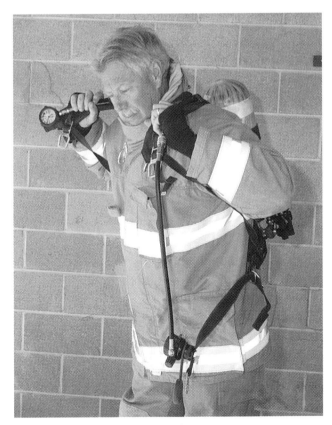

Figure K.11 Guide unit onto back.

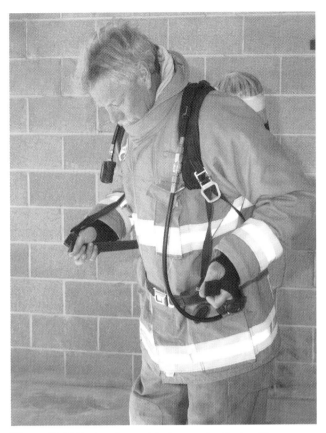

Figure K.12 Fasten the waist strap and adjust until snug.

Regular Coat Method

Self-contained breathing apparatus can be donned like a coat, putting one arm at a time through the shoulder strap loops. The unit should be arranged so that either shoulder strap can be grasped for lifting. Use the following steps:

Step 1: Check the unit.

    a. Crouch or kneel at the cylinder valve end of the unit, regardless of whether the unit is in its case or on the ground.

    b. Check the cylinder gauge to make sure that the air cylinder is full. Open the cylinder valve slowly and listen for the audible alarm as the system pressurizes. Then, open the cylinder valve fully. If the audible alarm does not sound, or if it sounds but does not stop, place the unit out of service by tagging and notifying an officer or supervisor; use another unit.

    c. Check the regulator gauge. Both the cylinder and regulator gauges should register within 10 percent of each other when the cylinder is pressurized to its rated capacity. If increments are in other measurements, such as fractions or minutes, they should correspond. If the unit has a donning switch, leave the cylinder valve open and the unit in the donning mode. If the unit is positive pressure only, refer to the manufacturer's instructions concerning the cylinder valve.

Step 2: Spread the straps out to their respective sides, and position the upper portion of the straps over the top of the backplate.

NOTE: By doing this, the straps are less likely to fall, and the arms can go through the straps with less difficulty.

NOTE: This procedure is written for those harnesses having the regulator attached to the left side of the harness. There are some SCBA that have the regulator mounted on the right. For these types, the right strap should be grasped with the right hand, and the backpack should be donned following the instructions in the next steps, but using directions opposite those indicated.

Step 3: Grasp the left strap with the left hand at the top of the harness. Grasp the lower portion of the same strap with the right hand (**Figure K.13**).

NOTE: When kneeling at the cylinder valve end, the left harness strap will be to the right hand.

Step 4: Lift the unit; swing it around the left shoulder and onto the back. Both hands should still be grasping the shoulder strap (**Figure K.14**).

Step 5: Continue to hold the strap with the left hand; release the right hand and insert the right arm between the right shoulder strap and the backpack frame.

Step 6: Lean slightly forward to balance the cylinder on the back; tighten the shoulder straps by pulling them outward and downward.

NOTE: It is sometimes necessary to lean forward with a quick jumping motion to properly position the SCBA on the back while tightening the straps.

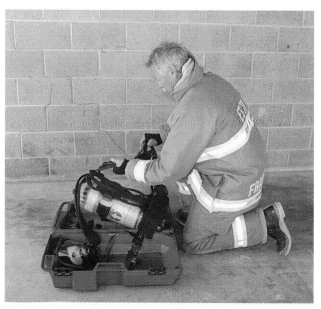

Figure K.13 Grasp the top of the left shoulder strap with the left hand. Grasp the lower part of the same strap with the right hand.

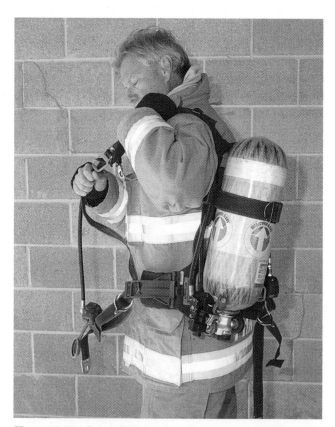

Figure K.14 Lift the SCBA by the straps and swing the unit around the left shoulder and onto the back while maintaining a firm grasp of the straps.

Step 7: Continue leaning forward, and fasten the chest buckle if the unit has a chest strap. Tighten the shoulder straps further if necessary.

Step 8: Fasten and adjust the waist strap until the unit fits snugly.

Step 9: Recheck all straps to see that they are correctly adjusted.

Step 10: Don the facepiece.

NOTE: This procedure is covered in the Donning the Facepiece section.

Seat Mount

Valuable time can be saved if the SCBA is mounted on the back of the emergency responder's seat in the vehicle (**Figure K.15**). By having a seat mount, fire and emergency services personnel can don SCBA while en route to an incident. If the SCBA is not needed upon arrival, it can be removed quickly and remain mounted in its support.

Seat-mounting hardware comes in three main types: lever clamp, spring clamp, or flat hook. A drawstring or other quick-opening bag should enclose the facepiece to keep it clean and to protect it from dust and scratches.

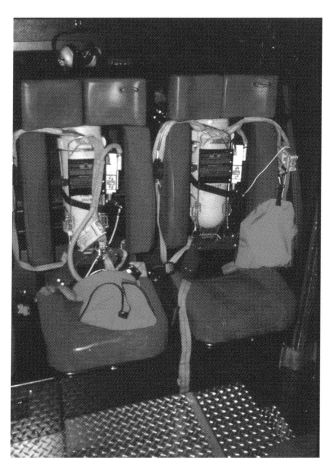

Figure K.15 Seat-mounted SCBA are shown in the fire fighting vehicle.

NOTE: Do not keep the facepiece hooked to the regulator during storage. These parts must be separate to check for proper facepiece seal.

Donning en route is done by inserting the arms through the straps while sitting with the seat belt on, then adjusting the straps for a snug fit (**Figures K.16** and **K.17**).

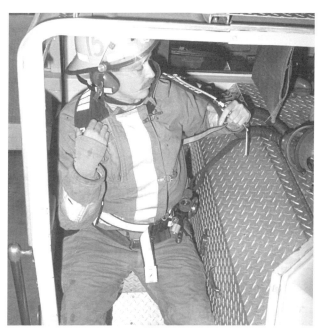

Figure K.16 Donning en route, the firefighter inserts both arms through the straps and carefully connects the waist belt to avoid entanglement with the seat belt.

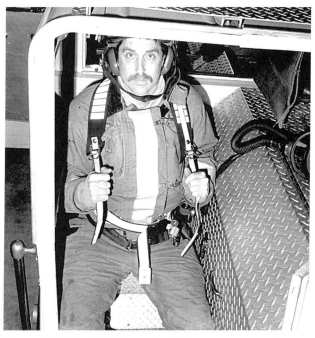

Figure K.17 The firefighter adjusts the straps as snugly as possible while seated. Upon leaving the apparatus, straps may be adjusted again as necessary.

The cylinder's position should match the proper wearing position for the emergency responder. The visible seat-mounted SCBA reminds and even encourages personnel to check the equipment more frequently. Because it is exposed, checks can be made more conveniently. Be sure to adjust the straps for a snug and comfortable fit when exiting the fire apparatus.

Side or Rear Mount

Although it does not permit donning en route, the side- or rear-mounted SCBA may be desirable. Time is saved because the steps needed to remove the equipment case from the fire apparatus, place it on the ground, open the case, and pick up the unit are eliminated. Current apparatus designs include mounting brackets inside weatherproof compartments (**Figure K.18**). However if the unit is mounted on the exterior of the apparatus, it will be exposed to weather and physical damage, in which case a canvas cover is desirable.

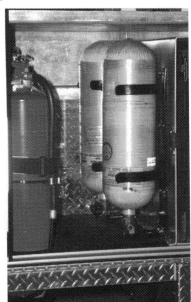

Figure K.18 In addition to storage for complete SCBA units, compartment brackets may also be used for storing spare breathing-air cylinders like the ones shown.

If the mounting height is correct, fire and emergency services personnel can don SCBA with little effort. Having the mount near the running boards or near the tailboard allows the emergency responder to don the equipment while sitting. The steps are essentially the same as those for seat-mounted SCBA.

Compartment or Backup Mount

SCBA stored in a closed compartment can be ready for rapid donning by using any number of mounts (**Figure K.19**). A mount on the inside of a compartment presents the same advantage, as does side-mounted equipment. Some compartment doors, however, may not allow an emergency responder to stand fully while donning SCBA. Other compartments may be too high for the emergency responder to don the SCBA properly.

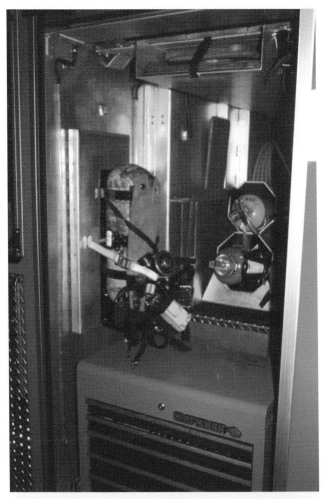

Figure K.19 These SCBA are stored in a closed compartment. While providing good protection, this compartment may not be the correct height for proper donning.

Other compartment mounts feature a telescoping frame that holds the equipment out of the way inside the compartment when it is not needed (**Figure K.20**). One type of compartment mount telescopes outward, then upward or downward to proper height for quick donning.

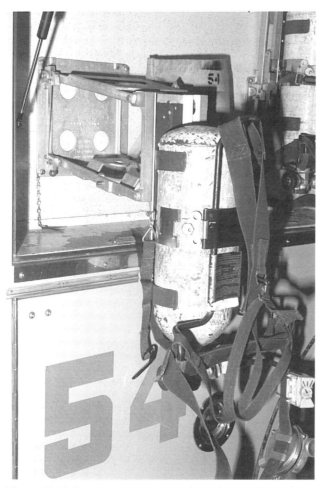

Figure K.20 A compartment mount featuring a telescoping frame to hold the equipment inside the compartment provides the proper height for donning.

The backup mount provides quick access to SCBA. Some high-mounted SCBA must be removed from the vehicle and donned using the over-the-head or coat method. The procedures for donning SCBA using the backup method, with slight variation for mounts from which the SCBA can be donned while seated, are as follows:

Step 1: Uncover the SCBA. Remove the facepiece and place it nearby.

Step 2: Check the unit.

    a. Open the cylinder valve slowly and listen for the audible alarm as the system pressurizes. Open the cylinder valve fully. If the audible alarm does not sound, or if it sounds but does not stop, place the unit out of service by tagging it and notifying an officer or supervisor; use another unit.

    b. Check the regulator gauge. Both the cylinder and regulator gauges should register within 10 percent of each other when the cylinder is pressurized to its rated capacity. If increments are in other measurements, such as fractions or minutes, they should correspond. If the unit has a donning switch, leave the cylinder valve open and the unit in the donning mode. If the unit is positive pressure only, refer to the manufacturer's instructions concerning the cylinder valve.

Step 3: Back up against the cylinder backplate, and place the arms through the harness straps (**Figure K.21**). While leaning slightly forward to balance the unit on the back, release the cylinder according to the kind of mounting device.

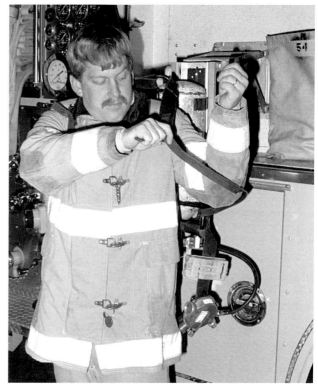

Figure K.21 Back up against the cylinder backplate, and place the arms through the harness straps.

Step 4: Step forward to clear the unit from the mount while fastening the chest buckle if the unit has a chest strap.

Step 5: Tighten the shoulder straps (**Figure K.22**).

Step 6: Fasten and adjust the waist strap until the unit fits snugly (**Figure K.23**).

Step 7: Don the facepiece.

NOTE: Donning the facepiece is covered in the following section.

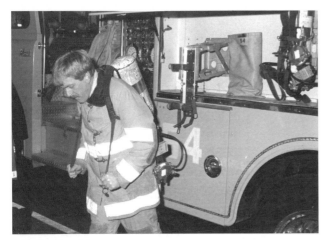

Figure K.22 With a slight jerk, pull the SCBA away from the bracket. Tighten the shoulder straps.

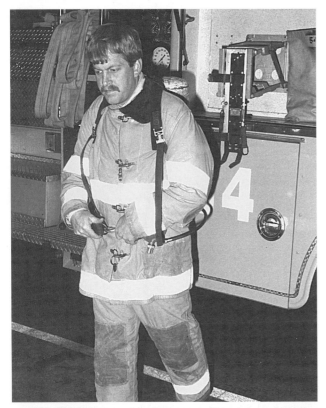

Figure K.23 Fasten and adjust the waist strap until the unit fits snugly.

Donning the Facepiece

The facepieces for most SCBA are donned similarly. One important difference in facepieces is the number of straps used to tighten the head harness (**Figure K.24**). Different models from the same manufacturer may have a different number of straps. Another important difference is the location of the regulator. The regulator may be attached to the facepiece or mounted on the waist belt. The shape and size of facepiece lenses may also differ. Despite these variations, the uses and donning procedures for facepieces are essentially the same.

> # WARNING!
> **Interchanging facepieces or any other part of the SCBA from one manufacturer's equipment to another voids any warranty and NIOSH certification.**

An SCBA facepiece cannot be worn loosely or it cannot seal against the face properly. An improper seal may permit toxic gases to enter the facepiece and be inhaled. Fire and emergency services personnel should not let long hair, sideburns, or mustaches interfere with the outer edges of the facepiece, thus preventing contact and a proper seal with the skin. OSHA and NFPA prohibit any facial hair, eyeglass frames, or other obstructions that might interfere with a complete seal.

An emergency responder should not rely solely on tightening facepiece straps to ensure proper

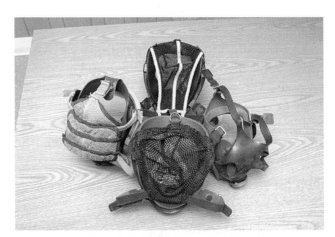

Figure K.24 Two types of head harnesses are depicted — a nylon mesh or hairnet model and a traditional style with five straps, sometimes referred to as a web-type harness.

facepiece fit. A facepiece tightened too much is uncomfortable and may cut off circulation to the face. Each emergency responder must be fitted with a facepiece that conforms properly to the face shape and size. For this reason, many SCBA are available with different-sized facepieces (**Figure K.25**). Nose cups, if used, must also properly fit the emergency responder.

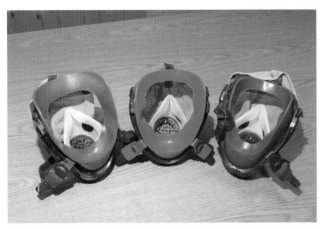

Figure K.25 To meet the requirements for complete facepiece-to-face seal, manufacturers provide respiratory protection facepieces in a variety of sizes.

Harness-Mounted Regulator

The facepiece for an SCBA with a harness-mounted regulator has a low-pressure hose, or breathing tube, attached to the facepiece with clamps or threaded coupling nuts. The facepiece may be packed in a case or stored in a bag or coat pouch. Wherever it is stored, the straps should be left fully extended for donning ease and to keep the facepiece from becoming distorted. The procedures for donning a facepiece having a low-pressure hose are as follows:

Step 1: Pull the protective hood back and down so that the face opening is around the neck. Turn up the collar of the turnout coat.

Step 2: If the harness is a web-type, grasp the harness with the thumbs through the straps from the inside and spread the straps (**Figure K.26**).

Step 3: Push the top of the harness up the forehead to remove hair that may be present between the forehead and the sealing surface of the facepiece (**Figure K.27**).

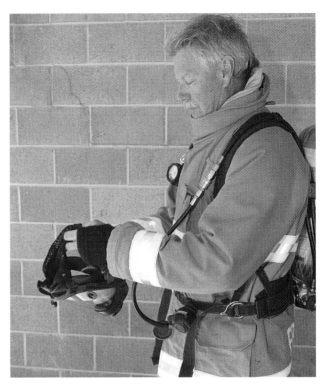

Figure K.26 When donning a web-type head harness, grasp the harness with the thumbs through the straps from the inside and spread the straps.

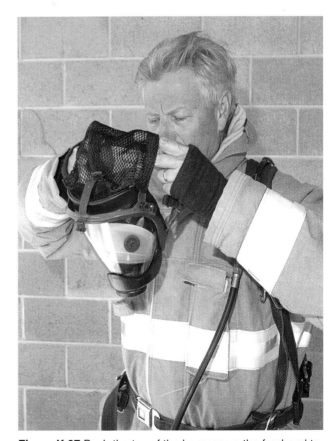

Figure K.27 Push the top of the harness up the forehead to remove hair that may be present between the forehead and the sealing surface of the facepiece. The web is contacting the forehead.

Step 4: Center the chin in the chin cup and position the harness so that it is centered at the rear of the head (**Figure K.28**).

Step 5: Tighten the harness straps by pulling them evenly and simultaneously to the rear. Pulling the straps outward, to the sides, may damage them and prevents proper engagement with the adjusting buckles. Tighten the lower straps first, then the temple straps, and finally the top strap if there is one (**Figure K.29**).

Step 6: Check the facepiece seal. Exhale deeply, seal the end of the low-pressure hose with a bare hand, and inhale slowly (not deeply) (**Figure K.30**). Hold the breath for 10 seconds. This action allows the facepiece to collapse tightly against the face. If there is evidence of leaking, adjust or redon the facepiece.

NOTE: Inhaling very quickly temporarily seals any leak and gives a false sense of a proper seal.

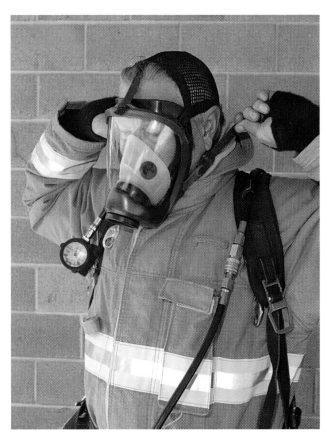

Figure K.29 Tighten the straps evenly and simultaneously, starting with the lower straps.

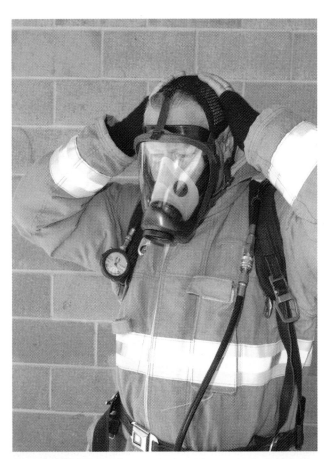

Figure K.28 Center the chin in the chin cup and position the harness so that it is centered at the rear of the head.

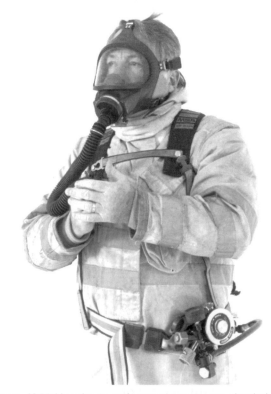

Figure K.30 Use the negative-pressure test to check the facepiece seal by sealing the low-pressure hose and inhaling slowly.

Step 7: Check the exhalation valve. Inhale, seal the end of the low-pressure hose, and exhale. If the exhalation does not go through the exhalation valve, keep the low-pressure hose sealed, press the facepiece against the face, and exhale to free the valve. Use caution when exhaling against a sealed facepiece in order to prevent discomfort and possible damage to the inner ear from exhaling forcefully. If the exhalation valve does not become free, remove the facepiece and have it checked.

Step 8: Put on the helmet, first inserting the low-pressure hose through the helmet's chin strap. The helmet should rest on the shoulder until the SCBA is completely donned.

> **NOTE:** Helmets with straps that completely disconnect may be donned as a last step.

Step 9: Connect the low-pressure hose to the regulator. If the unit has a donning switch, turn it to the PRESSURE, USE, or ON position. If the unit does not have a donning switch, open the mainline valve.

Step 10: Check for positive pressure. Gently break the facepiece seal by inserting two fingers under the edge of the facepiece. Air should be felt moving past the fingers. If air movement is not felt, remove the unit and have it checked.

Step 11: Pull the protective hood into place, making sure that all exposed skin is covered and that vision is not obscured (**Figure K.31**). Check to see that no portion of the hood is located between the facepiece and the face.

Step 12: Place the helmet on the head and tighten the chin strap (**Figures K.32** and **K.33**).

An alternative method is to wear the helmet while donning the SCBA. After donning the backpack, loosen the chin strap, allow the helmet to rest on the air cylinder or on the shoulder, and then don the facepiece. When the facepiece straps have been tightened and the hood is on, lift the helmet back onto the head and tighten the chin strap.

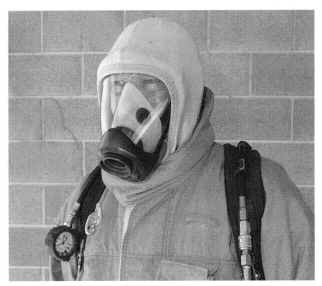

Figure K.31 Pull the protective hood into place, covering all exposed skin and being sure that vision is not obscured.

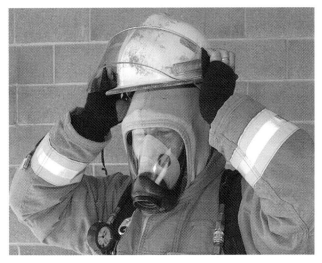

Figure K.32 Place the helmet on the head and ensure that the chin strap is under the chin and not tangled with the facepiece or hood.

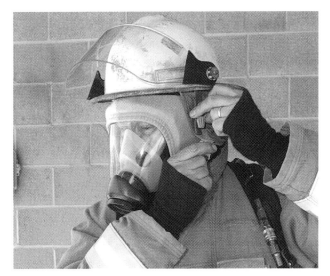

Figure K.33 Tighten the chin strap securely.

Facepiece-Mounted Regulator

Step 1: If using a protective hood, pull it back and down so that the face opening is around the neck. Turn up the collar of the turnout coat.

> **NOTE:** Depending upon the style of helmet used, it may be necessary to don the helmet now and allow it to rest on the shoulder.

Step 2: With the thumbs inserted through the straps, grasp the head harness and spread the webbing.

Step 3: Stabilize the facepiece with one hand, and use the other hand to remove hair that may be present between the forehead and the sealing surface of the facepiece.

Step 4: Center the chin in the chin cup and position the harness so that it is centered at the rear of the head.

Step 5: Tighten the harness straps by pulling them backward (not outward) evenly and simultaneously. Tighten the lower straps first, then the temple straps, and finally the top strap if there is one.

> **NOTE:** For two-strap harnesses, tighten the neck straps, and then stroke the harness firmly down the back of the head. Retighten the straps as necessary.

Step 6: Check the regulator to ensure that the gasket is in place around the regulator outlet port if the SCBA is so equipped.

Step 7: Attach the regulator to the facepiece (if is separated from the facepiece) by positioning it firmly into the facepiece fitting. Lock it into place (**Figure K.34**).

> **NOTE:** This procedure varies, depending upon the make of SCBA. Always follow the manufacturer's instructions.

Step 8: Check the facepiece seal. Make sure that the donning switch is in the DON position (positive pressure off). Inhale slowly (not deeply), and hold your breath for 10 seconds (**Figure K.35**). The mask should draw up to the face. Listen for the sound of airflow. There should be no sound and no

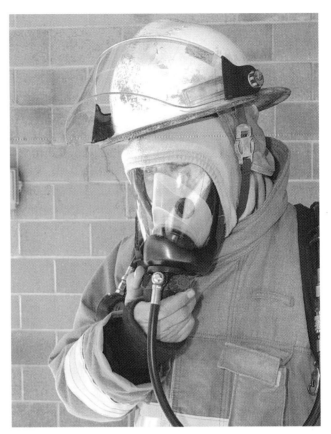

Figure K.34 If separated from the facepiece, attach regulator to the facepiece by positioning it firmly into the facepiece fitting and locking it in place.

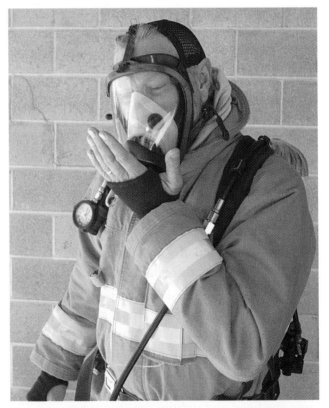

Figure K.35 Use negative-pressure test to check the facepiece seal by inhaling slowly and deeply for 10 seconds.

inward leakage through the exhalation valve or around the facepiece.

ALTERNATE METHOD: Another method for checking facepiece seal is to close the cylinder valve. Continue to breathe slowly until the mask collapses against the face, and hold the breath for 10 seconds. If the mask draws up to the face and no leaks are detected, reopen the cylinder valve. Adjust or redon the facepiece if there is evidence of leaking. If leakage persists, determine and correct the cause of the leakage. If unable to eliminate the leakage, obtain another facepiece and repeat the leak-check procedure. Use care with this method because it consumes some air.

Step 9: Check the exhalation valve. When exhaling during Step 8, make sure that the exhalation goes through the exhalation valve. If it does not, the valve may be stuck. To free it, press the facepiece against the sides of the face, and exhale to free the valve. Use caution when exhaling against a sealed facepiece in order to prevent discomfort and possible damage to the inner ear from exhaling forcefully. If the exhalation valve does not become free, remove the facepiece and have it checked.

Step 10: Check for positive pressure. Gently break the facepiece seal by inserting two fingers under the edge of the facepiece. Air should be felt moving past the fingers. If air movement is not felt, remove the unit and have it checked.

Step 11: Pull the protective hood into place, making sure that all exposed skin is covered and that vision is not obscured. Check to see that no portion of the hood is located between the facepiece and the face.

Step 12: Put the helmet back on the head and tighten the chin strap. Be sure to get the helmet strap under the chin.

NOTE: Helmets with a breakaway strap can be donned at this point.

ALTERNATE METHOD: An alternative method is to leave the helmet on while donning the backpack, then loosen the chin strap and allow the helmet to rest on the air cylinder while donning the facepiece.

Doffing the Open-Circuit SCBA

Steps are given in the following sections for both types of open-circuit SCBA: those with harness-mounted regulators and those with facepiece-mounted regulators.

Harness-Mounted Regulator

When you are in a safe atmosphere, take the following steps to remove SCBA having a harness-mounted regulator:

Step 1: Close the mainline valve and disconnect the low-pressure hose from the regulator.

NOTE: If the unit has a donning switch, make sure that it is in the donning mode.

Step 2: Take off the helmet or loosen it and push it and the hood back off the head (**Figure K.36**).

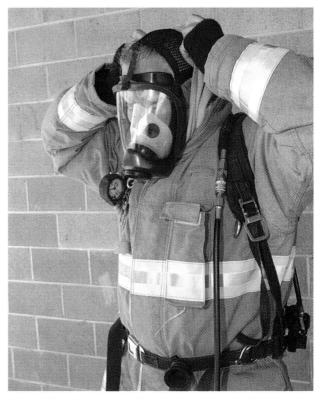

Figure K.36 Remove or slide the helmet back off the head and pull off the protective hood.

Step 3: Loosen the facepiece harness strap buckles. Either rub them toward the face or lift the buckles slightly to loosen them and to disentangle them from the hair (**Figure K.37**). Take off the facepiece, extend the harness straps fully, and prepare it for inspection, cleaning, sanitizing, and storage.

Step 4: Unbuckle the waist belt and fully extend the adjustment (**Figure K.38**).

Step 5: Disconnect the chest buckle if the unit has a chest strap.

Step 6: Lean forward; release shoulder strap buckles and hold them open while fully extending the straps (**Figure K.39**).

Step 7: Grasp the shoulder straps firmly with the respective hands. Slip off the shoulder strap from the shoulder opposite the regulator, and remove the arm from the shoulder strap. Grasp the regulator with the free hand, allow the other strap to slide off the shoulder, and lower the SCBA to the ground (**Figures K.40** and **K.41**). Do not drop the regulator or allow it to strike anything.

Step 8: Close the cylinder valve and then relieve the excess pressure from the regulator. If the regulator has been removed from the facepiece, recouple it, hold the facepiece against the face, and breathe until the remaining pressure is depleted. Another method is to open the mainline valve and allow the excess pressure to vent (**Figure K.42**).

NOTE: Do not use the bypass valve to relieve excess pressure.

Step 9: Remove the facepiece from the regulator and extend the straps fully. Prepare the facepiece for inspection, cleaning, sanitizing, and storage.

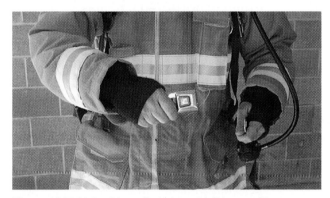

Figure K.38 Unbuckle waist belt and fully extend it.

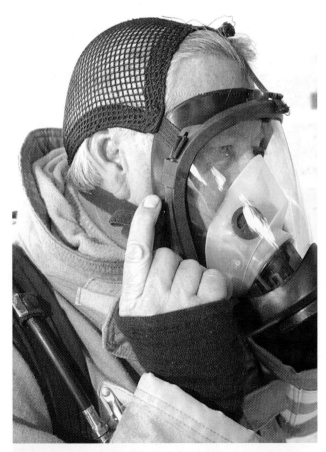

Figure K.37 Using the finger under the strap to maintain tension on the buckle, continue to rub the buckle using a scratching motion.

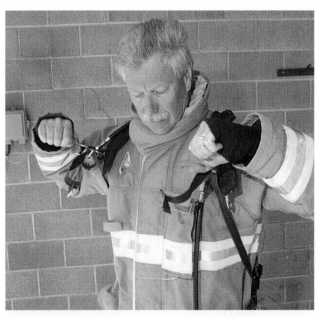

Figure K.39 Lean forward; release shoulder strap buckles and hold them open while extending the straps.

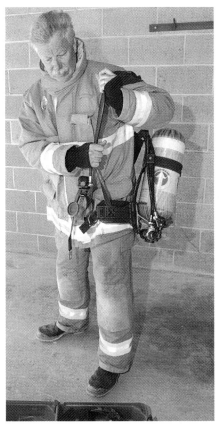

Figure K.40 Slip the shoulder strap from the shoulder opposite the regulator, and reach around to grasp the regulator with the free hand.

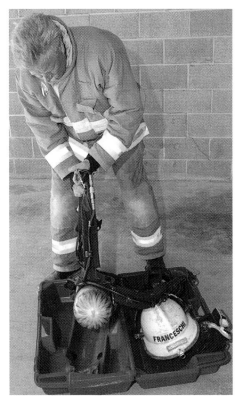

Figure K.41 Guide the SCBA to the ground while controlling the regulator.

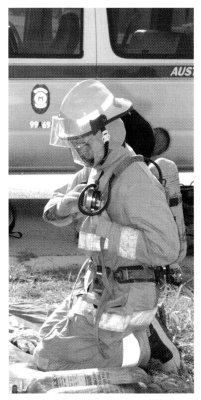

Figure K.42 Open the mainline valve to depressurize the system.

Facepiece-Mounted Regulator

When you are in a safe atmosphere, take the following steps to remove SCBA having a facepiece-mounted regulator:

Step 1: Take off the helmet or loosen it and push it and the hood back off the head.

Step 2: Turn the positive pressure off if the unit has a donning switch or place it in donning mode.

Step 3: Disconnect the regulator from the facepiece, depending upon the make of SCBA and the manufacturer's instructions.

Step 4: Loosen the facepiece harness strap buckles. Either rub them toward the face or lift the buckles slightly to loosen them. Take off the facepiece and prepare it for inspection, cleaning, sanitizing, and storage. Extend the harness straps fully.

Step 5: Unbuckle the waist belt and fully extend the adjustment.

Step 6: Disconnect the chest buckle if the unit has a chest strap.

Step 7: Attach the regulator to the harness clip if the unit is so equipped, or control the regulator by holding it while performing the next steps.

Step 8: Lean forward; release shoulder strap buckles and hold them open while fully extending the straps.

Step 9: Grasp the shoulder straps firmly with the respective hands. Slip off the shoulder strap from the shoulder opposite the regulator, and remove the arm from the shoulder strap. Grasp the regulator with the free hand, allow the other strap to slide off the shoulder, and lower the SCBA to the ground. Do not drop the regulator or allow it to strike anything.

Step 10: Close the cylinder valve and breathe down the pressure from the regulator by holding the facepiece against the face and breathing until the pressure is depleted.

NOTE: Do not bleed off air by operating the bypass valve.

Donning the Closed-Circuit SCBA

Donning a closed-circuit SCBA is basically the same as donning standard open-circuit models. However, there are differences in donning and using closed-circuit SCBA with which fire and emergency services personnel must be familiar.

The following steps may need to be adapted to the specific type of closed-circuit apparatus being used. Always refer to the manufacturer's instructions when donning and using SCBA. The inhalation and exhalation hoses must be kept sealed while the unit is stored. It is acceptable to store the unit with the facepiece hoses connected to the backpack hoses or with the hoses on the backpack connected to each other.

Step 1: Pull the protective hood (if used) back and down so that the face opening is around the neck (**Figure K.43**). Turn up the collar of the turnout coat.

Step 2: Check the turnaround maintenance tag. Never use a unit that does not have a completed maintenance tag attached (**Figure K.44**). Tear the turnaround maintenance tag from the oxygen cylinder and begin donning procedures.

Step 3: Place the unit on the ground, with the harness side up. Crouch or kneel so that the top is toward you, and fully extend the shoulder straps.

NOTE: If the unit has been stored with the low-pressure hoses connected to each other, they should be separated and attached to the facepiece at this time (**Figure K.45**).

Step 4: Spread out the shoulder straps.

Step 5: Grasp the body of the unit about 6 inches (150 mm) from its bottom, with the harness toward you and the top down, and lift (**Figure K.46**).

Step 6: Raise the unit over the head, and allow it to slide slowly down the back (**Figures K.47** and **K.48**). Place the arms through their respective straps.

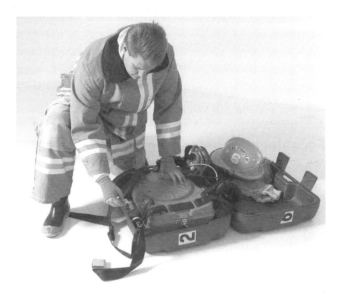

Figure K.44 Check the turnaround maintenance tag.

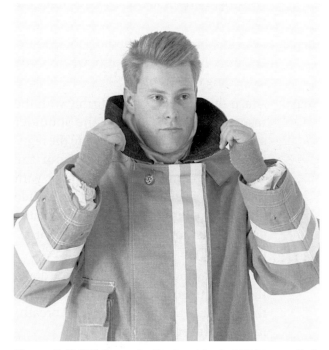

Figure K.43 Pull the protective hood back and down so that face opening is around the neck; turn up the coat collar.

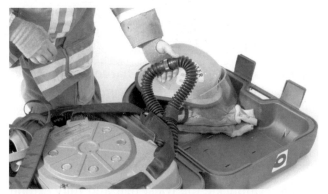

Figure K.45 Closed-circuit SCBA may be stored with the low-pressure hoses connected to each other.

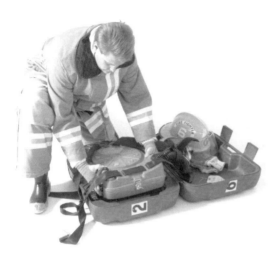

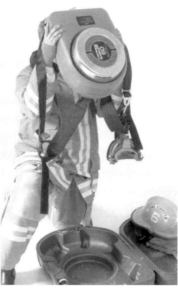

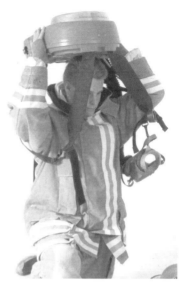

Figure K.46 With the harness toward the user and the top of the unit down, grasp the body of the unit about 6 inches (150 mm) from its bottom and lift.

Figure K.47 Lift the unit while allowing the harness to hang freely.

Figure K.48 With the elbows through the shoulder straps, allow the unit to slide down the back while firmly grasping the shoulder straps.

NOTE: This donning sequence is shown using the over-the-head method. The other methods described earlier in this chapter are also acceptable.

Step 7: Bend forward and grasp the free ends of the shoulder straps. Pull the straps outward and downward to tighten (**Figure K.49**).

Step 8: Secure the chest strap (**Figure K.50**).

Step 9: Fasten and adjust the waist strap (**Figure K.51**).

Step 10: Place the helmet over the head and let it drop onto the back, hanging by the chin strap. The helmet can then be placed back on the head after the facepiece has been donned.

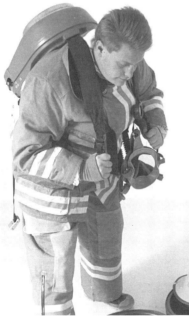

Figure K.49 Bend forward and grasp the free ends of the shoulder straps. Pull the straps outward and downward to tighten.

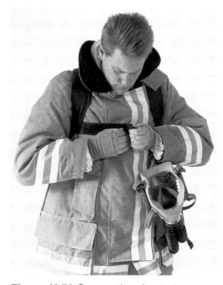

Figure K.50 Secure the chest strap.

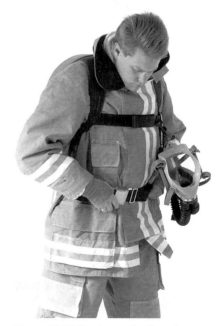

Figure K.51 Fasten and adjust the waist strap.

Step 11: Hold the facepiece about 1 inch (25 mm) from the face.

Step 12: Open the oxygen cylinder valve all the way and then turn the valve knob back one-half turn. Listen for a short chirp from the alarm whistle.

NOTE: This floods the facepiece with oxygen.

Step 13: Don the facepiece by holding the facepiece snugly against the chin and pulling the harness back so that it is centered at the back of the head. Tighten the chin straps, temple straps, and then the center strap (**Figures K.52** and **K.53**).

Step 14: Check the facepiece seal by tightly pinching the hoses closed and exhaling. Air escaping should not be heard or felt (**Figure K.54**).

NOTE: Pinching the hoses may require some effort.

Step 15: Momentarily open and close the bypass valve to be sure that it works. Close the bypass valve fully.

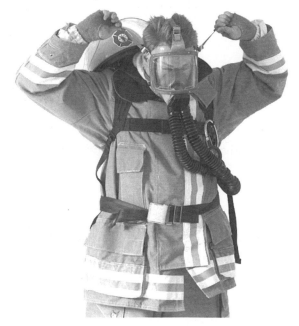

Figure K.53 Tighten the facepiece straps.

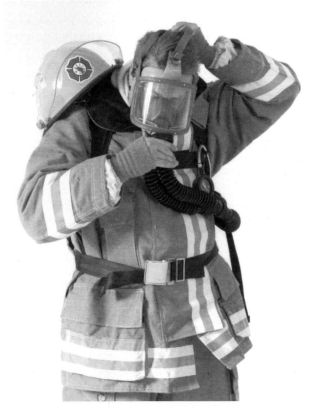

Figure K.52 Center the chin in chin cup and position harness so that it is centered at the rear of head.

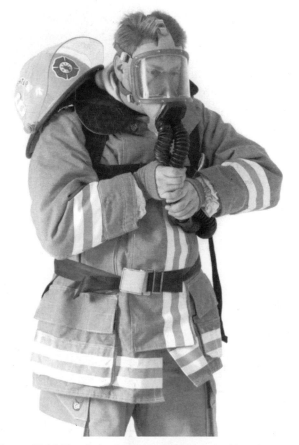

Figure K.54 Check the facepiece seal by pinching the hoses closed, inhaling, and exhaling. The user should not be able to hear or feel air escaping. Pinching the hoses on some models may require a lot of effort.

Step 16: Pull the protective hood into place, making sure that all exposed skin is covered and that vision is not obscured (**Figure K.55**).

Step 17: Place the helmet on the head and secure the chin strap under the chin (**Figure K.56**).

Step 18: Check the chest-mounted pressure gauge to verify cylinder pressure (**Figure K.57**).

An alternative method is to wear the helmet while donning the SCBA. After donning the backpack, loosen the chin strap, allow the helmet to rest on the air cylinder or on the shoulder, and then don the facepiece. When the facepiece straps have been tightened and the hood is on, lift the helmet back onto the head and tighten the chin strap.

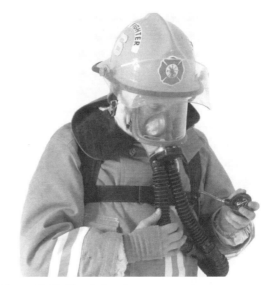

Figure K.57 Check the chest-mounted pressure gauge to verify cylinder pressure.

Doffing the Closed-Circuit SCBA

The steps for removing the closed-circuit SCBA are as follows:

Step 1: Reach back with the right hand and close the oxygen cylinder valve.

Step 2: Remove the helmet and hood, loosen the facepiece straps, and remove the facepiece. Clip the facepiece D-ring to the shoulder harness (**Figure K.58**).

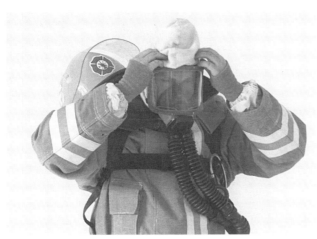

Figure K.55 Pull the protective hood into place, covering all exposed skin and making sure that vision is not obscured.

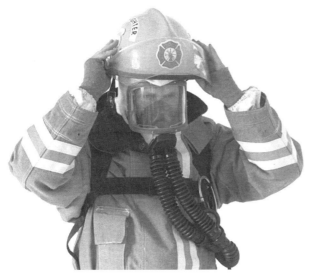

Figure K.56 Place the helmet on the head and secure the chin strap.

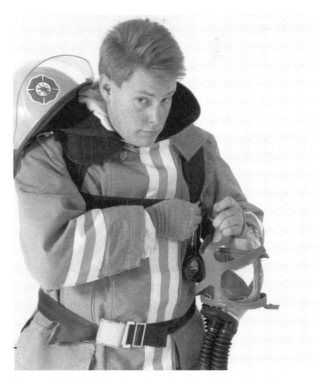

Figure K.58 Clip the facepiece D-ring to the shoulder harness.

Step 3: Release the chest strap. Loosen, unsnap, and fully extend the waist strap (**Figures K.59** and **K.60**).

Step 4: Fully extend the shoulder straps (**Figure K.61**).

Step 5: Grasp the left shoulder strap and allow the right shoulder strap to fall from the shoulder. Swing the unit around to the front and grasp the other shoulder strap; lower unit to the ground (**Figures K.62** and **K.63**).

Step 6: Fully extend all straps before storing the unit (**Figure K.64**).

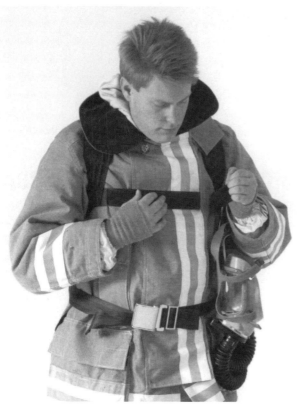

Figure K.59 Release the chest strap.

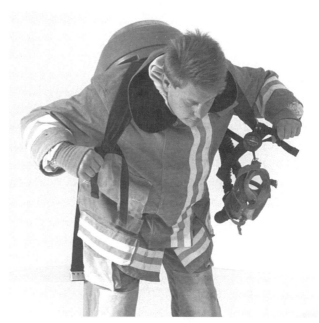

Figure K.61 Fully extend the shoulder straps.

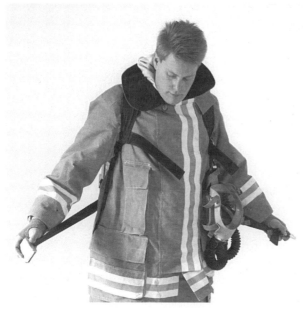

Figure K.60 Release and fully extend the waist strap.

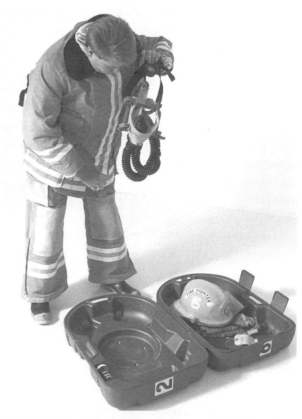

Figure K.62 Allow the shoulder strap opposite the facepiece to fall from the shoulder and then swing the unit around to the front.

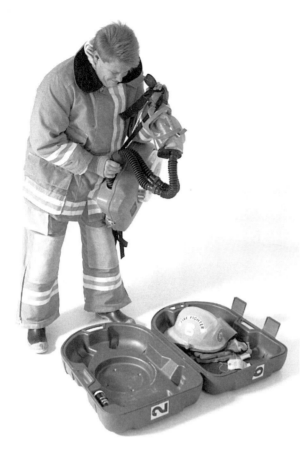

Figure K.63 Grasp the unit where the low-pressure hoses are attached and gently guide the unit to the ground.

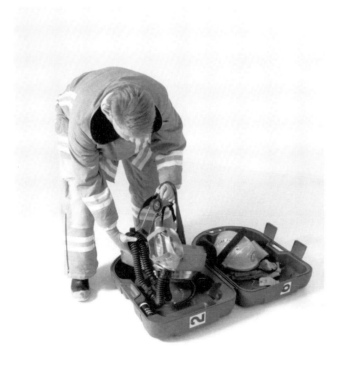

Figure K.64 Place the unit in the case and fully extend all straps before storing.

Changing Cylinders

Steps for changing the cylinders for both the open-circuit SCBA and the closed-circuit SCBA are given in the sections that follow.

Open-Circuit SCBA

With care and caution, an emergency responder can change an air cylinder at the scene of an emergency so that the equipment can be used again as soon as possible. Changing cylinders can be either a one- or two-person job. The one-person method for changing an air cylinder is described in detail as follows:

Step 1:   Doff the unit using the procedures described earlier.

Step 2:   Obtain a full air cylinder and have it ready.

Step 3:   Disconnect the regulator from the facepiece or disconnect the low-pressure hose from the regulator (**Figure K.65**).

Step 4:   Close the cylinder valve on the used bottle and release the pressure from the high-pressure hose. On some units, the pressure must be released by breathing down the regulator or opening the mainline valve. Refer to the manufacturer's instructions for the correct method for the particular unit.

NOTE: If the pressure is not released, the high-pressure coupling is difficult to disconnect.

Step 5:   Disconnect the high-pressure coupling from the cylinder (**Figure K.66**). Lay the hose coupling on the ground, directly in

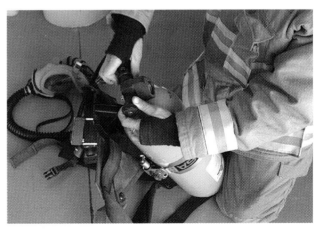

Figure K.65 Disconnect the low-pressure hose from the regulator.

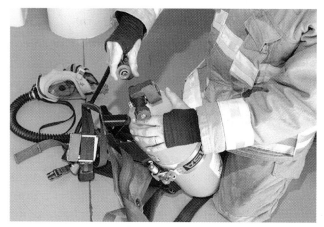

Figure K.66 Disconnect the high-pressure coupling from the cylinder.

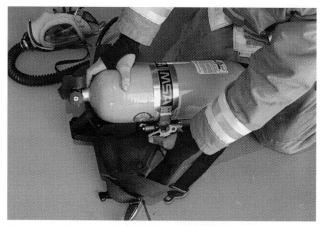

Figure K.67 Release the cylinder clamp.

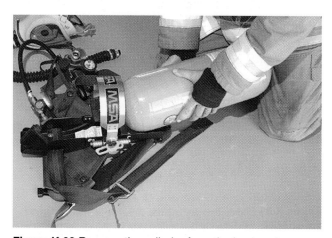

Figure K.68 Remove the cylinder from the backpack assembly.

line with the cylinder outlet, as a reminder so that the replacement cylinder can be aligned correctly and easily. Be sure that grit or liquids do not enter the end of the unprotected high-pressure hose prior to attaching it to the cylinder outlet valve.

NOTE: If more than hand force is required to disconnect the coupling, repeat Step 4 and then again attempt to disconnect the coupling.

Step 6: Release the cylinder clamp and remove the empty cylinder (**Figures K.67** and **K.68**).

Step 7: Place the new cylinder into the backpack, position the cylinder outlet, and lock the cylinder into place.

NOTE: For some cylinders, it may be necessary to rotate the cylinder one-eighth turn to the left; this protects the high-pressure hose by lessening the angle of the hose and preventing twisting.

Step 8: Check the cylinder valve opening and the high-pressure hose fitting for debris and the condition of the O-ring (**Figure K.69**). Clear any debris from the cylinder valve opening by quickly opening and closing the cylinder valve or by wiping the debris away. If the O-ring is distorted or damaged, replace it.

Step 9: Connect the high-pressure hose to the cylinder valve opening.

NOTE: Do not overtighten; hand tightening is sufficient.

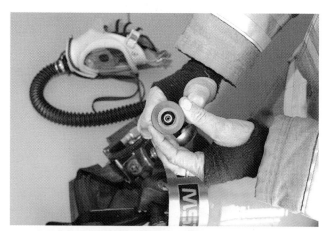

Figure K.69 Check the cylinder valve opening and the high-pressure hose fitting for debris and the condition of the O-ring.

Step 10: Open the cylinder valve and check the gauges on the cylinder and the regulator (**Figure K.70**). Both gauges should register within 10 percent of each other when the cylinder is pressurized to its rated capacity.

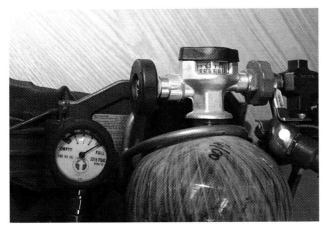

Figure K.70 Open the cylinder valve and check the gauges on the cylinder and the regulator.

If increments are in other measurements, such as fractions or minutes, they should correspond.

NOTE: Some units require that the main-line valve on the regulator be opened in order to obtain a gauge reading. Seal the regulator outlet port by placing one hand over it. On a positive-pressure regulator, the port must be sealed for an accurate regulator gauge reading.

When there are two people, the emergency responder with an empty cylinder simply positions the cylinder so that the other emergency responder can easily change it. Two methods for two people are shown in **Figures K.71** and **K.72.**

Closed-Circuit SCBA

When the oxygen supply of a closed-circuit SCBA is depleted, the empty oxygen cylinder cannot simply be exchanged with a full cylinder. The chemical scrubber unit as well as the oxygen cylinder must be changed. In other words, a complete inspection and turnaround maintenance must be performed before the closed-circuit SCBA can again be used. Refer to the manufacturer's instructions for recharging and maintenance procedures for closed-circuit SCBA.

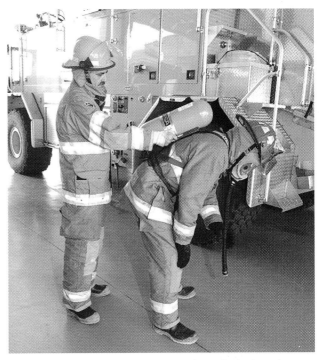

Figure K.71 One firefighter slides a full cylinder into the backpack assembly while the other firefighter braces to remain steady.

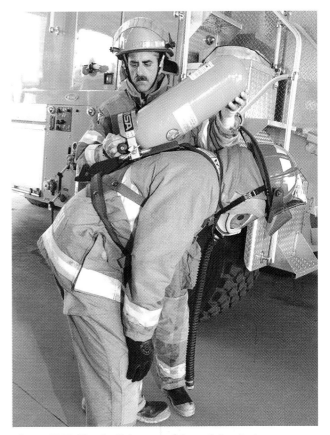

Figure K.72 The firefighter receiving a full cylinder may choose to kneel while the cylinder is being replaced.

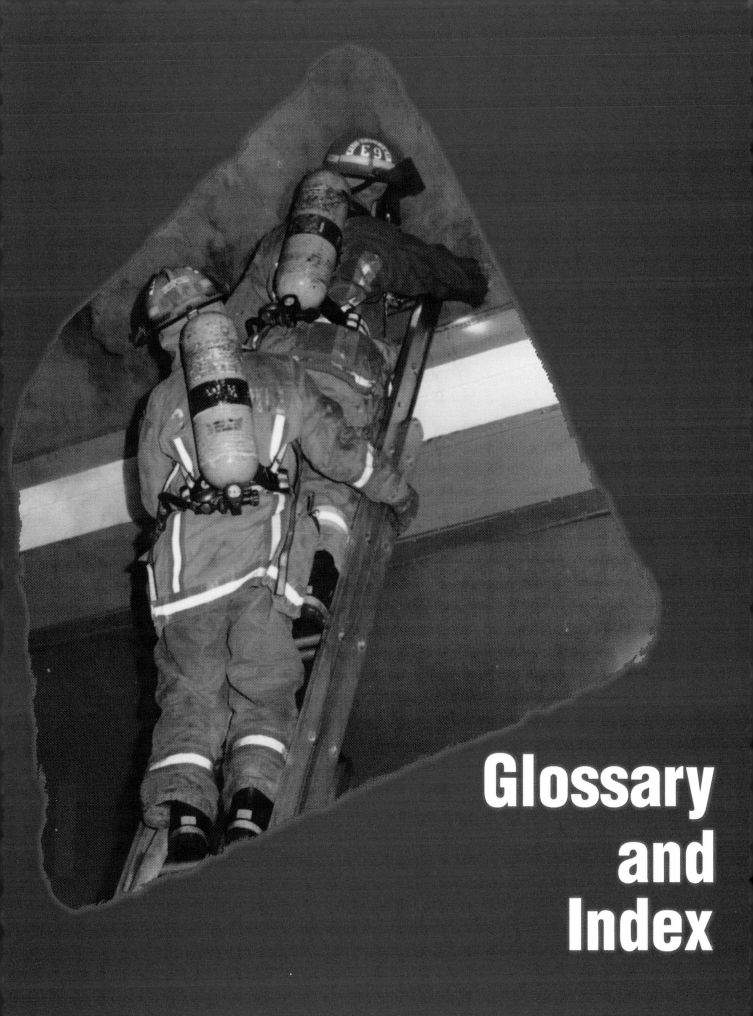

Glossary
and
Index

Glossary

A

Air-Purifying Respirator (APR) — Respirator with an air-purifying filter, cartridge, or canister that removes specific air contaminates by passing ambient air through the air-purifying element; may have a full or partial facepiece.

American Conference of Governmental Industrial Hygienists (ACGIH) — Consensus standards-writing organization that promotes worker health and safety through education and the development and dissemination of scientific and technical knowledge.

American National Standards Institute (ANSI) — Voluntary standards-setting organization that examines and certifies existing standards and creates new ones.

American Society of Mechanical Engineers (ASME) — Voluntary standards-setting organization concerned with the development of technical standards such as those for respiratory protection cylinders.

American Society for Testing and Materials (ASTM) — Consensus standards-setting organization that establishes testing procedures and minimum quality levels for manufacturing materials.

Atmosphere-Supplying Respirator — Respirator that supplies the user with breathing air from a source independent of the ambient atmosphere; includes SAR and SCBA units.

Authority Having Jurisdiction (AHJ) — Organization, office, or individual responsible for approving equipment, installations, or procedures.

B

Backdraft — Instantaneous explosion or rapid burning of superheated gases that occurs when oxygen is introduced into an oxygen-depleted confined space. It may occur because of inadequate or improper ventilation procedures.

Bloodborne Pathogens — Pathogenic microorganisms that are present in human blood and can cause disease in humans. These pathogens include (but are not limited to) hepatitis B virus (HBV) and human immunodeficiency virus (HIV).

Bureau of Mines — Former name for the Mine Safety and Health Administration. See *Mine Safety and Health Administration.*

C

Canadian Standards Association (CSA) — Canadian standards-writing organization.

Centers for Disease Control (CDC) — U.S. government agency for the collection and analysis of data regarding disease and health trends.

Closed-Circuit Breathing Apparatus — Respiratory protection system in which the exhalations of the wearer is rebreathed after the carbon dioxide has been effectively removed and a suitable oxygen concentration restored from resources composed of compressed oxygen, chemical oxygen, or liquid oxygen; usually long-duration device systems; not approved for fire fighting operations. Also called *oxygen-breathing apparatus (OBA)* or *oxygen-generating apparatus.*

Code of Federal Regulations (CFR) — U.S. government regulations that relate to various topics such as the use of respiratory protection or heavy equipment.

Compressed Gas Association (CGA) — Association that develops and promotes safety relating to the storage, use, and handling of compressed gases.

Condensation Nuclei Counter (CNC) — Quantitative fit-test protocol using a counting instrument that quantitatively fit tests respirators with the use of a probe. The probed respirator is only used for quantitative fit tests. A probed respirator has a special sampling device installed on the respirator that allows the probe to sample the air from inside the mask.

Consensus Standards — Rules, principles, or measures that are established through agreement of members of the standards-setting organization.

Control Zones — System of barriers surrounding designated areas at emergency incident scenes that are intended to limit the number of persons exposed to the hazard and to facilitate mitigation. At a major incident there are three zones: restricted (hot), limited access (warm), and support (cold).

Controlled Breathing — Technique for consciously reducing air consumption by forcing exhalation from the mouth and allowing natural inhalation through the nose.

Controlled Negative Pressure (CNP) — Quantitative fit-testing procedure that measures leak rates through the facepiece. It is based on the theory of exhausting air from a temporarily sealed facepiece to generate and then maintain a constant negative pressure inside the facepiece.

D

Demand-Type Breathing Apparatus — Breathing apparatus with a regulator that supplies air to the facepiece only when the wearer inhales or when the bypass valve has been opened; no longer approved for fire fighting or IDLH situations. Also known as *negative-pressure breathing apparatus.*

Department of Labor — Administrative body of the executive branch of the state/provincial or federal government responsible for labor policy, regulation, and enforcement.

Department of Transportation — Administrative body of the executive branch of the state/provincial or federal government responsible for transportation policy, regulation, and enforcement.

Deutsches Institut fur Normung (DIN) — Nongovernmental organization established in Germany to develop consensus standards to ensure quality and conformity in materials, testing, and processes; similar to ANSI in the United States.

Donning and Doffing Procedures — Standardized procedures recommended by the respiratory protection equipment manufacturer for putting the equipment on and taking it off. The authority having jurisdiction may also develop procedures as long as they do not violate the manufacturer's recommendation.

E

Emergency Breathing Support System (EBSS) — Escape-only respirator that provides sufficient self-contained breathing air to permit the wearer to safely exit the hazardous area; usually integrated into an airline supplied-air respirator system.

Emergency Responder — Qualified member of a fire and emergency services organization who is trained to provide search and rescue, fire suppression, medical, hazardous materials, or specialized protection services.

Emergency Services Organization — Emergency services organization that provides search and rescue, fire suppression, medical, hazardous materials, or specialized protection services. The organization may be publicly or privately managed and funded.

End-of-Service-Life Indicator (ESLI) — Visual indicator that alerts the user when the APR canister or cartridge has reached its limit and is no longer providing breathable air.

End-of-Service-Time Indicator (ESTI) — Warning device that alerts the user that the respiratory protection equipment is about to reach its limit and that it is time to exit the contaminated atmosphere; may be audible, tactile, visual, or a combination of alarms.

Environmental Protection Agency (EPA) — U.S. government agency that has the mission to protect human health and to safeguard the natural environment — air, water, and land. The EPA enforces regulations that restrict pollution of the environment.

Escape Time — Time required to exit a hazardous atmosphere without injury or death to the employee.

European Norm (EN) — Multinational organization intended to establish standards for materials, testing, and processes throughout the member states of the European Union and any nation providing materials to those members.

Exposure Limits — Exposure limits are the maximum lengths of time an individual can be exposed to an airborne substance before injury, illness, or death occurs.

Extrication — Removal and treatment of victims who are trapped by some type of man-made machinery or equipment.

F

Fight-or-Flight Syndrome — Psychological response to stress that creates a physiological effect on the human body in the form of increased heart rate and respiration. The individual must choose between the desire to run or to remain and face the hazard or threat.

Flashover — Stage of fire at which all surfaces and objects within a space have been heated to their ignition temperatures, and flame breaks out almost at once over the surface of all objects in the space.

Forcible Entry — Techniques used by emergency responders to gain entry into structures, vehicles, aircraft, or other areas of confinement when normal means of entry are locked or blocked.

Full-Facepiece Air-Purifying Respirator (FFAPR) — Filter, canister, or cartridge air-purifying respirator that covers the entire face from the forehead to the chin, providing protection to the eyes, nose, and mouth.

G

Guide — Document that provides direction or guiding information. Guides do not have the force of law but may provide the basis for what is reasonable in cases of negligence.

H

Hazard Assessment — Formal review of the hazards that may be encountered while performing the functions of a firefighter or emergency responder; used to determine the appropriate level and type of personal and respiratory protection that must be worn.

Hazardous Materials — Any substance or material in any form that may pose an unreasonable risk to health and safety or property when transported in commerce.

Hazards or Risk Analysis — Identification of hazards or risks and the determination of the appropriate response to that hazard or risk; combines the hazard assessment and risk management concepts.

Health and Safety Officer (HSO) — Member of the fire and emergency services organization who is assigned and authorized by the administration as the manager of the health and safety program and performs the duties, functions, and responsibilities specified in NFPA 1521, *Standard for Fire Department Safety Officer*. This individual must meet the qualifications or approved equivalent of this standard.

High Efficiency Particulate Air (HEPA) Filter — Respiratory protection filter designed and certified to protect the user from particulates in the air. The HEPA filter must be at least 99.97 percent efficient in removing monodisperse particles of 0.3 micrometers in diameter.

High-Rise Structure — Usually classified as a building of seven stories or higher above grade level.

I

Immediately Dangerous to Life and Health (IDLH) — Any atmosphere that poses an immediate hazard to life or produces immediate, irreversible, debilitating effects on health. A companion measure to the PEL, IDLH concentrations represent concentrations above which respiratory protection in the form of SCBA or SAR is required. IDLH is expressed in parts per million (ppm) or milligrams per cubic meter (mg/m^3).

Incident — For the purposes of this manual, an incident is defined as an unplanned, uncontrolled event resulting from unsafe acts and/or unsafe occupational conditions, either of which result in injury, death, or property damage.

Incident Commander (IC) — Person responsible for all operations at an emergency incident.

Incident Investigation — Act of investigating or gathering data to determine the factors that contributed to a fatality, injury, or property loss or to determine fire cause and origin.

Incident Management System (IMS) — Standardized system by which facilities, equipment, personnel procedures, and communications are organized to operate within a common organizational structure designed to aid in the management of resources at emergency incidents.

Incident Safety Officer (ISO) — Individual appointed to respond to an incident scene or who is assigned at an incident scene by the incident commander to perform duties and responsibilities specified in NFPA 1521, *Standard for Fire Department Safety Officer*. This individual must meet the qualifications or approved equivalent of this standard.

Incident Scene Rehabilitation — Procedures that are used to monitor the condition of fire and emergency responders at an incident and provide the rest, refreshment, and support to ensure that they are fit to return to duty.

International Organization for Standardization (ISO) — Standards organization that is intended to ensure quality in the manufacture of products that are produced in Australia, New Zealand, Europe, and North America. Some ISO standards have been adopted as part of the European Norm.

L

Lethal Concentration (LC) — Concentration of an inhaled substance that results in the death of 50 percent of the test population. (The lower the value, the more toxic the substance.) LC_{50} is an inhalation exposure expressed in parts per million (ppm), mg per liter, or mg per cubic meter (mg/m³).

Lethal Dose (LD) — Concentration of an ingested or injected substance that results in the death of 50 percent of the test population. (The lower the dose, the more toxic the substance.) LD_{50} is an oral or dermal exposure expressed in milligrams per kilogram (mg/kg).

Live Fire or Burn Exercises — Training exercises that involve the use of an unconfined open flame or fire in a structure or other combustibles to provide a controlled burning environment.

Loss Control — Encompasses the older concepts of salvage and overhaul. Loss control methods are intended to minimize damage to property and to provide good customer service to the incident victim.

M

Medical Evaluation — Annual evaluation performed by a physician or professional health-care provider to ensure that a fire and emergency services responder is physically fit to perform the duties assigned; required before a responder uses respiratory protection equipment.

Medical Examination — Complete medical examination by a physician or professional health-care provider for entry-level emergency personnel and periodically for all personnel during their service careers. It is mandatory for personnel who will be using respiratory protection equipment.

Member Organization — Organization formed to represent the collective and individual rights and interests of the fire and emergency services organization such as a labor union or fraternal association.

Mine Safety and Health Administration (MSHA) — U.S. government agency that regulates mine safety, including respiratory protection.

N

National Fire Academy — Educational arm of the Federal Fire Administration; provides courses in fire service topics.

National Fire Protection Association (NFPA) — Nonprofit, educational, and technical association devoted to protecting life and property from fire by developing fire-protection standards and educating the public.

National Institute for Occupational Safety and Health (NIOSH) — U.S. government agency that helps ensure the safety of the workplace and associated equipment by conducting investigations and making recommendations.

Negative-Pressure Breathing Apparatus — Open-circuit or closed-circuit respiratory protection breathing apparatus in which the pressure inside the facepiece, in relation to the immediate atmosphere, is positive (greater than) during exhalation and negative (less than) during inhalation. Also known as *demand-type breathing apparatus*.

O

O-A-T-H Method — Communications method used with tag lines when entering a hazardous environment. Each letter corresponds to a specific meaning and number of tugs on the line. One tug, *O*, means *Okay;* two tugs, *A*, means *Advance;* three tugs, *T*, means *Take-up;* and four tugs, *H,* means *Help.* Signals are answered with the same number of tugs on the line.

Occupational Safety and Health Administration (OSHA) — U.S. government agency that develops and enforces standards and regulations for safety in the workplace.

Open-Circuit Breathing Apparatus — Respiratory protection equipment that is designed to allow the user's exhalation to be vented to the atmosphere; usually SCBA or SAR units.

Overhaul — Searching for and extinguishing hidden or remaining fires.

Oxygen-Breathing Apparatus (OBA) — Alternate term for Closed-Circuit Breathing Apparatus. Also known as *oxygen-generating apparatus.*

Oxygen Deficiency — Atmospheres that contain less than 19.5 percent oxygen.

P

Parts per Million (ppm) — Ratio of the volume of contaminants (parts) compared to the volume of air (million parts).

Permissible Exposure Limit (PEL) — Maximum time-weighted concentration at which 95 percent of exposed, healthy adults suffer no adverse effects over a 40-hour workweek; an 8-hour time-weighted average unless otherwise noted. PELs are expressed in either ppm or mg/m^3.

Personal Alert Safety System (PASS) — Motion detector worn by emergency personnel while in hazardous environments to alert others in the event the user becomes incapacitated.

Personal Protective Equipment (PPE) — Equipment designed to shield or isolate a person from the chemical, physical, and thermal hazards that can be encountered at an emergency incident. Personal protective equipment includes both personal protective clothing and respiratory protection equipment. Adequate personal protective equipment should protect the respiratory system, skin, eyes, face, hands, feet, body, and hearing.

Personal Accountability System — System that readily identifies both the location and function of all members operating at an incident scene.

Point of No Return — Point at which the remaining operation time of breathing apparatus equals the time necessary to return safely to a nonhazardous atmosphere.

Positive-Pressure Breathing Apparatus — SCBA that maintain a slight positive pressure within the facepiece that is greater than the ambient atmosphere during both inhalation and exhalation. Also called *pressure-demand breathing apparatus.*

Powered Air-Purifying Respirator (PAPR) — Air-purifying respirator with a hood or helmet, breathing tube, canister, cartridge, filter, and a blower that passes ambient air through the purifying element. The blower may be stationary or portable.

Pre-Incident Planning — The process of gathering information on structures and target hazards, developing procedures for responses to the site, and maintaining an information resource system based on the potential hazards. The process requires inspections of the various sites, developing tactics and strategies for the specific site, and providing training based on the final strategies.

Pressure-Demand Breathing Apparatus — SCBA in which the pressure inside the facepiece, in relation to the immediate atmosphere, is positive during both inhalation and exhalation. Also known as *positive-pressure breathing apparatus.*

Products of Combustion — Materials that are produced and released during the burning process.

Q

Qualitative Fit Testing — Standardized fit test during which a person wearing a respirator is exposed to an irritant smoke, an odorous vapor, or other suitable test agent. If the wearer is unable to detect penetration of the test agent into the facepiece, the wearer has achieved a satisfactory fit.

Quantitative Fit Testing — Standardized fit test during which a person wears a respirator in a test atmosphere that contains a test agent in the form of an aerosol, a vapor, or a gas. Instrumentation that samples the test atmosphere and the air inside the facepiece of the respirator is used to measure quantitatively the penetration of the test agent into the facepiece.

R

Rapid Intervention Crew (RIC) — Emergency personnel who are equipped and designated to make an emergency entrance into the hot zone for the purpose of rescuing other emergency personnel. This crew has no other assigned tasks while assigned to this function; also known as *rapid intervention team (RIT)*.

Regulation — Authoritative rule issued by an executive authority of government; procedures, rules, or orders that have the force of law.

Request for Proposal (RFP) — Document that defines the specific requirements for an item that an organization intends to purchase through the bid process.

Respiratory Protection Program — Systematic and comprehensive program of training in the use and maintenance of respiratory protection devices and related equipment.

Respiratory Protection Specialist School — School that provides from 25 to 60 hours of additional or advanced training in the use of respiratory protection equipment. Also known as *smoke diver school.*

Respiratory Hazards — Any exposure to products of combustion, superheated atmospheres, toxic gases, vapors, or dust, or potentially explosive or oxygen-deficient atmospheres or any condition that creates a hazard to the respiratory system.

Respiratory System — System of organs that provide the function of respiration consisting typically of the lungs and their nervous and circulatory supplies and the channels by which these are connected with the outer air.

Risk Management Plan — Written plan that identifies and analyses the exposure to hazards, selection of appropriate risk management techniques to handle exposures, implementation of chosen techniques, and monitoring of the results of those risk management techniques.

Rollover — Condition where flames move through or across the unburned gases during a fire's progression.

S

Safety and Health Program Committee — Committee comprised of members of the fire and emergency services organization that is responsible for conducting research, developing recommendations, and advising the administration on safety-related matters.

Salvage — Methods and operating procedures associated with fire fighting that aid in reducing primary and secondary damage during fire fighting operations.

Self-Contained Breathing Apparatus (SCBA) — Respirator worn by the user that supplies a breathable atmosphere that is either carried in or generated by the apparatus and is independent of the ambient atmosphere.

Size-up — Mental evaluation made by the emergency responder to determine a course of action at an emergency incident. Size-up includes such factors as time, location, nature of occupancy, life hazards, exposures, property involved, nature and extent of the incident, weather, available resources, and respiratory protection requirements among others.

Skip Breathing — Emergency breathing procedure in which the emergency responder inhales normally, exhales, inhales then inhales again, and exhales; used to conserve air.

Smoke Diver School — *See* Respiratory Protection Specialist School.

Special Operations — Activities that require additional or specialized training and equipment in order to mitigate particular hazards

Standard — Criterion documents that are developed to serve as models or examples for desired performance or behavior. No one is required to meet the requirements set forth in standards unless those standards are legally adopted by the authority having jurisdiction, in which case they become law.

Standards Council of Canada (SCC) — Verification agency for standards-writing agencies in Canada; similar to ANSI in the United States.

Supplied-Air Respirator (SAR) — An atmosphere-supplying respirator for which the source of breathing air is not designed to be carried by the user; not certified for fire fighting operations. Also known as *airline respirator.*

T

Tag Line — Lifeline or rope that is attached to the waist, rescue harness, or respiratory protection harness when entering a hazardous environment.

Target Organ — Term referring to the body organ or system that a toxic gas will affect such as the eyes, respiratory system, or skin.

Thermal Hazards — Hazards that are created by the super heating of the atmosphere within a confined space such as a structure. Thermal hazards associated with fires include elevated temperatures, rollovers, flashovers, and backdrafts.

Threshold Limit Value (TLV) — Concentration of a given material that may be tolerated for an 8-hour exposure during a regular workweek without ill effects.

Threshold Limit Value/Ceiling (TLV/C) — Maximum concentration that should not be exceeded, even instantaneously.

Threshold Limit Value/Short Term Exposure Limit (TLV/STEL) — Fifteen-minute time-weighted average exposure. It should not be exceeded at any time and not repeated more than four times daily with a 60-minute rest period between each STEL exposure. These short-term exposures can be tolerated without suffering from irritation, chronic, or irreversible tissue damage or narcosis of a sufficient degree to increase the likelihood of accidental injury; impairing self-rescue; or materially reducing worker efficiency. TLV/STEL is expressed in ppm and mg/m^3.

Threshold Limit Value/Time Weighted Average — Maximum airborne concentration of a material to which an average, healthy person may be exposed repeatedly for 8 hours each day and 40 hours per week without suffering adverse effects. It is based upon current available data and is adjusted on an annual basis.

V

Vapor Density (VD) — Weight of a given volume of pure vapor or gas compared to the weight of an equal volume of dry air at the same temperature and pressure. A vapor density less than 1 indicates a vapor lighter than air; a vapor density greater than 1 indicates a vapor heavier than air.

Ventilation — Systematic removal of heated air, smoke, and /or gases from a structure and replacing them with cooler and/or fresher air to reduce damage and to facilitate emergency operations; may be vertical, horizontal, or forced.

Voice Amplification — Device attached to the full facepiece of a respirator to increase the volume of the user's voice; may be mechanical or electrical.

W

Weapons of Mass Destruction (WMD) — Explosive devices that can inflict extreme destruction and loss of life. They may be nuclear, chemical, etiological, or biological.

Index

Code of Federal Regulations (CFR). See OSHA (Occupational Safety and Health Administration) Code of Federal Regulations (CFR)
codes, defined, 46
communication
    in confined spaces, 191
    IC responsibilities, 194
    incident safety officer responsibilities, 88
    methods of, 85, 187–191
    personnel responsibilities, 187–191
    restrictions of equipment, 85
    training including information about, 159
Compressed Gas Association (CGA), 49–50, 205, 220, 224
condensation nuclei counting (CNC) tests, 137, 138–140
confined-space operations
    communication during, 191
    equipment used during, 79
    excavation sites, 246
    hazardous conditions, 32, 78
    rescues, 178, 245–246
    training, 159
contact lenses and eyeglasses, 66, 80–81, 159
contractors
    facepiece fit testing performed by, 146
    maintenance performed by, 219–220, 220–221
controlled breathing, 14, 263–264
controlled negative-pressure (CNP) tests, 135–136, 137, 139–140
control zones established by IMS, 263
cost/benefit analysis of risks, 62
costs of and funding for equipment, 63–64, 109, 114, 115–116
CSA (Canadian Standards Association). See Canadian Standards Association (CSA)
cylinders. See air and oxygen cylinders

D

data
    collecting and analyzing, 53, 64
    identification of risks using, 91–92
    keeping records of air consumption, 180
    reviewing while selecting equipment, 114–115
demand (negative-pressure) SCBA, 37–38
denatonium benzoate aerosol (Bitrex), 143–145
Deutsches Institut fur Normung (DIN), 57
Dumpster fires. See trash receptacle (Dumpster) fires
dust masks (particulate filters)
    acceptance testing, 121
    history of, 6, 8
    overview, 40, 41
    training for use of, 166–168

E

EBSS (Emergency Breathing Support System)
    APRs with, 263–264
    duration of cylinder operation, 171
    overview, 267
    SARs with
        amount of breathing air supplied by, 258
        controlled breathing techniques, 263–264
        inspection of, 210
        requirements, 84, 169–170
    SCBA with, controlled breathing techniques, 263–264
    situations requiring, 245, 246
    training for use of, 169–170
egress techniques, 264–265
Emergency Breathing Support System. See EBSS (Emergency Breathing Support System)
Emergency Information Bulletin on the use of SCBA in Low Temperatures, 251–252
emergency medical services (EMS) protocol, 15. See also medical responses
Emergency Response Guidebook, 33–34

emergency scene operations
    equipment
        air-replenishment methods, 259–260
        donning and doffing, 253–257
        end-of-service-time indicators and warnings, 86, 209, 258–259, 261–262
    exit indications and techniques, 261–271
    extreme temperatures, 251–252
    firefighter safety, 87–90
    fireground operations, 234–241
    hazardous materials incidents, 241–245
    high-rise structures, 249–250
    IC responsibilities, 192–195
    open-plan structures, 250–251
    operations mode changes, 262–263
    responder responsibilities, 185–191
    size-up, 233–234
    subterranean structures, 251
    technical rescues, 245–248
end-of-service-life indicators (ESLI), 212
end-of-service-time indicators and warnings, 86, 209, 258–259, 261–262
EN (European Norm), 57
environmental changes prompting operations mode changes, 262–263
Environmental Protection Agency (EPA), 242, 243
equipment carried by RICs, 269
equipment for respiratory protection. See also *specific types of equipment*
    acceptance testing, 121
    accessories, 113, 121, 122
    calibration during facepiece fit testing, 145
    care and cleaning
        cleaning and disinfecting, 215–217
        continuous use affecting, 172
        decontamination of respirators, 214–215
        frequency of, 214
        storage, 217–218
        training including, 163, 167, 170
    continuous use, effects of, 172
    costs of and funding for, 63–64, 109, 114, 115–116
    deciding to wear, 234
    disposal and end-of-service criteria, 67, 225, 226
    donning and doffing
        procedures for, 253–257
        training including, 162, 167, 170
    end-of-service-time indicators and warnings, 86, 209, 258–259, 261–262
    firefighter safety, 80–86
    fit testing, 146
    inspections and maintenance
        annual, 212–213
        continuous use affecting maintenance, 172
        costs of maintenance, 114
        daily or weekly, 207–212, 213
        disposal and retirement, 225–227
        postincident, 207
        record keeping, 213
        schedules for, 205–213
        testing procedures established by NIOSH, 53
        training including, 162, 167, 170
        written policies and procedures, 66
    limitations of, 84–86, 159
    physiological affects of wearing, 13–14
    products supporting, 121–122
    record keeping, 98–99, 120, 213
    selection and procurement
        conducting research, 110–112
        determining needs, 107–110
        evaluating equipment, 112–114, 311–312

NOTE: Page numbers in italics refer to illustrations.

Indexed by Kari Kells.

Respiratory Protection for Fire and Emergency Services
1st Edition

COMMENT SHEET

DATE _____ NAME _____

ADDRESS _____

ORGANIZATION REPRESENTED _____

CHAPTER TITLE _____ NUMBER _____

SECTION/PARAGRAPH/FIGURE _____ PAGE _____

1. Proposal (include proposed wording or identification of wording to be deleted),
   OR PROPOSED FIGURE:

2. Statement of Problem and Substantiation for Proposal:

RETURN TO: IFSTA Editor   SIGNATURE _____
            Fire Protection Publications
            Oklahoma State University
            930 N. Willis
            Stillwater, OK 74078-8045

Use this sheet to make any suggestions, recommendations, or comments. We need your input to make the manuals as up to date as possible. Your help is appreciated. Use additional pages if necessary.

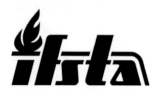
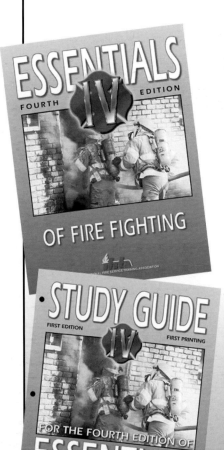
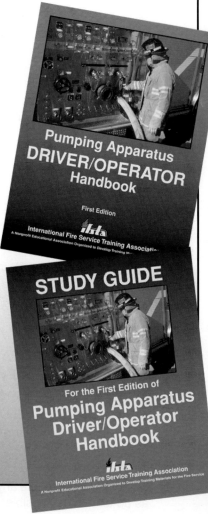
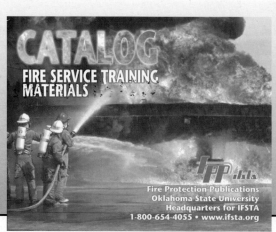